Vivien Thomas

The Man Who Overcame Racism to Save Millions of Lives

Also by Jan Pottker

Sara and Eleanor: The Story of Sara Delano Roosevelt and Her Daughter-in-Law, Eleanor Roosevelt
St. Martin's Press

Janet and Jackie: The Story of a Mother and Her Daughter, Jacqueline Kennedy Onassis
St. Martin's Press

Crisis in Candyland: Melting the Chocolate Shell of the Mars Family Empire
National Press Books

Celebrity Washington: Who They Are, Where They Live and Why They're Famous
Writer's Cramp Books

Born to Power: Heirs to America's Leading Businesses
Barron's Educational Series

Dear Ann, Dear Abby: The Unauthorized Biography of Ann Landers and Abigail Van Buren
With Bob Speziale; Dodd Mead

National Politics and Sex Discrimination in Education
With Andrew Fishel; Lexington Books, D.C. Heath and Company

Sex Bias in the Schools: The Research Evidence
Edited by Jan Pottker and Andrew Fishel; Associated University Presses

Vivien Thomas

The Man Who Overcame Racism to Save Millions of Lives

Jan Pottker

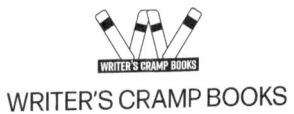

WRITER'S CRAMP BOOKS

Vivien Thomas: The Man Who Overcame Racism to Save Millions of Lives
©2024 Writer's Cramp, Inc. All rights reserved.

ISBN: 979-8-9893325-2-6 (hardcover)
ISBN: 979-8-9893325-1-9 (paperback)
ISBN: 979-8-9893325-0-9 (eBook)
Library of Congress Control Number: 2024900250

Names:	Pottker, Janice, author.
Title:	Vivien Thomas : the man who overcame racism to save millions of lives / Jan Pottker.
Description:	First edition. | Bethesda, Maryland : Writer's Cramp Books, [2024]
Identifiers:	ISBN: 979-8-9893325-2-6 (hardcover) | 979-8-9893325-1-9 (paperback) | 979-8-9893325-0-9 (ebook) | LCCN: 2024900250
Subjects:	LCSH: Thomas, Vivien, 1910-1985. | African American surgeons--Biography. | Biomedical technicians--United States--Biography. | Cardiovascular system--Surgery. | Racism. | LCGFT: Biographies. | BISAC: BIOGRAPHY & AUTOBIOGRAPHY / African American & Black. | MEDICAL / History. | SOCIAL SCIENCE / Cultural & Ethnic Studies / American / African American & Black Studies.
Classification:	LCC: RD27.35.T46 P68 2024 | DDC: 617.092--dc23

No part of this book may be reproduced in any form or incorporated into any information retrieval system without the permission of Writer's Cramp, Inc.

Published by Writer's Cramp Books, Bethesda, Maryland

All inquiries should be addressed to: writerscrampbooks.com

Additional photos and copies of archival documents about the life of Vivien Thomas may be found at VivienThomasBook.com

Cover photo courtesy of the Chesney Archives of Johns Hopkins Medicine, Nursing and Public Health

PRINTED IN THE UNITED STATES OF AMERICA

First Edition

For my father, Ralph Eugene Pottker, 1911–1988
Who treated every person with courteous respect and good cheer

CONTENTS

INTRODUCTION	The Man Behind the Medical Wonders	1
CHAPTER 1	Coming Up in Nashville	9
CHAPTER 2	The Turning Point	19
CHAPTER 3	Starting Off: Experiments in Traumatic Shock	26
CHAPTER 4	At Last, on His Way	33
CHAPTER 5	Coming Up Easy	39
CHAPTER 6	Staying Alive	44
CHAPTER 7	Outracing Death	49
CHAPTER 8	Caught Short	57
CHAPTER 9	Blalock, Thomas, and Henry Ford	67
CHAPTER 10	O Brother, Where Art Thou?	73
CHAPTER 11	Moving On Up?	84
CHAPTER 12	"Maryland, My Maryland"	88
CHAPTER 13	Putting Up and Doing Without	93
CHAPTER 14	Hoping to Do Good	100
CHAPTER 15	It's War!	106
CHAPTER 16	Blalock, Thomas, and Charles Drew, MD	114
CHAPTER 17	A Woman of Valor	118
CHAPTER 18	Thomas Decodes the Blue Babies	125
CHAPTER 19	A Black Man, a Blue Baby, and the Dawn of Heart Surgery	134
CHAPTER 20	A Vacation, at Last	159
CHAPTER 21	Clash of the Titans: Blalock vs. Taussig	166

CHAPTER 22	The Blue Baby Tour 171
CHAPTER 23	The Everlasting Salary Issue 176
CHAPTER 24	Hopkins's Greatest Surgeon? 181
CHAPTER 25	Theft and Deception. 187
CHAPTER 26	A Lulu of a Meeting 196
CHAPTER 27	Too Much Southern Comfort. 202
CHAPTER 28	Power Moves. 207
CHAPTER 29	The Headache Man 213
CHAPTER 30	Blalock's Nadir 218
CHAPTER 31	Betrayal at the Southern Hotel. 222
CHAPTER 32	Shattered Illusions 229
CHAPTER 33	The End of an Era. 234
CHAPTER 34	Token Recognition 240
CHAPTER 35	Vivien Thomas, LLD 248
CHAPTER 36	Pioneering Research in Surgical Shock and Cardiovascular Surgery. 254
CHAPTER 37	Stony Silence. 264
CHAPTER 38	Unsung Hero. 271

PHOTO GALLERY 143
ENDNOTES. 279
SOURCES. 325
ACKNOWLEDGMENTS. 331
ABOUT JAN POTTKER. 335
BIBLIOGRAPHY. 337
INDEX. 339

INTRODUCTION

The Man Behind the Medical Wonders

Nineteen forty-five was a hell of a year for headlines. Most Americans, kept in the dark about President Franklin Delano Roosevelt's declining health, were shocked by his death in March. Soon, though, good news prevailed: in April, Hitler committed suicide and the Jerries surrendered a month later. Americans and their allies celebrated in the streets; men wept openly and stranger kissed stranger. A sailor in Times Square firmly pressed his lips on those of a young nurse who swooned in seeming delight.

A few weeks later, to cap the month of May, Americans learned of the unbelievable blue baby heart surgery that could make dying newborns healthy again. The first surgery of this kind actually had taken place a half-year earlier in 1944 but had not been publicly announced until mid-May 1945.[1] Then, on August 14, came Victory over Japan Day, which ended the war in Asia. Peace and prosperity lay ahead in this auspicious year, and the successful life-saving operation was seen as another sign that nothing could beat America, this great can-do nation.

On the morning of that very first blue baby surgery, November 29, 1944, the mind of Mr. Vivien Thomas had no space for any thought except a dying baby girl, the emaciated fifteen-month-old Eileen Saxon, who was being prepped for her operation a few blocks away from the laboratory where he worked. Right or wrong, he felt full responsibility for her safety because he, a mere laboratory technician, was the one who'd created the surgery she was about to undergo. Only a few people at Johns Hopkins University Hospital in Baltimore, Maryland, knew of Thomas's pivotal accomplishments. These were kept anonymous: how could anyone in the medical establishment disclose that a Black man whose formal education ended with a high school diploma had accomplished all that he did?

At Hopkins's medical campus, people only knew that an incredibly innovative but also risky operation would take place that day. It already was dubbed the "blue baby" surgery (officially, the babies suffered from Tetralogy of Fallot). Eileen, like thousands of other blue babies born each year, had a heart defect that didn't allow enough oxygen to get into her heart and her blood circulation. She could barely breathe, didn't have the energy required to stand up, was woefully underweight, and her skin had a dark blueish tint (thus the term, blue baby). The operation, if successful, could be a medical game changer for two reasons.

At that time, any surgery at all on babies was rare but, more significant, there had been virtually no surgery on the heart in medical history.[2] The Hopkins health-care workers were abuzz with anxious questions about its chance of success due to this double risk. Thomas tried to clear his mind at least to pray God that this baby girl would not die on the operating table.[3] After all, he was the thirty-five-year-old father of two daughters, and he deeply empathized with the parents of blue babies.

Over at the hospital, spectators were eagerly jamming into the Halstead building's two-level gallery seats in Operating Room 706. These people understood that this could be a historic surgery that would result in either an awe-inspiring or a tragic ending.[4] If the upcoming surgery did not work, this infant would perish.

Some of the spectators watching looked hopeful and optimistic, but most were worried, questioning, and skeptical. People wondered whether a surgery on the heart was doable. Operating on the heart, even close outside it, was deemed disastrous and certainly immoral. No one could survive. This was virtually the first attempt at heart surgery, and it could jump-start an entire new era of cardiac care. Eileen was just an

The Man Behind the Medical Wonders 3

infant and the standard medical opinion at the time was that some babies would just die: there was nothing that could done about it, heartbreaking as it was.

The crowd whispered comments to each other as various doctors, surgeons, and nurses entered to take their places around the operating table. First entered Helen Taussig, MD, a tall pediatric cardiologist with bobbed hair that she would not bother to color, wearing clear-framed glasses and noticeable hearing aids. She was waiting calmly for her patient, Eileen, who lay ever-so-tiny on a child-size hospital cart being brought in by an attendant. Most observers knew that this pediatrician was the one who'd suggested that this lifesaving surgery might be possible. She would become a founder of the specialty of pediatric cardiology because of her diagnostic brilliance.

Taussig laser-focused on her patient and was unconcerned about what her male peers thought about a woman in medicine and, particularly, about her "demanding" ways.[5] She gently picked up this delicate fifteenth-month-old baby who, shockingly, weighed fewer than ten pounds and she placed the tiny girl on the operating table. You could hardly see the wee thing because Eileen was overwhelmed by the snow-like hills of white sheeting.

Now in came a young anesthesiologist, Merel Harmel, MD who, when not wearing scrubs, sported a jaunty ascot rather than a tie; in hushed tones, the spectators asked each other why, for such an important operation, why wasn't Austin Lamont, MD, chief of anesthesiology, present? They'd no idea that he'd refused to take part in what he predicted was an outrageous unknown heart procedure that would surely kill this baby. Harmel didn't want to be there, either, but Lamont had assigned him to the surgery and, as a junior anesthesiologist, Harmel could not refuse.[6] Although his nerves were a-jitter, he was comforted seeing that Olive Berger, an experienced nurse anesthetist, was close by his side. Scrub nurse Charlotte Mitchell was also present. The tall blonde surgery assistant resident, Denton Cooley, MD, was calm and collected,[7] but the dark-haired chief resident surgeon with sunken brown eyes, William P. Longmire, MD was anxiously shifting from one leg to another. He didn't see how this could end in anything but tragedy.[8]

In stepped Alfred Blalock, MD, the star of this operation who was the chief of surgery at Hopkins. He was easily identified by his pitch-black hair and clear-framed glasses, balanced precariously above his face mask. Despite the odds, this risk-taking surgeon had agreed to perform the first operation that might give life to thousands of blue babies with malformed hearts. He knew with certainty that Eileen would die without any surgical attempt to improve her health. More than anything, he understood that if he were successful, he'd be responsible for virtually beginning the age of heart surgery. For Blalock, who had already attained the position he'd coveted, chief of surgery at Hopkins, it was worth the gamble.

Blalock, though, looked distraught as he scanned the people at the table. His frown indicated that someone was missing. Then he looked up, hoping this man was among those in the gallery. Almost no one at this segregated university could have guessed that he was seeking out Vivien Thomas, who was Hopkins's sole Black laboratory technician. When he spotted Clara Belle Puryear, Thomas's chemical lab tech, he called, "Miss Puryear, I guess you better call Vivien."[9] Then he whispered to someone at the table and soon an orderly appeared with a step stool that he placed slightly behind and to the side of the surgeon's shoulder, at Blalock's specific direction.

Now, everyone on the floor waited, self-consciously swaying slightly in the silence. Suddenly, into the gallery above the operating theater, strode a distinguished and intelligent-looking tall man wearing a coat and tie. Vivien Thomas, Blalock's lab assistant who rarely left his laboratory several blocks away, was walking into the observation balcony above. Blalock caught his breath, relieved to see him enter the room, and then spoke loudly: "Vivien, you better come down here."[10]

Now the heads of the spectators bobbed back and forth, questioning each other why the surgery director would bring his lab assistant—and a Black lab worker, at that—down to the theater. Within minutes, Thomas emerged from the back, scrubbed and ready for surgery. Alfred Blalock directed Thomas to stand on the step stool so nothing could impede his view of the surgeon's hands. This caused another buzz from the audience. After all, it was 1944 and the Hopkins medical staff had never yet allowed

The Man Behind the Medical Wonders   5

an African American surgeon to operate at its surgical table, much less a Black man who wasn't a physician.[11]

This day was the dawn of heart surgery, and it could not begin without Vivien Thomas.

The medical miracles of Thomas neither began nor ended with this blue baby surgery. Earlier, while working with Blalock at Vanderbilt University hospital in the thirties, Thomas performed hundreds of Blalock's experimental dog surgeries to find remedies for traumatic shock, which had been a leading cause of death throughout all of history. The initial theoretical framework was Blalock's, but it was Thomas's experimental surgeries at both Vanderbilt and Hopkins that proved the theoretical hypotheses were correct. The lab assistant had become such an expert on traumatic shock that when Blalock was writing articles for publication, he would call Thomas to review and verify what he was writing. At that time, Thomas never received credit from Vanderbilt or Johns Hopkins universities, Alfred Blalock, or anyone else for these life-saving experiments.

Then, the blue baby surgery became a dramatic news-wire story in 1945; "New Operation Helps Doomed 'Blue' Babies," was a typical headline.[12] There had been no photographs taken of the first surgery of Eileen Saxon because no one knew how it would turn out. Later, nearly two years after Blalock and Taussig became famous for the blue baby operation, Thomas appeared fleetingly in a blue baby still-shot photo that was taken from Hopkins's first black-and-white closed-circuit film in 1947. He stood respectfully in the background with his hands crossed and idle. The usual step stool had been removed for the camera. His face was completely blocked by a standing spotlight that made it difficult to determine his race. He was only partly scrubbed, wearing his street clothes under his white coat and his hands were bare whereas everyone else is gloved.[13] Johns Hopkins hospital never identified him on their press release, which gave the names of only the white people present. It was as if Vivien Thomas didn't exist.

The favorable blue baby surgery publicity made Blalock eager to press for continued surgical research on the heart.[14] Again, it was Thomas who took the challenge and advanced heart surgery a step forward by creating a second cardiac operation technique in 1946. He was able to lessen the symptoms of a different kind of a congenital heart malformation where babies were born with transposed (wrongly placed) arteries in their hearts, another disorder that made newborns' blood short of oxygen. The congenital circulatory problem was solved by Thomas's creation of an opening in the heart wall that allowed these sick newborns a chance at life.[15] What he created became the first palliative treatment for transposition of the great arteries (TGA). Once again, he received no credit whatsoever for the operation because it went to others. Just as the blue baby operation is named the Blalock-Taussig surgery, the TGA operation is known as the Blalock-Hanlon surgery.

Medical historians have named several of the most important early cardiac surgeries and among them, two were created by Vivien Thomas; first, the blue baby heart surgery and then the TGA atrial septal defect operation.[16] Despite his being responsible for both these surgical breakthroughs, he remained uncredited and anonymous for decades after. One surgeon described him: "For decades, Thomas was the world's most skilled and innovative surgeon in the nascent fields of cardiothoracic and vascular surgery."[17]

With others at Hopkins in the 1950s and beyond, Thomas investigated how to restart hearts that had stopped beating, sometimes by directly massaging the heart to keep it pumping, a technique that eventually became known as cardiopulmonary resuscitation (CPR). Later, in the seventies, he assisted Levi Watkins, MD (the first Black medical resident at Hopkins) when, in 1980, Watkins became the first surgeon to implant an automatic heart defibrillator, a device that corrects irregular heartbeats.[18]

This is the only biography of Vivien Thomas written for adults rather than young people. It is a provocative narrative of race, medicine, and ethics that provides a new paradigm for an analysis of the life and work of this medical pioneer. The complete story of Vivien Thomas has never been told; most of his accomplishments remain unrecognized and his ability to persevere in the face of institutionalized and social racism has never been adequately examined. The biography contradicts, in large part, the comfortable yet destructive myth that Vivien Thomas was treated well and befriended by his highly lauded Southern white supervisor of more than thirty years, Dr. Alfred Blalock. It exposes how both Vanderbilt and Johns Hopkins universities have sugar-coated the treatment of this extraordinary Black man.

This true story is more than a narrative of Vivien Thomas's medical miracles. It is the tale of a kind and gentle man who, while living in vicious discriminatory environments, only wanted to use his considerable talents to keep people healthy. Although he never reached his own childhood dream of becoming a physician, he managed to heal other people's patients. It's the story of a man who, somehow, managed not to call anyone or anything "racist," despite how he was treated because of his skin color. It is the untold and painstakingly researched story of a man with grit, a survivor who could forgive nearly everyone their trespasses against him. All his life, he took full responsibility for his work with no exceptions. He showed himself capable of thinking and working through nearly insurmountable challenges. Although he endured emotional pounding over the years, his character allowed him to successfully navigate the choppy waters of his life and times.

This book illuminates what it was about Vivien Thomas and his environment that infused him with an unusual resiliency in the racially biased world in which he worked. You will see how the lessons his parents taught him as a child, and the support of his talented Black community while growing up in Nashville, allowed him to be the rare man who was victimized but never saw himself as or behaved as if he were as a victim. Throughout his life, Thomas was battered, time and again, but remained unbroken.

As a sociologist with a PhD from Columbia University who worked in civil rights for many years in the federal government, I was able to ferret out a treasure trove of Thomas's previously unseen writings, notes, and letters at more than a dozen medical archives, not merely his papers at the Hopkins archives. There were thousands of documents to peruse. Meticulously and at great depth, I interviewed his family, colleagues, and friends. Literally years of research went into this effort to learn and write the story of Vivien Thomas with truth and accuracy. What you will read here has never been told before—the story of Vivien Thomas will surprise you, anger you, and hold you spellbound. What follows is an unblinkered look at the life and times of a remarkable man, a true American unsung hero.

CHAPTER ONE

Coming Up in Nashville

Vivien Thomas was born on August 29, 1910, in Louisiana, and spent his first few years in a small town named Lake Providence in the northeast corner of the state, which is the heart of the Mississippi Delta cotton kingdom. It had been less than fifty years since the end of the Civil War and slavery was still a living memory for older folks in his community. Throughout the South, enslaved men and women had spent generations working on white men's plantations, slouched over low cotton plants on flat fields without shade, long heavy burlap sacks tied around their waists that weighed up to sixty or seventy pounds, their slow inching progress abruptly stalled when saw briers and cockleburs grabbed at the sack, jerking them backwards, or slicing into hands and fingers like razors. After the Civil War, many of these freed men, women, and children had no other option but to remain on the land and become sharecroppers, working just as hard, yet never able to get out of debt to the plantation's owner.

The Lake Providence of Thomas's childhood remained resolutely segregated, split down the middle by its oxbow lake of the same name, with the better-off white community living on the north side of the lake and the poorer Black families on the south side. The year Thomas was born, Lake Providence still lacked clean water and electricity. Even as recently as the late 1990s, Lake Providence was known not only as the poorest town in the nation—with 70 percent of its children living in poverty—but also as "the most unequal town in America" because of the vast disparity in wealth between the haves and the have-nots.[1]

Life on the banks of the lake town was harsh. In the summer, temperatures often climbed as high as 110 degrees, with the intense humidity turning regularly, and without warning, into drenching rain. The mosquitoes swarmed so thick they'd block the sun and sang so high around your ears that you thought you could lose your mind. In *Life Along the Mississippi*, Mark Twain had written that if you lived in Lake Providence, you needed to buy an extra life insurance policy that covered death by mosquito.

Worst of all was the flooding. Each spring, the nearby Mississippi River tipped its alluvial waters into Lake Providence, splitting its banks, the overflow streaming into any and all houses in its path, including the Thomas house. "Lake Providence was one of those places where when the waters came up, you ran," Thomas remembered.[2] With the spring rain, families like the Thomases had to flee to higher land, returning home to the back-breaking work of shoveling out wet silt and soil, some of which had been dragged by the river all the way down from northern Minnesota. There was a reason they called the Mississippi "Big Muddy."

Lake Providence, then and now, held no future for Black people. In 1920, eight years after the Thomas family had left town for Nashville, the percentage of tenant farmers—that's the modern word for "sharecroppers"—grew to 95 percent of those working the land. These sharecroppers were left mired in both mud and everlasting poverty, for the Southern landowners had successfully rigged up a system that kept you in debt owing money, with your red numbers getting higher the longer and harder you worked for them.[3] The odds of being a Black child whose parents could escape this rigged game were slight. But William Maceo Thomas, Vivien Thomas's father, a master carpenter, would never accept the subservient role of tenant farmer. He could look ahead and plan for a brighter future whereas so many other families had no option but to stay in Lake Providence, which meant you'd abandoned hope, not just for yourself but for your children, too. Who would ever have guessed that the miraculous story of Vivien Thomas started in the muck of Lake Providence?

COMING UP IN NASHVILLE

William Maceo Thomas and Mary Eaton Thomas, Vivien's parents, already had three children by the time he came along. His older sister Olga was born in early 1906 and later that same year, Vivien's eldest brother Harold came along. Then another boy, Maceo, was born the next year. When Mary became pregnant in late 1909, she and William were so certain they would be having another girl that they picked out her name, Vivian. To their surprise, the daughter they'd expected was instead a son, born on August 29, 1910. They used the English style to masculinize his name with a spelling sleight of hand, calling him "Vivien." Although little Vivien never much liked his first name, he did have the good fortune to be born to parents who were determined to make a better life for their children than the one offered by Lake Providence.[4]

It was essential to the family's well-being that William Thomas was a master carpenter, a skilled worker in a trade that had been taught to him by his own father, and he became well known around town for his meticulous handiwork and the sturdy houses that he built. The Thomas children grew up playing with wooden toys their father made for them and it was his reputation as a craftsman and builder that helped the family make the slow climb into the middle class—and gave them an escape from Louisiana against considerable odds. When Vivien Thomas was two years old, the family got out of Lake Providence and didn't look back.

Thanks to their hard work and planning, William and Mary were able to take their savings and move their family to thriving Nashville, Tennessee, some 400 miles to the northeast. Friends had told them about Nashville, its strong Black middle class and their leaders, its progressive spirit, and the opportunities it would offer Black residents in the form of access to land, livelihood, and education.[5] Most important was that the city was "vitally aware of the need for higher education for negroes."[6] Unlike other southern cities, Nashville offered a high school education to Black adolescents as far back as 1897, whereas the larger Atlanta, Georgia, for example, did not open a high school for its Black youngsters until 1924, nearly thirty years later.

Nashville was the perfect place for the aspiring Thomas family. There was no doubt about it. The city offered opportunities to "colored people," as they were called back then by both Blacks and by Southern whites when the whites were being polite. "Nashville was a bastion of aspiring opportunity," said Reavis Mitchell, PhD a Fisk University sociology professor whose father had worked with Thomas's older brother, Harold. Mitchell recalled that the Thomas family had been "ambitious."[7]

Black Nashville, by the late 1800s, had adopted Booker T. Washington's philosophy of hard work and self-help.[8] Toward the end of that decade, W. E. B. Du Bois arrived from Massachusetts to attend Fisk College, the first Black university with a million-dollar endowment from such Northern philanthropists as Carnegie and Rockefeller. Du Bois, who became a professor of sociology at the University of Pennsylvania in the 1890s and one of the founders of the NAACP, was amazed by the progress of African Americans in Nashville and their sense of security and self-assurance. In Nashville, for example, the Thomases could buy land and enter the middle-class world of homeowners, whereas in Louisiana, owning land would have been unreachable.[9] "Perhaps no Americans better understood the meaning of property ownership than those themselves who had been considered 'a species of property' themselves," said one commentator.[10]

The city had two African American-owned banks that would lend them mortgage money to do so.[11] William and Mary Thomas quickly bought three city lots on which to build their own residence: a good-size stucco house at 2007 Albion Street. To this day, the city is known as "the Athens of the South" to its white citizens because of its fine public schools and its thirteen colleges and universities, including Vanderbilt University. Similarly, its Black residents deemed Nashville "the Black Mecca,"[12] because young Black high school graduates could choose from its historically strong Black colleges, including the Ebony League's Fisk College (currently Fisk University), the Meharry Medical College, and the publicly supported Tennessee A&I State Teachers College (currently Tennessee State University).

The city's river trade and railway hub made Nashville home to a lively economy, and William soon began growing his carpentry business into that of a small housing contractor and real estate investor. He would purchase maybe a half-acre of land, build a nice house on it, and then sell it, with the profits going toward the next piece of property. "You could not buy a white man's house and, as a result, we built our own," said Thomas.[13]

Nashville gave the Thomas family access to a solid Black middle-class way of life.

According to the *Nashville Black City Business Directory,* around the time the family moved to Nashville, the city's Black community boasted fifty-two physicians, thirty-five Black-owned grocery stores, twenty-six restaurants, seven brick and carpentry contractors, eighty-nine churches, and two hospitals.[14] If the churches and hospitals hadn't done the trick, there were also nine Black undertakers. Nashville's daily newspaper, *The Tennessean,* covered this community in a daily column called "Happenings Among Colored People." A more conservative paper, the *Nashville Banner,* ignored Nashville's African American population except to criticize it. The Nashville Public Library was open to people of color—so long as they visited the Negro branch.

The Thomases made a deliberate choice to build their house in the Fisk neighborhood. An additional benefit was that Meharry Medical College was considering moving its campus a few blocks from the Thomas household, which it subsequently did.[15] It was a lovely neighborhood, advertised by one housing developer as "Fisk University Place, the beautiful Colored subdivision."[16] The Thomas parents wanted their children to see, every day, the young Black Fisk undergraduate students so that the next generation of Thomases would know that they, too, could have an authentic future. Meharry moved so close that today, the medical school currently owns the land on which the Thomas house stood. In this Nashville environment, the Thomas children understood that further education was both possible and expected.

The Thomas parents could also offer their offspring the advantage of an early childhood education. Although Tennessee did not begin public school for any child until age seven—and offered no public kindergarten whatsoever—William and Mary paid private-school tuition to send their children to Fisk College Training School, a preschool and kindergarten run by faculty and undergraduates in the college's teacher training program. Kindergarten was a new German concept, advanced at Fisk by

W. E. B. Du Bois, its former student.[17] This way, Vivien and his siblings were given the advantage of a strong grounding in education even before starting public school.

In later years, Thomas remembered his time growing up in Nashville fondly. "Segregation? Yes, plenty of it," he wrote, "[but] Nashville, even then, was a good place for Negroes, or anyone else, to live and work. We, as a race, in Nashville have never been afraid to get our hands dirty. We'd paint our own house, fix our own fence, cut our own grass—and all the houses had lawns—no row houses."[18]

In many ways, the Thomas household was conservative and upheld strong beliefs that are now less popular. Vivien Thomas recounted that his father "worked endlessly to supply the family needs."[19] As for his mother, he acknowledged her constant chores, too, done without the convenience of modern appliances. Mary Thomas sewed all her children's clothes, including their suits and coats. If she had time, she occasionally made clothes for other people's families and added to the family income.[20] She tended the vegetable garden on their half-acre piece of land. She cooked all the meals for the seven-member family and, when the boys were teenagers, she learned to put her husband's supper aside if he were late or else "the wrecking crew," as William called his sons, would have eaten that, too.[21]

The year after the Thomas family arrived in Nashville, in 1913, Mary gave birth to a baby girl, Melba, the only one of the children to be born in Tennessee. With William's steady income, Mary did not need to hold a job outside the home as so many other Black women did and so she was kept busy taking care of her five children and their household. William had built the house, but it was Mary who turned it into a home. Vivien's earliest memories were formed in that house. When it came time, he walked by himself to Fisk for kindergarten and then, with his siblings, to the elementary school. The Thomas family attended the nearby United Methodist church and on Sunday, the five Thomas children dressed in their best outfits—the three boys in suits and ties, the two girls in their prettiest starched dresses—and would go with their parents to church.

Vivien's religious beliefs, passed down by his parents and his church, also influenced his interest in medicine. Years of Sunday school had taught him about the important of service and helping others. What's more, the path of doctor was one that he felt he could easily find and follow. After all, by 1920, the nation could boast of nearly 4,000 Black physicians, and the majority had graduated from either Howard University medical school or from Meharry, right on his doorstep.[22] Thomas was perfectly content to receive his medical education within his Black local community, having no interest in enrolling in a mostly white medical school, which was a typical attitude of many Black students of that time, as a medical historian notes.[23]

When he was thirteen, Thomas started at the nearby Pearl High School, following in the footsteps of his older sister and two older brothers. Founded in the late nineteenth century as a high school for African American students, Pearl (now known as Pearl-Cohen High School) had a longstanding reputation for educational excellence.[24] Not only did Pearl prepare its students for college—rather than assuming they were only destined for manual or vocational work—it was also responsible for educating generations of leaders of Nashville's Black community. The school's motto was, "We finish in order to begin."[25] Former Nashvillean Afi-Odelia E. Scruggs wrote in her memoir, "When you couldn't identify a person by church or neighborhood, one question placed him among friends and relatives: 'When did he finish Pearl?'"[26] Pearl is such a celebrated high school that, more than one hundred years after its founding, the top hip-hop singer, Drake, arranged to speak to its students.[27]

Pearl's reputation for excellence was solidly earned, even though public schools in Tennessee were notoriously poorly funded and under-resourced, even for white kids. Although few Northerners knew this, a number of urban Southern schools that served African American students were able to supplement their budgets with funds and equipment from such Northern philanthropic organizations as John D. Rockefeller's General Education Board and the Julius Rosenwald Fund. Unitarian and Quaker congregations, too, raised money for Black segregated Southern schools.[28] In fact, in 1928, a full half of all Southern African-American children attended schools that were financially supported by the Rosenfeld Fund, established by the founder of Sears, Roebuck and Co.[29]

In Tennessee at the time, there was less difference in quality between the urban public schools for white and Black children than there was between the rural public schools and urban public schools for either race.[30] This in a state where only 74 percent of children had enrolled in school at all, and 95 percent of these students never went beyond the elementary school level. In the 1920s, relatively few students in Tennessee, Black or white, rural or urban, made it through twelfth grade; graduating with a high school diploma put you in the upper tier of Tennesseans.[31]

Lessons at Pearl High were taught by its excellent teachers, some of whom had master's degrees but ended up in education because they lacked other professional options due to their race.[32] These dedicated men and women instilled self-worth in their students, something that Black students would not necessarily receive from white teachers after school desegregation many decades later. "The teachers were concerned and dedicated," remembered Thomas. "They were determined that children would learn whatever they were supposed to learn while attending their classes. By today's standards there was an almost unbelievable cooperation between parents and teachers."[33] One of the school's first principals was G. E. Washington, who went on to become president of Lincoln University. He would also be the maternal grandfather of civil rights leader Julian Bond.

The teachers were hard graders. There was no sloughing off in a school like Pearl, where the graduating valedictorian in Thomas's class earned only an 88 percent average.[34] Nor was there grade inflation; parents would have laughed at that unfamiliar concept. What would be the point of grades, then? As Melvin Black, the director and curator of the Pearl Museum, said, "Pearl represents an important and difficult road to reach success, one that was traveled by so many individuals."[35]

Thomas chose college prep classes and, with his interest in science, enrolled in all its science lab courses. Having outgrown his earlier gawkiness, he grew into a tall and good-looking student with a mellifluous baritone voice and a quick sense of humor, accompanied a hearty laugh. Thomas did well in school and, though quiet and reserved, he was well-liked by his peers. He had a rich baritone voice, and sang in his church choir, performing for groups around town as a good deed.

Besides his duties to church and school, he was also kept busy helping his father in the family business. For about three hours each evening, and for eight hours on Saturdays, Thomas worked alongside his brothers in their father's workshop. He later remembered, "If you could do nothing but drive a nail, you'd drive that nail."[36]

It wasn't that William expected or even wanted his sons to go into a trade; instead, the elder Thomas wanted to make sure that his boys gained an idea of the work world and, at the same time, gave them no time to get into trouble. The boys contributed some of their earned money toward household expenses. While they might spend a few dollars on shoes or a shirt, they saved the rest for college. Meanwhile, the Thomas girls also enrolled in college-prep classes at Pearl and, at home, their mother taught them skills in home economics that they could put to good use when they were older and married.

In the spring of 1929, Vivien Thomas proudly graduated high school. The Pearl ceremony took place at Nashville's Ryman Auditorium, later known as the Mother Church of Country Music. The girls wore white dresses and the boys wore navy blazers, white flannel pants, and neckties. In his graduation photo, Thomas looked particularly smart in his outfit, standing head and shoulders above many of his peers—by now he had grown to over six feet. He looked like a quintessential college man, polished and preppy, ready to attend some Ivy League university if he'd had enough tuition money. A female valedictorian was introduced and a male salutatorian spoke on "Chemistry in Everyday Life." Thomas had done very well and had earned academic credits beyond the school's graduation requirement, but he was not one of its several honors students, as others have claimed.[37] There were only ninety graduates in Thomas's class, but the African American community in Nashville was so supportive of the excellent Pearl High School that 4,000 *people* turned out to watch the ceremony that day.[38]

Like his older siblings, Vivien Thomas was expected to go to college. At the time of his Pearl graduation, his older sister Olga was married and working as a nurse at a hospital in Detroit. His older brother, Harold, was still at Fisk, and only Maceo, the middle son, had a yearning for independence, and so had dropped out of high school and was working as a driver for a wealthy Nashville family. Thomas, meanwhile, had his heart set on medical school. His role model was the family physician, who took careful care of the young Thomases and had a special talent that made them feel better, no matter the illness or ailment. He was a kindly man who "knew all about you, from head to foot," as Thomas recalled. "You always called anytime you needed him... He just sort of impressed me that it would be a nice thing to do, go around and see sick people and make them well."[39]

He took a summer carpentry job at Fisk University and, in August, was the only summer hire asked to stay on. He was delighted with his well-paying job and decided that "times were so good"[40] he would keep working and wait until January 1930 to enroll at the tuition-free Tennessee State University, which had the low costs per quarter of $10 dollars for registration and $10 for textbooks.[41] His only financial hurdle would follow college graduation because Meharry Medical School charged a tuition of $250 a session, with additional costs of fees and textbooks.[42]

He knew that he would be well-prepared for Meharry by studying at A&I: there were a number of A&I graduates who went on to Meharry to get their MD degrees. In fact, the American Medical Association rated A&I as one of the top ranked liberal arts colleges that trained pre-med majors.[43] His goal was realistic and well within his reach. Now, with his job at Fisk and by living at home, he knew he could save money for college and medical school. He had plenty of time, he assured himself.

CHAPTER TWO

The Turning Point

Working at Fisk, Thomas kept busy repairing objects around campus, anything from cabinets and doors to floors and desks.¹ Thomas had acquired his dad's skill with tools as he quickly and deftly used his long, elegant fingers. The young Thomas excelled in his work and, after the summer was over, he was the only seasonal worker paid $20 a week who was asked to stay into the winter.² Each week, as soon as he received his paycheck from his carpenter's job, he went to the Nashville People's Bank to put as much of the money away as possible for his education. He already had set aside $350, a good sum for nineteen years old. After all, going to college was expected by his parents: his oldest sister had attended A&I and his oldest brother, Harold, was an undergraduate at Fisk and planned to continue with a master's degree. Thomas fully intended to follow them by starting college in the spring semester of 1930.

He thought he had it made until the stock market crashed on September 29, 1929, when Fisk laid off all nonessential workers, including Thomas. It was a serious blow, especially for someone with goals that went far beyond carpentry. He was still optimistic that he could put off college for a few years, not realizing that his future could get bound down as if he'd tied it to a cement block. The news from an upbeat White House, desperate to minimize the Depression, was that "good times are just around the corner," and Thomas knew if he could just locate that corner, he'd be fine. Until then, he was caught in a maze, shouldering through tight turns and getting nowhere. He needed a job, but jobs were scarce to nonexistent. Even his carpenter father couldn't help him out—William Thomas didn't need an extra pair of hands during a time when his clients were already halting construction on their houses, wary of the economic strictures to come.

Out of options and worried sick, in February of 1930, young Thomas turned to Charles Manlove, his good friend who was a little older. Manlove worked as a diener, or assistant, in the Bacteriology and Immunology lab at Vanderbilt University's medical school, where the lab was working toward culturing vaccines in chicken embryos, which would lead to the mass production of vaccines.[3] The role was as close to professional as one could get without a college degree, and Manlove had managed to remain at Vanderbilt when others were being laid off.

Vivien Thomas and Charles Manlove had first met as boys, in 1922, when Vivien was twelve and Charles was thirteen. Vivien had gotten involved in a scuffle with two other kids from the neighborhood. Charles didn't like bullies and when he spotted some big boys shoving around a tall but spindle-legged kid who showed no interest in fighting back (or perhaps no one had taught him how to spar with fisticuffs), he was jolted into action. "Hey, cut it out!" he yelled, as his right foot pushed him up and off the sidewalk to run toward trouble.[4] As quick as a fireball, he shoved off, pushing the hooligans away. The bullies scattered, as bullies will do when the odds are no longer in their favor, and Charles introduced himself to the skinny boy. Since then, Thomas and Manlove had become closer than brothers.[5]

Now that Thomas was struggling to find work, it was only natural for him to ask Charles Manlove to come to his rescue again. Could he help him find a job at Vanderbilt?

"You don't want to work out there," was Manlove's immediate response.[6] Unlike Fisk, Vanderbilt was for white students and professors only, and Manlove knew from personal experience that it was not a friendly or even approachable environment for a young Black man trying to make his way in the world. Thomas replied that he couldn't be particular about whom he worked for or where he worked; he just needed a job.

Manlove said he would do what he could. People at the university respected Manlove, they knew the quality of his character and his work, but even so, it was going to take some courage to advocate on Thomas's behalf. A Black man approaching his white supervisors to ask for support for another Black man might easily be interpreted as audacious, "uppity" even.[7]

Despite the risk, Manlove asked around and returned to Thomas with mixed news. "There's a lab job but you'd have to report to Dr. Blalock," he explained, describing him as "a son of a bitch."[8] These were strong words from Manlove, who, like Thomas, was a churchgoing man. Despite these warnings, Thomas urged his good friend to recommend him for the job. As a young Black male in the segregated South in the early months of the Great Depression, he knew any job opportunities were rare and that he couldn't risk throwing away this chance.

Based on Manlove's recommendation, Blalock agreed to interview Thomas for the position of lab assistant at Vanderbilt University's medical school in Nashville—and Thomas, only nineteen years old, was determined to look like a professional at this meeting. He was a handsome young man, with medium-length hair, a wisp of a mustache on his upper lip and a look of intelligent purpose in his eyes. Having carefully dressed in his Sunday suit and tie, he strode out of his family's neighborhood in Nashville, making his way to the bus stop where he met his friend Charles Manlove. They climbed aboard a passing city bus heading southeast, paid their fares, and walked to the restricted back section for African Americans where they sat down, Thomas awkwardly squeezing his long limbs into the narrow seat as the vehicle expelled exhaust, laboriously jolting and belching its way through town. He must have felt nervous, although he always tried to keep his cool.

When the two young men climbed down from the bus, they walked through a quadrant of campus buildings toward the impressive arched entrance of Vanderbilt's medical school. As they approached, Manlove nudged him to the right, away from the majestic entrance. "We go through the back door," he said, and Thomas needed no explanation of why this was. He followed his friend down the hallway to the experimental surgery laboratory where Charles introduced him to assistant professor Alfred Blalock, who was slugging down an ice-cold bottle of Coca-Cola.[9]

In the years to come, Blalock would gain a reputation as a titan of the medical field, but for now, he was just a young doctor at a then-mediocre medical school with only a handful of research publications to his credit. Thomas was awfully surprised when he sighted Blalock because he'd been expecting the "son of a bitch" to be older, more distinguished, a tweed-suited professor.[10] Instead, Blalock could easily have been mistaken for a letter-sweater undergraduate, his dark wavy hair slicked back, jug ears sticking out, and black-and-white saddle shoes on his feet. In fact, at thirty, Blalock was only eleven years older than Thomas.

Blalock invited Thomas into his "office," made up of a makeshift desk and chair in a small area in Vanderbilt's experimental surgery laboratory. Blalock offered Thomas one of the lab's high stools for a seat and pulled up another for himself. The doctor was shorter, so the straight-backed Thomas self-consciously towered over him as they perched on their lofty stools.

Blalock pitched questions to Thomas about his prior education, his work experience, and his family, putting down his Coke bottle and picking up a Pall Mall cigarette, offering one to Thomas, who accepted, using each draw of tobacco as a few seconds of opportunity to think about his responses. Nodding sympathetically while Thomas talked, Blalock gave the appearance of supporting Thomas's goal to become a physician. The surgeon was a keen listener and, with the perspicacity for which he would later become known, he quickly sized up Thomas, assessing this young man for his full worth. The young surgeon possessed an uncanny ability to detect people who could be of genuine assistance to him.

As the men spoke, the applicant described his job experience, pointing out the dexterity he had gained from working with carpentry tools and he also emphasized his solid science and math background in high school. He recited all his impressive courses: biology, physics, chemistry, geology, geometry, and advanced algebra. He let Blalock know that his older sister was a nurse and that his brother would be starting a master's degree in biology. About his own plans and ambition, Thomas was candid from the beginning. "I told him that I would like to go on to medical

THE TURNING POINT

school," he said, and that he had put a freeze on his savings until he could add to it.[11]

He recounted his beloved family doctor, someone who had inspired his early interest in medicine. That's how he saw himself too, he explained. He just needed to save more money before he could complete his education. Blalock appeared interested, nodding at his word as if in affirmation of the young man's goals, which appealed to Thomas, who was wondering why the stories about the surgeon were so negative. For his part, Blalock described his ideal candidate for the job.

"I want someone in the lab whom I can teach to do anything I can do and maybe things I can't do," Blalock told Thomas. "I want someone who can get to the point that he can do things on his own even though I may not be around."[12] Thomas swallowed hard when he realized the level of responsibility Blalock demanded from him.

After the interview, Blalock was eager to show Thomas around the lab. Thomas was unimpressed when he saw the long narrow and dingy space. He surveyed the dreary room's five wooden operating tables, with an old metal double sink and a single light hanging from the ceiling. His thoughts were interrupted when Blalock introduced him to two other Black lab techs, Samuel Waters, who was fifty-four, and Isaac Body, who was about ten years older than Waters. The pair looked up from their work to briefly greet Thomas before returning to their tasks.

Watching Thomas closely, Blalock intuited he might just prove to be instrumental to his new findings on the deadly effects of traumatic shock, which was one of the major medical problems throughout the world. The surgeon-researcher had published his first article on fatal traumatic shock in 1927.[13] Three years later, when he met Thomas, he was awaiting the publication of his second journal article on traumatic shock that pointed toward a viable solution or "cure" for treating shock.[14] Blalock had a feeling—call it a hunch—that the reserved young Black man would be capable of assisting him on his momentous shock research. "He saw something in Vivien," related Dan Blalock, his youngest child.[15]

Now that Blalock was satisfied that he'd found the right man, he offered Thomas the lab research job on the spot. Thomas's spirits lifted immediately but when Blalock explained that Vanderbilt's surgery department would pay him only $624 a year (currently $11,570) he was shocked.[16] He had been earning $1,040 (currently $19,300) as a carpenter at Fisk.[17] He wondered if the surgeon was purposely undercutting his salary because he knew that Thomas, like so many others in 1930, was desperate for a job. That he was a Black man made it easier for Blalock to undermine his earnings.

Thomas was caught short. Couldn't Vanderbilt do better? Blalock's proposed salary would mean a 40 percent pay cut, which didn't make sense. Surely the university had a heftier budget than Fisk? After all, the role of an assistant in a laboratory conducting independent medical surgery experiments required far more responsibility than a carpentry job fixing squeaky doors and building bookcases.[18] Blalock insisted that the pay was fair; then hemmed and hawed, saying that Thomas could receive a pay raise in April or May, which was three to four months away.

Faced with Blalock's salary proposal, Thomas was in a dilemma. Should he take the job or walk away? His father had schooled him in "the economics of life" and so he knew that such low pay would barely cover his daily expenses and leave him with no money to save.[19] On the other hand, he was out of work and had no other job offers on the horizon. At least working in a medical research lab would give him a solid foundation for admission to medical school. What's more, if he took the Vanderbilt job, he could always return to better paid carpentry work later in the spring when, he hoped, construction would pick up. Then, with more money saved, he could finally start college. Trusting the surgeon's word to improve his pay within a few months, Thomas agreed to Blalock's thirty-cents-an-hour wage.

Blalock told him to arrive the next morning at eight o'clock sharp. With that, the surgeon nodded and went on his way. Thomas stayed on at the lab, watching how the other lab staff worked, asking them about what they were doing and why, and about Blalock's reputation as a supervisor. The other lab technicians didn't go as far Manlove had done in his description, but neither were they particularly enthusiastic. "He's all right," was their highest endorsement.[20]

When Blalock returned some hours later, he was surprised to see Thomas still there, conscientiously preparing himself for this first day on the job. The two men were unaware that this brief twenty-minute interview would reconfigure both their lives.

CHAPTER THREE

STARTING OFF: EXPERIMENTS IN TRAUMATIC SHOCK

After being hired on the spot by Alfred Blalock, Thomas was expected to appear at work the very next day, Tuesday. Once again, he left his family's home to make the journey to Vanderbilt University. This time he did not take the bus because he knew he could no longer afford the luxury of a bus token on his Vanderbilt salary. Instead, he walked the several miles from his home to campus, aiming to arrive at the university for his appointed start time of eight in the morning. With his long-legged strides, Thomas managed to get to Vanderbilt early, but as he walked into the lab, he found to his great embarrassment that Professor Blalock, dressed in his white lab coat, was already there, eager and ready to start an experiment.

To prepare Thomas for the surgical work ahead, Blalock proceeded to explain to his new assistant what was known about shock. Simply described, he said, traumatic shock is the body's natural reaction to being physically injured. Shock, not the injury itself, often caused death. The most common reasons for traumatic shock included heavy bleeding, cardiac arrest, crushing, severe allergic reactions, burns or an infection. Even such minor injuries to the body as dehydration can result in lethal shock if not properly treated.

Starting Off

Although Blalock never elucidated his motivation for studying shock, it wasn't long before Thomas realized that the professor was working to address one of the most consequential unsolved medical mysteries of the times. If Blalock could only crack the problem, doctors and surgeons around the world would be able to save millions of human lives every single year—and Blalock's reputation would be secured forever in medical history.

For traumatic shock was a god-awful thing, a killer. For thousands of years of human history, physicians had observed traumatic shock and described its symptoms in the medical literature, but no one had been able to understand what caused it or how to treat it. Now we know that shock is caused by a certain type of fluid, rich in protein, that has been redirected from general circulation and sent to the injured area. Because there is far less circulating fluid throughout the body because of this redirection, the fluid loss typically precipitates a dangerous loss in blood pressure. Today, traumatic shock is treatable using extra fluid and blood infusions into the body and is no longer a danger to the vast majority of us. But when Blalock first began studying the condition, traumatic shock was both untreatable and, typically, fatal.

The first person who is credited with defining shock was the "highly inventive" Hippocrates, born in 460 BCE.[1] Shock was called *extremia* to indicate that once patients began to show symptoms, death was sure to follow. About 700 years later, a surgeon to Roman gladiators, Claudius Galen of Pergamon (CE 129–200), declared that shock should be treated by bloodletting, which in fact only worsened the problem and resulted in more deaths. Still, this method dominated medical treatment for the next 2,000 years or so, until nearly the beginning of the twentieth century.

William Harvey, an Englishman in the early 1600s, was the first to identify the basics of blood circulation. His discoveries significantly improved knowledge of how the heart worked as a pump to drive the body's blood circulation but he never made the direct connection between it and shock. It wasn't until the 1700s that the French physician Henri-François Le Dran first coined the term shock (*saisissement* or "stunned") to describe the body's response to injury.[2] Firearms and other weapons of war became more sophisticated throughout the eighteenth and nineteenth centuries, and the need to understand the body's reaction to wounds became all the more pressing.

Samuel D. Gross, MD, a nineteenth-century professor at Thomas Jefferson Medical College in Philadelphia, dramatically and accurately described shock as "the manifestation of the rude unhinging of the machinery of life."[3] In other words, shock caused death. Before Gross, physicians had always associated shock with traumatic physical injuries; however, he made a significant breakthrough when he established that shock could be caused by mere illnesses, too. Severe dehydration, allergic reaction, heart conditions, internal bleeding, infection, and spinal injuries can all put the body into shock. (Gross was the subject of Thomas Eakins's great representational American 1875 painting, *The Gross Clinic*, which depicted the gruesome realities of surgery. The painting is at the Philadelphia Museum of Art.)

Most of Gross's firsthand experiences were with external injuries because he had been a surgeon in the American Civil War, which, by its end, had killed 600,000 soldiers and injured many times that number. As the author of several medical manuals for military surgeons serving in that war, Gross recommended a few basic treatments: mostly keeping patients warm and having them drink such stimulants as coffee, alcohol, and, in small amounts, ammonia.[4] In many instances, Gross's stimulants did help, but no one knew why. By the end of the nineteenth century, a handful of doctors tried administering epinephrine (the hormone adrenaline) because it constricts blood flow during hemorrhage. However, an older generation of surgeons soon quashed that idea, convinced that bloodletting was the only valid treatment.

In the late 1890s, the Italian physician Scipione Riva-Rocci developed a new medical instrument, the mercury sphygmomanometer, to measure brachial (upper arm) blood pressure. The device gave a more accurate metric to evaluate blood pressure; it was an important indicator because physicians wondered whether low blood pressure was causing shock.[5]

Another important advance was made by George Washington Crile, MD when he performed the first human blood transfusion in 1914.[6] His technique enabled transfusions to be given during operations to prevent

Starting Off

shock, and these became known as shockless surgery. Crile thought that the problem of traumatic shock was caused by experiencing too many sensory inputs to the body. He disagreed with Gross's use of stimulants to ameliorate shock, arguing that stimulants would not raise blood pressure and therefore could not help a patient undergoing shock.

Then, in 1917, a leading medical researcher named Walter Cannon, MD joined the list of eminent medical minds to take on the problem. The Great War, as World War I was still known, was in its third year and the US had just entered the European conflict. Cannon was asked straight-away to join the Army's research laboratory as a member of the Harvard Hospital Unit and he was dispatched to Belgium to serve as a surgeon on the Western Front. At the time, Cannon was already considered a giant in the field of physiology, having been the first to describe the interaction between the nervous system and adrenaline, becoming famous for coining the term "fight or flight."[7]

Cannon was convinced that there had to be a better cure for shock than bloodletting. In this, he was not alone. During the war, English, French, Belgian, and American physicians began working cooperatively to conquer shock. After all, the Great War introduced vicious new weapons—including machine guns, hand grenades, poisonous gas, tanks, and airplane bombers—into the international arsenal. These horrific instruments of death made Allied research on shock nothing short of vital. On the Belgian Front, Cannon had plenty of opportunity to observe its effect on human subjects and became convinced endogenous toxins were to blame. These "histamine-like substances" are released by the body itself.[8] Shock, he reasoned, was entirely the result of these toxins being released in the body after an injury.

As Cannon and other medical researchers continued their work, the Great War wore on. By the time the conflict came to an end in 1918, every town and village throughout Europe was affected, with an estimated eighteen million casualties. On the battlefield, lives were lost; at home, hearts were broken. So many of those fatalities were due to wounds, burns, or injuries that led to traumatic shock. If only an authentic treatment had been found, many of those millions of deaths could have been avoided.

Five years after the end of the war, in 1923, Cannon published *Traumatic Shock*, a book that advocated his toxicity theory.[9] Cannon's lab results were inconsistent, but, at the time, he stubbornly adhered to his hypothesis. Almost no physicians disagreed with him because his reputation was so stellar. The medical community wholeheartedly endorsed his assertion that toxemia was the major reason for shock.

At the time Cannon published his book, twenty-four-old Alfred Blalock was merely a recent graduate of Johns Hopkins University medical school. Within a few years, he'd decided that the older man's methodology was wrong as well as the earlier theories on what caused shock. This young and unknown surgeon set out to disprove Cannon's shock theory, backing his thoughts up with the lab work that supported his findings. He was taking a tremendous risk by challenging the esteemed older man. Later, when Blalock was at Vanderbilt, Blalock's department head, Barney Brooks, MD asked him if he really wanted to challenge Cannon: "Are you sure, Al, really sure? You know, this can make you or break you."[10] After all, Cannon was an icon at that time. Undeterred, Blalock was keen to identify the authentic cause of shock and to devise a medical treatment for it.[11] Blalock already had his first two articles of four pivotal journal publications on shock finished by the time he'd hired Vivien Thomas.

That day, without further ado, Blalock started Thomas on shock experiments by showing him how to prepare a dog for surgery. He told him to record his observations by taking detailed notes. In fact, Blalock was a stickler for quantitative accuracy. Thomas pulled out a black-and-white speckled composition book he had thought to bring with him. The men walked to the rows of cages where the captive lab dogs were constrained. Thomas found himself faced with dozens of stray dogs that had been purchased from the local animal pounds for medical experiments. Initially, he felt torn at the very thought of inflicting harm on these creatures but as he said, "Fortunately, Dr. Blalock had explained the need for these experiments in such detail that I soon overcame my reluctance to inflict the trauma."[12]

STARTING OFF

At this time in 1930, lab dogs were widely used to advance medical breakthroughs through experimentation. In fact, dogs had been used in scientific research as far back as the days of antiquity because of their relatively small body size and their physiology, which is very similar to that of humans. Autopsies on human beings—other than convicted criminals—were taboo in classical ancient Greece; dissecting animals was the closest anyone could come to understanding the human body.[13] Then, after a long lull in animal research that continued throughout medieval times, it returned during the Renaissance period starting in the 1500s, with no real thought for the animals' suffering.[14] It wasn't until the 1700s, roughly, that people began considering the pain inflicted on animals and the ethical treatment of animals.[15] By the 1850s, a medical revolution was taking place in north Germany with a new focus on scientific findings that derived from observation and analysis of animal experiments. Still, there were no laws yet that protected animals. Doctors justified animal experimentation by the idea that saving human lives was more important than the suffering of animals.

In the coming years, Blalock would be forced to participate in a very public battle with animal rights protesters who opposed his use of these animals in his research. At the time, he and his work were little known, and he remained convinced that the medical insight gained from experiments on these animals was worth their sacrifice. Thomas had to rapidly come to grips with his discomfort at imposing harm on dogs. Thoughtfully taking care of the lab dogs so they remained as comfortable as possible, Thomas saw to it that his lab colleagues also treated them with care.

On that January morning, Blalock selected a dog and brought it into the main lab area to be weighed, ushering it onto a long metal scale. Once the dog's weight in kilograms was determined, Blalock showed Thomas how to use the weight metric to calculate the precise number of milligrams of barbital sodium needed to anesthetize the animal. Next, Blalock demonstrated how to fill a glass tube, known as a burette, with a powerful mix of the diluted barbital sodium. Then, the men lifted the dog up onto the table, and Blalock asked Thomas to restrain the animal while he showed him how to inject a shot of Novocain, a local pain killer, into its thigh.

Once the area was numb, Blalock cut down a vein with a scalpel and inserted the burette, slowly letting the sodium barbital and saline solution drip into the open vein until the dog became unconscious.[16]

Thomas stood at Blalock's side as he waited for the dog on the lab table to be fully sedated. The experiment Blalock was about to perform concerned the shock consequences of such crushing injuries as blunt force, rather than a burn or a bullet injury. Once the dog was fully unconscious, Blalock reached for a hammer and, without blinking an eye, bludgeoned the sleeping dog repeatedly. This way, he successfully induced traumatic shock. Thomas stood by, taking copious notes. He was to spend the rest of the day observing the animal and recording its vital statistics.

Finished with his instruction session, Blalock gave Thomas an assignment for the next morning. He wanted Thomas to have another dog anesthetized and ready for surgery: this time, before Blalock arrived at the lab. Thomas had taken plenty of notes. He was smart, diligent, and a quick study, but even so, Blalock's high expectations and his demand left him "speechless."[17] He had only just started at the lab. He had never seen any surgical instruments before, yet alone used them, and now he was supposed to prep a dog for surgery?

As soon as the professor departed, Thomas turned to Sam Waters, another one of the lab technicians.

"Is he serious?" Thomas asked.

"He won't show you but once," Waters replied.[18]

CHAPTER FOUR

AT LAST, ON HIS WAY

The next morning, Thomas again walked several miles to work. This time, he arrived before Blalock and apprehensively looked around the unfamiliar lab filled with the many tools and instruments he'd yet to use. Sam Waters was also early at work and took it upon himself to help Thomas with his surgery prep, reminding Thomas how to repeat the steps that the "professor," as Thomas would call Blalock, had shown him the day before. When Blalock walked in, he was pleased to see that the dog was indeed sedated and ready for surgery, exactly as he had instructed.

Soon Blalock put on his white coat and gathered his surgical tools, then stepped in to take over. As he started the operation, the surgeon explained what he was doing and why he was doing it. "Keep your eyes open and write things down," he told Thomas, who was faithfully writing down each individual step of each procedure in his composition book.[1] If these first days with Blalock were any indication of what was to come, Thomas knew he would need to watch, listen, and learn, fast, on his feet.

After the crushing experiment done on the previous day, Blalock worked with Thomas on shock experiments that involved burning the anesthetized animals. Thomas felt better knowing that the experiments were the only means available to find a solution to shock, but he admitted that the burn experiments, with their flesh-scorched smells, did not "make me particular for lunch," as he told a friend.[2] As the days progressed, the new lab assistant was never told beforehand exactly which experiment Blalock would want him to perform. Thomas familiarized himself with the necessary lab instruments: the mercury manometer with a spring motor that measured blood pressure, a Van Slyke-Neil blood glass measurement apparatus that measured carbon dioxide and oxygen content, a Benedict-Roth spirometer that measured oxygen consumption, and a Salhi hemoglobin meter that measured hemoglobin.[3]

Less than a month later, Blalock casually informed Thomas that he would be delayed the following morning and Thomas should complete the surgery on his own, without supervision. This was a daunting prospect for someone who had no prior formal training and was barely in his second month on the job. Thomas decided to use his lunch breaks to study both traumatic shock and the methodology of operating on small animals. He wrote formulas and equations in his trusty composition book, which he guarded as carefully as his wallet. He was complimented that Blalock had enough confidence to leave him alone to perform these experimental surgeries, but he still felt under significant pressure.

He needn't have worried. After only a short time on the job, Thomas began to handle the once unfamiliar surgical equipment with a surprising level of skill. It occurred to him that his lab work might accomplish something important, and this pleased him, not for his own glory, but simply because he felt such a strong calling to help others.[4] Maybe he could even save some lives.

The subject of his pay, however, continued to prove distressing and particularly stressful for him. Thomas never knew where he stood. When April arrived, Blalock's promise of a salary adjustment failed to materialize. Thankfully, Thomas was able to add some carpentry work on Saturdays to make a little extra money.[5] In late May, he finally approached Blalock about his promised raise, confident that he deserved it because of his exemplary work. Blalock seemed less sure.[6] Appearing confused, the professor cocked his head, looking like a confused basset hound trying to perk up one ear. Thomas, new to Blalock's manipulative games, didn't know whether Blalock really had forgotten about his promise or if he was he simply pretending. It was hard to tell. The meeting ended with Blalock assuring Thomas that he'd get back to him.

Coincidentally, Thomas received a phone call from Fisk: the college wanted to rehire him for a full time position the very next day at the galvanizing pay level of twenty dollars a week. Not having heard a word from Blalock about his salary and with his new Fisk job offer in hand, Thomas went back to Blalock and simply resigned.[7] He was tired of waiting and he thought he was being jerked around. He did appreciate his job, but he knew he needed to keep his primary goal in mind, which was to save whatever money he could for his further education.

When he told the professor that he was leaving, Blalock seemed genuinely surprised and somewhat offended that Thomas could command twenty dollars a week somewhere else. "We can't pay that kind of money," the surgeon whined. Then he quickly added, "How much will you stay here for?"[8]

Thomas was bewildered. He had just given notice and never anticipated that quitting a job would make Blalock so perturbed; in no way was he prepared for the arguments and negotiations that followed. Blalock seemed annoyed and began lecturing Thomas on the advantages a lab job had over carpentry work. He first mentioned the relatively short (eight hour) workday, without acknowledging that Thomas daily stayed late. Then Blalock appealed to Thomas's ego and cleverly pointed out that he was now working with people with a higher level of education and greater intelligence than carpenters.[9] This seemed clearly designed to appeal to Thomas's own desire to become a physician. He added that lab work was done inside, not outside in all types of weather, and he reminded him of Vanderbilt's generous one-week paid vacation.[10] The surgeon seemed prepared to rebut Thomas on every point, all the while claiming that he remembered nothing about a promised raise.

Thomas, though, had to wonder. How could the small undergraduate Fisk College be able to pay him more than Vanderbilt University, with its multimillion dollar gifts from the Rockefeller foundation? In any case, Blalock added that any pay raise needed approval from Barney Brooks, who was Vanderbilt's surgery head and Blalock's boss. This was inauspicious news given Brooks's reputation for refusing to talk with or even acknowledge any staff member who was Black. If you were a Black member of Brooks's staff and said, "Good morning" to him, he would cut you dead. You just didn't exist."[11] A few weeks later, Blalock told him that Brooks didn't seem to have any time to meet to discuss his salary. Therefore, claimed the professor, the salary issue was out of his hands. He shrugged. Thomas just had to learn to be more patient.

Worried about losing the twenty-dollar-an-hour job at Fisk, Thomas quit, once again. He was serious. Immediately, Blalock agreed to a slightly improved salary of $17.50 per week or $884 annually (currently $18,000 a year).[12] Thomas was surprised, feeling caught and uncertain, because the offer was still less than he would have received as a carpenter at Fisk. As he hesitated, the professor tried to hold out another promise, "One day, I'll have my own surgery department and no one will be able to tell me how much I can pay people."[13] Thomas had no reason not to believe him.

In his first six months on the job, Vivien Thomas had not been listed on Vanderbilt's surgery staff list. On July 18, when his pay raise went into effect, Thomas appeared for the first time on the fiscal year 1930 surgery budget, although not as a lab technician. He didn't know this at the time, but he was listed as a "janitor in experimental surgery to be paid from Supplies and Equipment as a temporary salary item."[14]

Of course, the salary issue was not whether the surgery department had enough money to pay Thomas a fair wage but rather how it wanted to allocate its resources. Black hires at Vanderbilt were receiving lower wages than white staff. Tinsley Harrison, MD, also a surgeon at Vanderbilt, for example, had hired a young white female lab tech, Minnie Mae Timms, who, like Thomas, had only a high school diploma; she was paid 50 percent more than Thomas. Harrison also acknowledged Timms's lab contributions by including her as last author on his articles, after his own name and those of his physician colleagues.[15] Of course, this information was never given to Thomas who, like other Black employees, was purposely kept ignorant by Vanderbilt.

In 1932, Blalock and Brooks used grant money that had been specifically designated for Thomas but was not included in his wages: presumably, they diverted this extra money into the general surgery budget.

AT LAST, ON HIS WAY

This is how they carried out their deception: the department was receiving fluid research grant funding from the General Education Board, the same Rockefeller philanthropy for Southern education that had already given a million dollars to Vanderbilt. In his application for the grant, Blalock specifically requested an annual salary of $1,000 for "my present excellent technician, Vivien Thomas." He continued, "My technician has been most satisfactory and it would handicap me greatly to lose his services which, I realize, would be necessary if this grant is not obtained."[16] Blalock received the grant money, yet Thomas never received a penny more than his usual $884. This chicanery continued for several of the most devastating years of the Depression.

The story gets more unappealing. Blalock, Brooks, and Vanderbilt also chose to take advantage of the liberal New York philanthropy with its deep pockets by claiming in their grant application that Thomas's title was "laboratory technician."[17] Yet the department and the university's personnel rosters listed him as a janitor in his beginning year of work. The next year, his status was inexplicably downgraded to assistant janitor. The year after that and for the rest of the decade, he went back to being listed as a janitor again.[18] Thomas didn't know any of this until 1937, when he and his fellow lab techs did some sleuthing and finally determined that "he and the all the colored men" were listed as janitors by Vanderbilt, no matter what their actual job entailed.[19]

At that point, Thomas had worked at Vanderbilt for seven years and he wanted to talk the problem through with the professor, by himself. Discussions of pay and job titles should take place one-on-one, between the supervisor and the worker, he thought. He said of Vanderbilt, "Had there been an organized complaint by the Negroes performing technical duties, there was a good chance that all kinds of excuses would have been offered to avoid giving us the technician's pay and that leaders of the movement or action would have been summarily fired."[20] Thomas, ever practical, realized that his pay was more important than his title.

This time, he told Blalock that he would not remain at Vanderbilt unless his salary was raised. In response, Blalock immediately wrote Brooks, "I am afraid of losing him unless his salary can be increased."[21] Then Blalock suggested that the surgery department pay his talented lab worker "an extra $72 a year," beginning in 1938. It meant that Thomas began to earn $956, which was only $44 less than the money that was allocated for him by the grant.

Thomas never learned that Blalock and Brooks deceived him by using his allocated GEB salary to increase the surgery budget rather than paying the sum designated for him. How could Blalock have been so indifferent to Thomas's needs, especially during the Depression? To answer that question, it's important to understand the degree to which Blalock's worldview was shaped by his family and his Southern upbringing.

CHAPTER FIVE

Coming Up Easy

Alfred Blalock was born at home on April 5, 1899, in Culloden, Georgia, a sleepy town a long 350 miles farther south than Nashville, to Martha (Mattie) Davis Blalock and George Zadock Blalock. During Mattie's labor, word came of an approaching storm, so George moved her to a safer location, which was a good decision: the blustering storm blew the roof off their house. Alfred's birth was thirty-four years after the end of the Civil War, and if cotton was King, then Blalock was born into an aristocratic family of former Confederate plantation owners, businessmen, and bankers. Alfred's mother even claimed to be related to the president of the Confederacy, Jefferson Davis, and although her lineage proved putative, Alfred believed it and the entire family esteemed her purported antecedents.[1]

As it happened, Mattie Blalock, through her paternal Thomas Warren line, was an authentic descendant of colonists from Jamestown, Virginia's first colony, which was far more prestigious for Southerners than even being kin to Davis. Warren had built a fifty-foot brick house back in 1652, which remains the oldest residence still standing in the state, and it is open to visitors.[2] That property was purchased so long ago that Mattie's antecedent Thomas Warren had bought its land from the son of Pocahontas (Rebecca) and John Rolfe.[3]

On the father's side, the Blalock family first came to the US from the Scottish Highlands and eventually settled in Georgia. Before the Civil

War—or the War of Northern Aggression, as the Blalocks would likely have called it—Alfred's grandfather, Zadock Blalock, lived in a large white plantation house, supported by eight Tuscan columns on the front porch of the two-story Greek revival. Here he ran the family cotton plantation, relying on the toil of enslaved people to plant and pick the crop. Though the Blalocks were not the top tier of the richest Southern plantation owners, they nevertheless did very well indeed.

King Cotton was the crop to which the state of Georgia owed its accelerating growth throughout the 1800s. After the invention of the cotton gin (gin for engine), which speedily separated out the seeds and unwanted parts from the desired fine lustrous fibers, King Cotton became the state's number one commodity, outweighing in importance tobacco, sugar, and rice. The plantation owners wanted more land for planting cotton and then more slaves to pick it. The explosion in the demand for land ultimately led to the expulsion of American Indians from their traditional lands. The Trail of Tears, as it was later named, ejected and relocated the Chickasaw, Choctaw, Creek, Seminole, and Cherokee people. Part of its path ran through Nashville. With more land, more slaves, and the gin mill, plantation owners became obscenely rich. With their wealth came the need for institutions in which they could place their money.[4] The Blalocks founded several banks in which they and their friends could deposit their own riches, thus becoming members of an elite group of plantation owners/bankers.

The Bank of Jonesboro (formerly spelled Jonesborough) was founded and owned by Alfred's uncle Alfred C. Blalock, who also had served as the town's mayor and councilman and, who, as a state senator, voted to remove Georgia from the Union. Another uncle, Eugene M. Blalock of Jonesboro, founded the Atlanta Loan and Banking Company in 1851, a farm-loan lending bank that charged lower interests rates made possible through Blalock connections. Atlanta Loan grew to serve four Southern states. William Blalock, yet another relative, founded Atlanta's Fulton National Bank and Aaron O. Blalock, although not a banker, was Georgia's tax collector.[5] "The Blalocks were considered one of the best families in this region," said the historian Joe Moore. "Making money came as natural to the Blalocks as breathing air."[6]

Alfred had four siblings: Edgar, Elizabeth, Mary, and Georgia (note her name) and they lived in a two-story, twelve-room house on three acres of land. Mr. Blalock, as Mattie always addressed her husband George, was the autocratic head of a joyless home. Alfred's sister Georgia described her father as "hard to please."[7] He oversaw everything from child-rearing philosophy (strict) to their social life (virtually nonexistent). "The only show of love or tenderness that I ever saw between my parents was shown by Mother as Father lay dying," Georgia said.[8]

Despite the house's gloom, Mattie always deferred to her husband in all matters, including his decision to forbid the family's celebration of holidays and birthdays.[9] As a result, the children avoided their father whenever possible. He seemed impervious to humor and few ever caught him smiling. He also forbade laughter during meals. Alfred, as a young child, responded by being a very conscientious student in elementary school and stayed up past his bedtime to study his spelling lists and multiplication tables.

Perhaps their father's day-in and day-out stomach and intestinal problems contributed to his continual air of displeasure. Eventually, George's health became so troublesome that he elected to undergo an operation in the early 1900s, at a time when most people saw hospitals as the last step before the morgue. The surgery was done at Johns Hopkins University Hospital in Baltimore, Maryland, and George became a living witness to the superiority of Hopkins and its physicians at the beginning of the twentieth century. In a rare instance of praise, he told his family that Hopkins was "a fine place" and "the best medical facility in the world."[10]

George's surgeon recommended that he leave the countryside to be closer to Atlanta's superior hospitals. When Alfred was eleven, the family moved north to Jonesboro and his father built a clay court on their property where Alfred played tennis as often as he could. Alfred noted that there were other reasons for his father to choose a new location. "A good number of my father's relatives lived there, and, furthermore, he was anxious to retire from business," which he did at the enviable age of forty-four.[11]

Jonesboro, where Alfred spent most of his childhood, may not be a household name but the town holds a special place in our collective

American popular culture because of a fellow Georgian who was born a scant seven months after Blalock, and only sixty-four miles away. Her name was Margaret Mitchell and she wrote *Gone with the Wind*. The novel depicts a nostalgic Old South, brilliantly pictured, and Mitchell carefully selected Jonesboro as the location for Tara, the cotton plantation that was her heroine Scarlett O'Hara's beloved home.[12] The portrayal of the heroic Confederate South, no matter how false, has influenced Americans for years, despite the efforts of frustrated American history teachers who tell students that it is not a true representation of life in the slave-holding South.

Fiction aside, during the Civil War, the Battle of Jonesboro included a skirmish at Blalock's Gap, right on the family's cotton plantation. Their house also served first as a commissary and then as a field hospital for Southern wounded during the War.[13] Following the Civil War and the abolishment of slavery, planters were typically land rich and cash poor. Not the Blalocks. Their banking connections provided access to authentic federal dollar bills rather than worthless Confederacy currency. In addition, Alfred's grandfather, Zadock, who was one of the last Blalock slaveholders, signed the Confederate Reconstruction Oath Book on July 31, 1867, two years after the end of the War.[14] True Southern patriots scorned this oath (as did the fictional Scarlett O'Hara) and many refused to swear allegiance to the US Constitution and to the Emancipation Proclamation because it required them to state that, "I have never… engaged in insurrection or rebellion against the US, or given aid or comfort to the enemies thereof…." By signing this oath, however, Zadock Blalock could vote and run for office. It also meant that he was able to receive cash repayment for damage done to his property during the 1864 Battle of Jonesboro. With the cash, he restored his 250-acre plantation, and even purchased fifty more acres, bringing his plantation size up to 300 acres.[15]

As the Blalock plantation continued to prosper, sharecroppers, the same people who had worked on the plantation while enslaved, continued to harvest Blalock cotton. Georgian sharecroppers were typically given free rent for the shacks in which they lived and received in return, at most, one-third of the profits. As the sharecroppers were never paid in money, they had to buy life's necessities, including seeds for planting, on credit and often from the owner himself, who saw to it that the sharecroppers never got out of debt.[16] This system lasted for nearly one hundred years past the Emancipation Proclamation.

Alfred spent much of his childhood hearing about the Civil War from his parents, and as a result, took away a particularly nostalgic and romanticized view of the vanquished South. His father had been born only a year after the war ended and grew up hearing sentimental tales from grandparents and uncles and aunts about their antebellum way of life. As a child, Alfred had seen, firsthand, families of field hands on Blalock land, backs twisted over cotton plants. Instinctively, he understood the status quo: one for you, the laborer, and two for me, the owner. He saw this as the natural order and kept this value set through his lifetime, blinkering his eyes from the changing world about him.

No doubt his fellow high school students at Georgia Military College and later, the undergraduates at the University of Georgia, reinforced his sense of white superiority. When he graduated in 1918, Alfred decided to go to medical school and set his eye on Hopkins because his father venerated its physicians and surgeons. Although it was in the waning days of the war, young men still had to register for possible conscription, but Blalock was given an exemption that allowed him to go to medical school because the military needed physicians. With his connections, Blalock was easily admitted to the Johns Hopkins School of Medicine. He was quite pleased; it seemed that his life was moving along smoothly on its righteous course.

CHAPTER SIX

Staying Alive

In the fall of 1919, twenty-year-old Alfred Blalock entered Johns Hopkins medical school with eighty-some other students. He already knew that the Hopkins hospital had opened in 1889 and the medical school four years later, in 1893. The Founding Four were the distinguished physicians William H. Welch, MD, William S. Halsted, MD, William Osler, MD, and Howard Kelly, MD. These men followed the German model of medicine that integrated teaching, research, and patient care, and they initiated those standards at Hopkins, just as Yale University and the University of Pennsylvania had already done.[1] In turn, Johns Hopkins University Medical Institutes, now Johns Hopkins Medicine, set the template for modern hospitals well into the twenty-first century by restructuring the major practices and tenants of medical training that were imitated by other American medical schools and hospitals. Its founders believed that students should learn by doing rather than by memorizing, they updated old autocratic teaching methods and they decreed that medical research was a key mission.[2] Their perspicacity of including a hospital within its medical campus was visionary: most other universities did not have their own hospitals and needed to scramble to place students in whatever nearby hospital that would take them.[3]

Perhaps Hopkins's greatest contribution, say medical historians, was its focus on empirical research.[4] By the time Blalock began medical school, the results of research had spawned the exponential growth of medical discoveries in the US, which topped other nations to become the first in the world in health innovations. Hopkins medicine fast gained the reputation of being an exciting place to study or work.[5]

Hopkins is, of course, located in Baltimore, Maryland, which falls just below the Mason-Dixon line, the traditional border separating the North and the South. At that time, Baltimore's ambience was of a Southern mentality and nearly half of Blalock's American classmates were fellow Southerners.[6] In his first year at Hopkins medical school, Blalock, as a member of the Student Army Training Corps, was required to wear a uniform and live in one of the dormitories newly designated as Army barracks, complete with Reveille and Taps. Nearly 75 percent of Hopkins medical students were in the same situation, which served as consolation to him because he would have preferred more freedom than the barracks gave. Another plus—and this was an important one—was that the government covered his tuition and gave him a soldier's salary, paid in cash with new jingly silver dollars handed out on campus.

Out of the barracks during his second year, Blalock roomed with fellow medical student Tinsley Harrison of Alabama, whose physician father, Groce Harrison, MD, had studied under Hopkins's William Osler a generation earlier and was consequently a graduate of Hopkins's first medical class. Tinsley Harrison, a Southerner himself, said that Blalock had "an accent so thick you could cut it with a knife." He claimed that Blalock had introduced himself this way: "Mah name is Alfred Blalock and Ah'm from Jonesboro, Georgia."[7]

Although Harrison was only sixteen years old, he was already a second-year student, having transferred to Hopkins from the University of Michigan. (In the 1800s and early 1900s, medical schools enrolled much younger students than they do currently. Many had not even a college degree.) The two men joined the same fraternity and were doubles tennis partners. While Harrison worked hard at his studies, Blalock was not your typical cloistered medical student: instead, he spent many hours on the tennis court by day and by night he was carousing and raising hell until close to dawn. Blalock had also bought the rights to run the student bookstore and he put a lot of energy into his profit-making enterprise.

Despite their differences, Harrison soon considered Blalock the best friend he ever had outside of his own four brothers and sisters.

When not playing tennis or running his store, Blalock dated almost compulsively even as Harrison worried that he was shortchanging his studies. "Alfred Blalock was a Casanova," he later asserted. "He was Don Juan."[8] Goucher College, then a college for bright and socially prominent women, was nearby and Blalock could be found on campus three or four nights a week, driving the car he shared with Harrison. At first glance, you would never guess that Blalock was a ladies' man: he was average height, skinny, not particularly handsome. In Baltimore, he had lost whatever tan he had, and his complexion looked fish-belly white, despite his time on the tennis courts. He liked to slick back his coal-black hair and added a part that was a little too close to the middle of his scalp for the fashion of the time. He looked intelligent, although his ears comically stuck out and when he spoke, his Georgia accent oozed from his mouth like molasses. Still, he had a charm that he used to his advantage all his life with both men and women.

Despite his superficial charisma, or maybe because of it, Blalock did well in some of his courses but if he was not interested in a subject, he saw no reason to do any more work than required. Harrison said that getting good grades held little interest for Blalock. In 1922, he graduated from Hopkins medical school at the bottom of the upper half of his class.[9] He'd completed what's known as being an "undergraduate" medical student and now would move on to his "graduate" medical education, which meant a residency in a specialized field.

That spring, however, Blalock's dreams of a great surgical career at Hopkins were shattered. Now a resident house officer, Blalock coveted the general surgery residency, but, because of his grades, he didn't make it. Hopkins placed him as an assistant dispensary urologist.[10] In 1924, he was allowed to become one of five assistant resident surgeons; however, four of the five men kept this position the following year, but Blalock was not retained. Against his wishes, he was moved to the role of an extern in urology.[11] He was crushed and doubly embarrassed because Tinsley Harrison, MD, gained a top surgical internship at Peter Bent Brigham Hospital in Boston under an eminent former Hopkins neurosurgeon, Harvey

Staying Alive

W. Cushing, MD, who had left Hopkins and was now at Harvard University. In contrast, the postgraduate training positions that came Blalock's way were unimpressive, at least to a man whose mediocre grades did not prevent him from envisioning himself as a great surgeon.

Although he was only in his mid-twenties, Blalock began to show signs of ill health that would plague him for the rest of his life. One day, he was on the tennis court with Harrison when he developed a rather painful blister on his heel that quickly became infected. Antibiotics would have been a quick remedy, but these were not yet available. Soon enough, Blalock had a headache, fever, and pain in his sternum, or breastbone, and so he was admitted to the hospital. Released a few days after admission, he returned with a noticeable swelling on his chest and underwent surgery for osteomyelitis, a torturous bone infection. His surgeon cut away parts of Blalock's breastbone and ultimately detected a small abscess caused by a staph infection.

Blalock returned to the Hopkins hospital a few months later, in January 1923, and was diagnosed with hematuria, or blood in the urine. He returned for another exam in February, when his doctor could feel a mass near his left kidney. During yet another operation, the surgeon confirmed that he had a very large hydronephrosis, or distended kidney. The kidney came out along with a liter of clear fluid, but, as it would turn out, the surgeon left Blalock's ureter stump at bit longer than it should have been. The following year, 1924, Blalock went back to Hopkins's hospital for treatment of a nasty sinus infection and facial nerve palsy.

Finally, after two years of being in and out of work and the hospital, Blalock seemed to be healthy again, but he felt adrift: very few senior physicians recognized his potential, even though he'd managed to publish five studies at Hopkins in 1924 and 1925.[12] He had applied for an appointment in general surgery at Hopkins and yet again he was denied. It seemed time for Blalock to move on and leave Hopkins if he were ever going to advance his surgical career. He only had one prospect through a former supervisor, who finally convinced Cushing to let Blalock train at Peter Bent Brigham Hospital in Boston in 1925. Cushing agreed, albeit reluctantly, to try to find a place for him.[13]

Thanks to his friend Harrison, who was now an internal medicine resident at Vanderbilt in Nashville, Blalock also had a connection at that university. Though unexcited about either option, he prioritized going to Vanderbilt to work in surgery over a questionable placement in Boston. Harrison also wanted Blalock to join him as a resident in general surgery. Blalock went along with the idea; it would put him back in surgery and he imagined himself, perhaps unreasonably, becoming head of Vanderbilt's surgical laboratory despite his weak surgical background.

Barney Brooks had recently been named chairman of surgery at Vanderbilt and in a stream of letters written throughout the early winter of 1924 and spring of 1925, Blalock implored Brooks to hire him. He knew that Brooks, a Texan, would be sympathetic to his preference for the South and expressed this in a four-page note, "I hope you will pardon me for writing you in person. I am very anxious to locate in a Southern city."[14] The correspondence stopped just short of begging, but it worked.

Despite his ardent wooing of Brooks and even as he made his way South, Blalock couldn't help but be awash in disappointment. "I thought I was finished, going down to nowhere, to that school in the backwoods," Blalock lamented.[15] In his view, Vanderbilt was not in the same league as Hopkins. One of his sisters later wrote, "I did not know until many years later how much he hated leaving Hopkins."[16] He remembered his father's high opinion of Johns Hopkins and now that he'd failed to make his career there, Blalock characterized himself as "a loser."[17]

CHAPTER SEVEN

OUTRACING DEATH

Al Blalock's first impressions of Vanderbilt did nothing to change his opinion of the place. When Blalock arrived on its Nashville campus, he was horrified to see that Vanderbilt's old hospital had a rodent problem. Harrison called it a "pest house, full of [Norwegian] rats" that were up to eighteen inches long and he remembered that Blalock was bitten by one.[1] To add to their misery, the summer-long heat wave was accompanied by equally high humidity. And, perhaps most notably, Vanderbilt medical school was in chaos with both financial problems and a low rating from the American Medical Association.

Rockefeller's General Education Board philanthropy donated more than three million dollars to build a new Vanderbilt hospital. The facility was designed with a series of very small labs which, the GEB noted, "makes it possible to teach students in small groups and also to meet the conventional requirements of segregation of the races."[2] Harrison, who, though younger, was fast becoming Blalock's mentor as well as friend, tried to buck Blalock out of his slump, pushing him to do his research, insisting that Blalock verify his experimental medical findings by using modern scientific methodology, reiterating what the two men had learned at Hopkins.[3] One colleague later described Harrison as "a kind of 'burr under the saddle' of Al Blalock, stimulating or pushing him in his investigative work."[4] Most of the articles that Blalock had published at Hopkins had not been based on surgical experiments, which Harrison kept emphasizing. The men focused their research on the heart, with Harrison choosing heart failure as his primary interest while, said Blalock, "I selected shock or peripheral circulatory failure as mine, although I had no preconceived ideas regarding etiology (origin)."[5]

Despite Blalock's close friendship with Harrison, it's worth noting that they differed greatly in their outlook when it came to bigotry. Harrison was progressive and at least tried to rise above his Southern background, perhaps because his family's values were different from those Blalock's parents had passed down to their children. In Nashville, when Harrison saw a wooden sign that read "Gentiles Only" nailed to the outside of a bar near Vanderbilt, he and a colleague tore the sign off the building, stormed into the saloon and shoved the plank at the owner, who angrily threw it back. The two physicians then seized the sign to sweep the bar's counter clear of all glassware, to the amazement of the bar customers. "As both were formidable physical specimens," said a colleague, "no attempt was made to delay their leaving."[6]

Still, Harrison and Blalock grew closer and with Harrison's encouragement, Blalock did indeed begin to focus more attention on his own experiments on traumatic shock. He was resolutely self-confident in applying sound, systematic, and orderly research techniques in his experiments. He persevered, diligently experimenting on shock in Vanderbilt's experimental lab, and, slowly, a more mature Blalock began to labor harder, smarter, and longer than ever and became increasingly ambitious. He knew that any breakthrough in the intricate physiology of shock would boost his status in the medical world. Similarly, a major failure might doom him. Only his belief in himself kept him balanced on the high wire, with no net beneath him.

Blalock's background—his sense of entitlement and security in his position in the world—gave him a natural self-confidence, an important quality for any scientific researcher. In a 1927 paper, he had reviewed the established theories about what caused trauma.[7] Then, as the original experiments he began conducting on shock showed promise, he grew increasingly assured that he was perhaps not "a loser," that perhaps he had a real future in front of him. That notion was confirmed when, in

1927, Dean Robinson promoted him to assistant professor at an annual wage of $3,500.[8]

Of course, he had just published that first important article on traumatic shock resulting from hemorrhage, or severe bleeding. His paper, "Mechanism and Treatment of Experimental Shock: Shock Following Hemorrhage," would be the first in a series of four groundbreaking shock studies.[9] He knew his research was not yet definitive, but his article established him as a serious thinker, even if his conclusion was not proven to everyone's satisfaction, including his own. Still his study had power and influence in the medical community, and it showcased, for the first time, Blalock's sophisticated analytic methodology.

However, the momentum in his career and research came to a crushing stop when, at what he assumed was just a routine regular checkup, he was diagnosed with tuberculosis, at the time often a deadly disease. Blalock had a lesion in his lung's left apex that was visible in an X-ray and his sputum showed acid-fast organisms.

Reluctantly, he packed up and left Nashville for the well-regarded Trudeau Sanatorium in Saranac Lake, in the cool and dry Adirondack Mountains of upstate New York. Ever loyal, Harrison traveled on the train at his side to provide emergency medical intervention, if needed, and emotional support.

Arriving at Trudeau, Blalock was devastated at being told he was forbidden to work; he had brought all his latest shock research results that he had performed after his 1927 article was printed and he yearned to write his newest results up for publication. Harrison, generous as always, told him not to worry; he would ghostwrite the article, making clear to others that "I didn't really do the work."[10]

Stuck in the TB asylum, unsure if he would live or die, he initially was relegated to his assigned infirmary bed. He wrote Walter E. Dandy, MD at Hopkins, "It is my sole ambition in life now to be able to become active in surgery again."[11] Instead, he was shut away in the mountains, feeling smothered and claustrophobic. He fretted that his first paper on shock would be read by another physician who might use his initial results to advance his own career, to the detriment of Blalock.

He also exchanged a flood of letters with Barney Brooks, always mentioning his frustration at being sick and suggesting that he return to work. Also, knowing Brooks would be sympathetic, he complained of his fellow patients, writing "practically all of the people here are either Jews or Catholics."[12] The sanitarium started him on a regimen of fresh air, sunlight, cold weather, isolation, and rest in the infirmary, which was a large room filled with others who were hawking up blood and bacteria-filled sputum. Blalock was so ill that he was not allowed to shift his body and, instead, lay flat on his back. Always with his eye to his work and his future, Blalock practiced crocheting to keep his fingers nimble.[13]

During the dark nights, he was required to sleep outdoors in the cold, constrained by his tight sheets and tautly secured blankets, standard treatment at the time. There were no effective anti-tubercular drugs then available. Blalock's declining health did not stop him from smoking, though he reduced his habit to four cigarettes a day, down from his usual two packs. Nor did it deter him from sneaking out on Saturday nights to drink at the Bear Club, near Lake Placid, and flirting with any female company he could find. Blalock wrote Brooks again, claiming that he could return to Vanderbilt in the fall if he first was given a two-month vacation at home, but Brooks refused to be swayed by any of Blalock's emotional ploys. Later that year, though, in a sign of support, Brooks named Blalock the chief resident surgeon and an instructor even though he was still absent and had been on paid sick leave for more than a year.[14]

After spending about ten months in the infirmary, Blalock was happy to move from the general ward to Lea Cottage, where he roomed with four men, including three other physicians. However much he enjoyed their company, he found the mood in the cottage gloomy. One of his housemates was the Canadian Communist Henry Norman Bethune, whose own father had died of TB. Bethune later became a thoracic surgeon and patterned himself after his grandfather Norman Bethune, a physician, and, as a child, dropped his first name, Henry, and insisted that he be called Norman. He spent his life in the service of others: he gave medical care to those fighting Franco during the Spanish Civil War; he organized medical services in China for the Mao-Tse Tung army. In Canada, he fought for socialized health care. He died at age forty-nine from sepsis, which developed from an abscess on his finger after he operated, barehanded, on a Chinese soldier.[15]

More than ten years earlier, while he was in Lea Cottage with Blalock, Bethune drew a gruesome mural about tuberculosis, taping five-feet-high brown wrapping paper that spanned sixty feet around the walls of the small cottage. He titled it, "The TB's Progress—A Drama in One Act and Five Scenes."[16] In the last scene, the Angel of Death clutches at Bethune, who is surrounded by the gravestones of his cottage mates. Each man predicted the year of his death. Blalock decided to give himself another year of life and inscribed "Alfred Blalock, 1899–1929."

Despite the hospital's rule of silence for its TB patients, the men discussed their treatment and other medical topics when they could get away with it. When they couldn't, Blalock used his quiet time to think further about his recent research on traumatic shock. Eager to step up his treatment, he wanted to try a new and a more progressive TB therapy that was only available in Europe and, while he was there, to study thoracic medicine. When his Trudeau doctors refused to discharge him, Blalock—headstrong and confident as ever—pushed forward with his plan. Brooks supported him by renewing Blalock's leave of absence, now at half-salary, and by arranging an additional $1,000 fellowship from Rockefeller's General Education Board, to study thoracic medicine.[17] Blalock easily borrowed another thousand dollars from the family bank in Jonesboro, with the loan conveniently signed off on by his sister, and he cashed in his life insurance policy.

Although he was finally escaping from the TB asylum, he remained frightened by Bethune's Angel of Death. Harrison was by his side to remind him that he was no longer "Al the Unbreakable who can burn candles at both ends without paying the price."[18] Still, Blalock felt defeated by the disease, which would smother him, he thought, before he had made his mark on medical history. Harrison, who was never too reverential to poke fun at him, claimed that the first thing Blalock did with his extra money was to buy "a sporty new Chrysler convertible coupe, and began to work harder and live faster than he had ever done before," as if a Chrysler coupe were fast enough to outrun death.[19]

In Germany and England, however, Blalock's time was well spent. He became a private patient of Ferdinand Sauerbruch, MD, a famous Munich surgeon. (A decade later, Sauerbruch became infamous for allocating funds for the Third Reich's "medical research" atrocities on concentration camp victims, many of them children.[20]) When he felt that Sauerbruch did not pay him enough deference as a fellow doctor, however, he left him to seek treatment in England and, at the same time, worked at the Physiological Laboratories in Cambridge. A few months later, he found a Trudeau physician willing to try pneumothorax treatment, which involved collapsing his left lung so it could rest and heal, a relatively new approach that would be popular for the next twenty years. Blalock continued his "collapse therapy" in New York, and then at Vanderbilt, for another eighteen months until the cavity in his left lung finally closed and he could stop treatment.

Blalock finally returned to work at the end of 1929. Upon his return from more than a year's worth of sick leave, Brooks generously promoted him to associate professor of surgery and increased his pay to $4,600.[21] Brooks also nominated Blalock for membership in the American Society of Clinical Surgery, then located in the South, and noted his very first qualification: "He is a native of Georgia."[22]

Acting heedlessly, Blalock once more resumed his frenetic pace of playing hard and working hard. Now that he had skirted death itself, he was willing to take risks and he worked hard and long. Back in Vanderbilt's lab, he doubled down on his research despite an offer of an internal medicine practice in Atlanta where he could make "a lot of money."[23] He said that he was not interested in getting rich, although thanks to his privilege and the easy availability of Blalock money, he must have known he would never want for material comforts.

Research was now his complete focus. He understood that his work on shock would be pivotal to his career, and he was determined to make his mark. His 1930 article was called "Experimental Shock: The Cause of the Low Blood Pressure Produced by Muscle Injury," and it garnered attention and established him as a serious thinker by offering a new perspective on how blood volume loss produces hypovolemic shock, a theory validated over the years.[24] Blalock argued for the importance of the circulatory system to shock and boldly announced that traumatic shock's best remedy was to administer a dramatically increased volume of saline solution and blood.

Never tiring of female company, Blalock had begun courting a dark-haired and dimpled twenty-year-old Mary O'Bryan, a local girl known for her vivacity, who worked in the hospital's admissions office. With Al continuing to see other women, Mary left for a trip to Europe to put some distance between herself and her beau. When she returned, Blalock impetuously asked her to marry him, and she said yes. He persuaded her parents to announce the engagement with the wedding date only fifteen days away. In late October, as the Monday wedding date neared, Blalock asked Thomas, as a favor, to drive his car to the church so it could be waiting there after the ceremony. Thomas, ever obliging and perhaps even pleased to play a part in the ceremony, said yes.

On the wedding day, Thomas picked up the car from a service station and parked it in front of the church during the ceremony. Blalock told him, specifically, to let it run with the keys in the ignition and to keep an eye on it. As instructed, Thomas was waiting outside of the church. After the ceremony, neither the bride nor groom showed much interest in going to their reception: halfway down the aisle toward the church door they started to run.[25] To the surprise and definite displeasure of the bride and groom's parents—and to the disappointment of their guests—the couple jumped in the getaway car and drove off, leaving their wedding party in the dust. It was the honeymoon, not the reception, that interested them most. The next day, the Nashville papers carried the O'Bryan-Blalock wedding story just as Mrs. O'Bryan had submitted it the week earlier containing references, now proven false, to the bride and groom greeting guests at their reception.[26]

While the new Mr. and Mrs. Blalock were away on their eagerly anticipated honeymoon, events at home took a more devastating turn. On November 14, 1930, Tennessee's largest bond trading house, Caldwell & Co., collapsed, a full year after the New York crash.[27] One short week later, in a vicious game of dominoes, it brought down the Thomas family's bank, Peoples Savings and Loan.[28]

Thomas's savings disappeared, as did the rest of his family's money. The bank, Thomas later said, "caught me and mine." On his meager salary, there was no way he could save that kind of money again. "I knew I was sunk right then and there."[29]

CHAPTER EIGHT

CAUGHT SHORT

Given the circumstances, Thomas felt that his safest and best option was to continue working for Blalock. With his tuition savings vaporized like steam in a chemistry experiment, college and med school were definitely on hold. He was stunned at the unjustness of it; he felt a real anger that a bank could snatch all his hard-earned money just as quickly as if he'd been mugged in the street.

The Great Depression was a difficult time for many, but it was worse for some: in Nashville, African Americans' jobless rate rose to 25 percent.[1] Suddenly, there were 10,000 more relief applicants in Davidson County alone. To make matters worse, an appalling drought unexpectedly set in—and lasted for the next three years—turning cotton and tobacco fields barren. "For Black Tennesseans, the outlook was especially bleak," was everyone's take.[2]

The entire Thomas family was in financial trouble because very few Black families choose to commission a new house at this time. Vivien's father, such a hard worker, now had nothing to do except insubstantial repair jobs. Their house was cozy and snug, without guestrooms, but for extra income the Thomases took in an adolescent boarder whose parents wanted her to have the advantages of a Pearl High School education. As for Vivien, he had a small wad of cash that he had yet to deposit in the bank, and his father asked if he could borrow it. It wasn't that much, but William told Vivien that without it, the family might lose their home.

Vivien felt trapped. Without his money, his chances of becoming a doctor were just about gone. Ever since he'd attended kindergarten at Fisk, his parents had drilled into him the importance of education. Now, he felt, his father was asking him to give up his dreams after having encouraged him to pursue them. Reluctantly, he lent the money to his father. It was never repaid.

Thomas grew to resent all his parents' admonitions about getting a good education. He was ensnared by an economy he didn't understand and wondered if he was ever going to get to college. One of the hit songs of the early 1930s was the poignant, "Brother, Can You Spare a Dime?" Bing Crosby sang a line that followed Thomas, no matter how hard he tried to shake it out of his head: "They used to tell me I was building a dream...."[3]

A gloom descended on the Thomas household. Some days more than others, Vivien struggled to accept that all his money was simply gone, and that his family was fraying. On those days he would want to just give up. Although his parents had had many good years together, after they lost all their money, the marriage suffered. They eventually divorced and his father moved out of the house he had built for his family.

If nothing else, Thomas had his work with Blalock to keep him busy. Blalock was accelerating his research on traumatic shock and the experimental surgery lab was brimming over with activity and innovation. Blalock was pushing hard to counter the toxemia theory of the acknowledged shock expert, Walter Cannon, and to prove his own ideas about shock. He pursued it diligently. According to Thomas, "There was no one who spent as much time in the laboratory as Dr. Blalock."[4]

Thomas never complained about his own long hours and hard work; on the contrary, he rose to the challenge and absorbed all the exposure he possibly could to this world of scientific research. At Vanderbilt, the two men fell into a pattern: Blalock would meet with his lab assistant to talk over the background of what was to be done so that Thomas could then return to the lab to work it out in practice, with Blalock stopping by once or twice a week to see how things were going and, perhaps, to make suggestions.[5] When Thomas completed enough experiments, Blalock would gather the data, notes, and individual file cards, and bring them home. After calling Thomas and reviewing the quantitative data with him over the phone, he'd write into the night and, by dawn, the professor would have a publishable journal article ready to send off in the mail.

To measure the effect of temperature relative to shock, Blalock and Thomas often worked in the "cold room," which had a dropped ceiling lined with cooling coils. It was a tiny, refrigerated, four-by-five-foot space that was smaller than a walk-in closet. At the professor's request, Thomas somehow found room in it for Blalock's cases of Coca-Cola, which he tucked neatly under the shelving unit. The professor would swill between four and eight Cokes a day and he wanted them cold, nearly freezing. Thomas was perfectly happy with a mug of aromatic steaming black coffee. No cream, no sugar. Soft drinks were for kids, he thought.

Blalock's long hours didn't mean he worked without respite. Ignoring Prohibition, which had been federal law since 1920, Blalock kept a five-gallon keg of whiskey on a high shelf in the laboratory's locked closet, draped under an old white gown. Everyone knew where the whiskey was hidden; despite this, Blalock kept a proprietary key in his pocket. He saved the whiskey for after work hours and, at Vanderbilt, was not known to drink during the day when he saw patients. He showed no reluctance in asking Thomas for help taking down the heavy keg every evening or putting it back up but did not offer him a collegial drink. Thomas said that they drank together only on "two or three occasions" total,[6] certainly not often, as some surgeons would later claim.[7]

During his first few years at Vanderbilt, Thomas rigged together various creative fixes to compensate for working alone, which both he and Blalock preferred him to do. He became so efficient at operating without an assistant that he could drape medical tubing around himself, like multicolored lights around a Christmas tree. Or, if there was more tubing than his tall body could support, he'd bring a wooden coat rack and drape the tubing on it.

Initially, Blalock couldn't fathom how Thomas was able to carry out so many challenging experiments without assistance. After all, he figured Thomas had only a high school education from a segregated school for Black students, which in Blalock's estimation must mean that his education had been inferior. Additionally, the tasks Blalock assigned were extremely difficult for a single person. If he, a surgery chief, couldn't operate solo, how could his lab assistant? He must have recognized then that his lab tech was more dexterously skilled of the two of them, which might have been a painful realization.

As time went on, Thomas became so skilled at administering the experiments and performing surgeries that he worked without Blalock's supervision and soon was performing them by himself, without an assistant. One time, Blalock walked in just as Thomas was closing the last incision on a dog after surgery.

"Sorry, I got busy," was Blalock's usual greeting. He walked over to the table and inspected the dog.

"Who helped you with this?" Blalock asked.

"No one," replied Thomas.

So perfect were Thomas's incisions that Blalock was surprised. He turned to Sam Waters, the other lab worker there.

"Did he really do this by himself?"

Waters pushed the tobacco cud to the side of his mouth, and he told Blalock yes, Thomas had.[8]

At work, Blalock never mentioned Thomas's superior surgical skills in public and seemed to take care not to praise his underpaid and underpromoted assistant. His own slow, workmanship surgical skills were criticized by Tinsley Harrison, who often reminded Blalock—in front of other people and in a very loud voice—that Thomas was a better surgeon than Blalock.

Harrison needled Blalock over his cavalier attitude about his taking advantage of Thomas by describing Blalock's stages of research. First, said Harrison, was the planning stage, when Blalock would say, "We need to do [this]." Then, for the actual work that needed to be done by Thomas was, 'You do this.' When the research report was written up, Blalock would say, 'I did this.'"[9]

Although Harrison's candid comments about Blalock were amusing, they put Thomas in a precarious position. His job at Vanderbilt was at the whim of Blalock and his moods. If Thomas's presence threatened his white supervisor, he might have lost his precious job. Blalock needed Thomas's lab discoveries, but the surgeon would neither go so far as to demonstrate his appreciation of Thomas or to encourage him to rise higher.

Fortunately, a few months after Thomas began working in the lab, a surgical fellow, Joseph W. Beard, MD, arrived to work with Blalock. Thomas seemed to inspire in Beard an interest and desire to support and develop the younger man's craft and knowledge of chemistry. Beard lent Thomas his own physiology and chemistry textbooks and he set up regular study sessions with Thomas as well. Beard had an infectious enthusiasm for chemistry, which Thomas enjoyed. With Beard's help, he was getting a small taste of what concerted study into a scientific discipline might have been like had he been able to attend college and medical school. Thomas appreciated his experimental work the more deeply he understood it and was always grateful to Beard for his tutoring, for Blalock never took any interest in his education.[10]

Beard taught Thomas how to use a slide rule, which was created several hundred years ago, although it was just starting to be used for calculating various math equations and functions. For his part, Blalock refused to learn how to use the newly popular device, preferring to steer clear of it, convinced that his penciled arithmetic was more accurate than that "slip slide." Whenever Blalock's calculations varied from Thomas's, Beard and Thomas would exchange furtive smiles and Blalock would call Tinsley Harrison to come in and mediate. This happened so many times that eventually Harrison became peeved and took pleasure in pointing out when Blalock's figures were incorrect. Thomas later noted of Harrison, "He seemed to thoroughly enjoy seeing Dr. Blalock squirm."[11]

Thomas always attributed his lifelong desire to stay in pioneering research to Beard's support and interest, and never to Alfred Blalock. The effort that Beard put into tutoring him puzzled Thomas, who couldn't figure out Beard's motivation for giving up his own precious leisure hours. Certainly, the physician's interest seems unusual given that Beard was an active supporter of segregation. Three decades later, when Beard was teaching at Duke University, he noticed that someone had used a solvent to erase the "Whites Only" sign above the washrooms in his building. He made sure to have the segregation signs repainted.

The next morning, he saw that the new paint had been removed once more. Beard had it painted a second time. The day after, the signs had disappeared again. What he didn't know was that his colleague, William S. Lynn, MD, a chemist and a Southern integrationist, was using his specially mixed solvent to remove the signs. This Scarlet Pimpernel game went on for months, until a frustrated Beard finally gave up.[12] It's not clear why Beard decided to tutor Thomas, but it's most likely a testament to Thomas's keen intelligence and his eagerness to learn that he did.

Had Blalock only been able to see Thomas's potential as a medical researcher and recognize the oceanic depth of his character, as Beard did, then cardiac and thoracic or other medical discoveries might have accelerated so much more quickly. No one, no matter how great their praise for Thomas, ever considered how much more Vivien Thomas could have accomplished had he become an actual physician-scientist.

At the same time, Thomas's talents were so obvious he was increasingly given additional responsibilities. Before long, he began making all the experimental chemistry determinations and producing the measurements typically completed by a chemistry technician. He did this work by hand because commercially available instruments did not yet exist, nor were there any standardized chemical reagents (substances used to measure components) available for purchase. Instead, Thomas had to figure everything out by himself.

With Thomas's help, Blalock was able to ramp up his experiments and, in 1932, Blalock purchased additional dogs to create different types of injuries. Thomas designed and constructed a pneumatic cup or boot that applied great pressure to body tissue without causing bone fractures. Then, after imposing these crush injuries, he took blood from the dog's injured area to compare its chemical composition to the blood that was circulating throughout the rest of the body, measuring hemoconcentration and other chemical substances, including toxins. He demonstrated that injecting plasma to treat the injured dogs caused their death rate to plummet from 95 percent to 25 percent.

One day, Blalock gave Thomas a bottle of Nembutal capsules to sedate the dogs. This new drug from Abbott Laboratories was an improvement over the barbital nitrate they'd been using because it didn't keep people under sedation quite as long. But it had never been tried on dogs. Moreover, Nembutal was sold only in powder form inside of capsules meant to be swallowed whole. Dogs, of course, would prove an extra challenge regarding dosage. Thomas had to determine the correct amount of Nembutal and then add it to a liquid solution for canines of various weights.

He felt under terrible pressure as he worked out the dosage metric. Most of the dogs were also being used for other trial experiments in shock and hypertension and he was worried sick at the prospect of getting his dosages wrong. If he accidentally administered a lethal dose, that dog's death would mean that he would jeopardize his research and the status of Blalock's future publications. Blalock did not ease Thomas's nervousness when he told him, "Don't you kill any of those dogs."[13]

An interesting assignment came Thomas's way when Vanderbilt's new postdoctoral fellow, Stanford Leeds, MD joined the surgery department. Stanford's last name was Levy when he was at Vanderbilt, but he changed it to "Leeds" to escape the virulent anti-Semitism of medical schools and hospitals, and their physicians. For example, when Barney Brooks later wrote a favorable job recommendation for Leeds, he began "Although a member of the Hebrew tribe...."[14] Leeds must have wondered what he'd gotten into by coming to Vanderbilt when Margaret Mitchell's bestselling book, *Gone with The Wind*, was published in 1936, and won a National Book award and a Pulitzer Prize. For many days in the doctor's dining room at lunch, Leeds had to listen to Blalock's domineering conversations about the book. After all, Blalock had lived in Jonesboro just like the fictitious Scarlett O'Hara. Then, in 1939, when the famous movie was released, Blalock's favorable commentary on the Old South began once again. Leeds told people that he thought he'd go out of his mind.[15]

Still, a new experiment that Thomas conducted with Leeds proved critical to Thomas's career—and Blalock's. The professor wanted Thomas and Leeds to begin experiments on high blood pressure (pulmonary hypertension) that focused on the role of the kidneys. Thomas and Leeds transplanted a dog's kidney, including the vein, artery, and ureter, to its neck. Thomas removed the kidney and connecting material while Leeds opened the neck muscles to receive it. Within a half-hour, the kidney was circulating normally and the dog was urinating out of its neck. It was a failure so far as proving any theory about pulmonary hypertension, but later it would be used in Thomas's creation of the blue baby surgery.

While Thomas became ever more reliable and accomplished, Blalock was not quite so consistent. Notwithstanding his recent marriage to Mary, his nighttime drinking was prodigious, and many early mornings, Thomas's lab colleague Waters would warn Thomas, telling him "You better watch yourself with that man today."[16]

Blalock's varying moods and outbursts could be hard to predict. Thomas found it difficult to believe that such a well-educated individual could act so childish. On one occasion, Thomas made a mistake in the lab as the professor watched, and Blalock became furious. He threw a proper temper tantrum, cursing at Thomas, while the lab tech stood there silently, before the professor stormed out of the lab. "His profanities," said Thomas, "would have made the proverbial sailor proud." He, hurt and insulted, went back to his locker, to change into his street clothes. He had never heard his father swear. Now fuming, he headed to Blalock's office and firmly told him, "Don't come try to yell down my throat and slam and cuss at me."[17] He told Blalock that he had not been brought up to suffer or use that kind of language and that if he continued to act like this every time Thomas made a mistake, it would be better for both if he left now. Blalock was flabbergasted when Thomas offered his resignation, and he apologized and promised not to repeat his verbal abuse.[18] Indeed, this time he kept his word.

In June 1933, Thomas had the bittersweet experience of attending his older brother Harold's commencement ceremony at Jubilee Hall on the Fisk campus. Vivien was pleased for Harold, but watching his brother receive his BA must have been difficult. Harold had now achieved what Vivien had always hoped to accomplish for himself, and he was headed straight to graduate school. Now two of Vivien's older siblings, both Olga and Harold, were pursuing careers in science. There was real talent for this in the Thomas family. The only difference between Vivien and his older siblings' ambition was that they had managed to start college before the crash that had destroyed their younger brother's financial foundation.

Shortly before his brother's graduation, Thomas traveled to see friends in Macon, Georgia, about a six-hour bus ride from Nashville. There, he was introduced to Miss Clara Beatrice Flanders, a young lady of Jamaican ancestry on her mother's side. Clara's parents were Leonard Flanders, who was a skilled car mechanic, and Mary Gross Flanders, who made a little money from home by doing the laundry for another Macon family. (Clara's maternal grandfather, whose surname was Gross, was European and had married an African Caribbean woman, therefore the US Census bestowed upon young and pretty Clara its official racial designation of "mulatto."[19]) At first, Thomas saw Clara only at her house with both parents in attendance. Then he was asked to join her family for meals when he was in town and the number of his weekend visits increased. Finally, he was invited to join the family at church.

There was a special something about Clara besides her sweet looks. She had a good mind and was capable of a sharp comment delivered so ingenuously that you didn't realize you'd been cut until later. When they met, Clara was twenty to Vivien's twenty-three years. Her homemaking skills in sewing and cooking rivaled even those of Thomas's mother. She had plans to go to Freedman's Hospital's School of Nursing in Washington, DC, but when Thomas proposed, she decided that her future lay with him. This suited Thomas just fine. Her burgeoning interest in health care would make her an excellent wife for someone who planned to become a physician. They married on December 22, 1933, and his new bride moved into his mother's house.[20]

Thomas didn't discuss his upcoming marriage with any of the surgeons at Vanderbilt: he considered this information private and personal. He did not want her discussed by people who so clearly exhibited a belief in white superiority. On the rare occasions when he mentioned Clara after their marriage, he referred to her always as "Mrs. Thomas." The surgeons understood this intuitively and, though they always called Vivien by his first name, to them she always was "Mrs. Thomas," whether consciously or unconsciously. Thomas was successful in protecting his wife from the firsthand discrimination he faced every day at work.

CHAPTER NINE

BLALOCK, THOMAS, AND HENRY FORD

In 1934, Vivien and Clara welcomed their first child, Olga. Clara had a dainty foot but when she learned she was pregnant, she put it down so hard that even her husband heard it. She did not want to continue living with her mother in-law because she had to spend every long day listening to the older woman's suggestions of doing things "the right way."[1] Clara wanted a home of her own.

Thomas's bank had repaid him 35 percent of his savings that he'd thought he'd lost in 1930. With this money and the cash they'd saved through their frugality, they could now afford to buy a house on Elm Hill Road. It was small yet attractive, with a spacious front porch on a large, appealing yard "with lawns and trees" where their baby could play. It had "what I called a little elbow room," said Thomas.[2]

Finally, Clara could be mistress of her own home and she enjoyed her traditional marriage.[3] When Theodosia, their second daughter, was born four years later in 1938, they considered their family complete. Clara was busy laundering cloth diapers and sewing all the girls' clothes—and her own, too—except for the personal items. She was said to be just about the best home cook in Nashville. Every morning, the family awakened to the tantalizing aroma of her fresh-baked bread and, for their evening meal, she could take a half-teaspoon of drippings and make of it a generous amount of tasty gravy.[4]

By now, Blalock also had two children: his first son, William Rice, was born in 1931 and the couple's daughter, Mary Elizabeth, was born in 1932. (In the 1940s, they would have a second son, Dandy, whom they named after Walter Dandy, the esteemed neurosurgeon at Hopkins.) Their mother, too, stayed at home while Blalock concentrated on his career. Mary Blalock, however, did not enjoy the long days and nights without her husband, having only her young children for companionship, and she took solace in a drink or two in the daytime and perhaps more in the evening. Nor did it help that Blalock was perpetually cross because he needed to pass more than forty painful kidney stones and feared that he'd never be free of his many ailments, on top of these constant kidney stones.

Blalock's mood improved considerably when he was given a chance to face off with Walter Cannon and directly refute Cannon's toxicity theory on the etiology and treatment of shock at the annual surgeon's meeting in Chicago in 1934. To prepare, he needed Thomas; he was the one who'd performed the surgical experiments and knew their exact metrics. With Thomas coaching him, he practiced his talk over and over until he felt he'd be presenting accurate data. As Thomas put it, this was his "big chance."[5] The surgeons anticipating this showdown expected high drama and were thrilled by the thought of explosive pyrotechnics, at least figuratively.

Cannon, in his sixties, spoke first and, although he never contradicted his toxemia work, he did incorporate some of Blalock's research. Blalock, in his thirties, was the young Turk having to establish the superiority of his work; he was the long shot in this race. He strode to the podium, asserting as much gravitas in his youthful demeanor as he could. He tried to restrain his Georgia drawl, knowing that it could harm his presentation, as he asserted his own findings and minimized those of his opponent. When he ended, he was grateful and a little surprised at the decibel level of the audience's applause.

"The surgeons of the day were vehement in their support of Blalock's position," said one.[6] He had convincingly and soundly refuted Cannon's old theories about a mysterious toxin issue and instead pointed to fluid loss. As he continued to stand as tall as he could, chin high, he finally felt as if his colleagues had just placed a floral bouquet on his back. He had just set the new standard for treating shock and, when he learned that the mechanics of his ideas would be added to "The Johns Hopkins Hospital Surgical Routine" in 1937, he felt partly vindicated for having to leave Hopkins.[7]

His victory was fleeting, though, for Blalock was mercurial and always looking toward his next big score, frustrated after stagnating for eight years as an associate professor. Having wanted a promotion to a full professor for so long that he could feel it, he hoped that he, and not Tinsley Harrison, would be the first to receive this advancement. Their friendship did not dampen Blalock's ambition. He'd even considered leaving Vanderbilt a few years earlier when the University of Louisville offered him its surgery chief position, but demurred because it was a lower-ranked department at the time.[8]

Finally, the opportunity for promotion to a full professorship at Vanderbilt—and before Harrison attained this, too!—arose when he received a job proffer from the Henry Ford Hospital in Detroit (currently the Henry Ford Health System). Blalock crafted a way to turn this offer from its surgery chief, Roy B. McClure MD, into a promotion by telling everyone, including Thomas, that he was considering leaving Vanderbilt to become *surgery chief* at Ford.[9] Everyone knew he'd already been offered the same post at Louisville and assumed that Blalock's description of the Ford proposition was factual.

However, the truth is that McClure had never offered him the top surgery job. McClure's unambiguous letter to Blalock reads, "I am writing you at this time to offer you a position as *associate surgeon* on our staff."[10] (Emphasis added) The associate status would have made Blalock the head of the experimental lab, which was one of several at Ford. This meant that he would have to report to the director of the Ford labs and not directly to McClure, who would have become his second-level supervisor. The offer was not at all a promotion, much less a request for

Blalock to take McClure's job. Why would it be? McClure was not considering leaving Ford, where he retained his high position from 1916 to 1951, when he died in his sleep. Blalock, though, puffed up his offer to the Vanderbilt staff in the hope of gaining a promotion there.

In doing so, Blalock told Brooks that he was traveling to Detroit to discuss the offer with McClure and, separately, Edsel Ford, the hospital's chairman. When he met with these men, he did his best to indicate sincere interest in the position and used his natural charm to his advantage. Mr. Ford even gifted Blalock an expensive watch to help seal the deal.

To Thomas, Blalock said that if he accepted the Ford job, he would bring him along. As it happened, Olga Thomas Calhoun, Vivien's oldest sister, was a nurse at a different Detroit hospital who, said Thomas, "told me not to get my hopes too high, that Henry Ford Hospital was strictly lily white, and that it was worse than anything she had seen, even though she had grown up in the South."[11]

Calhoun was not entirely correct, in that there were African Americans employed in the hospital; still, they were in custodial positions and were not professional staff.[12] It was true that Henry Ford was one of the country's most pernicious bigots, but he was growing older—in 1937, he was seventy-three years old—and he was always a businessman first. At this point, his son Edsel Ford, age forty-four, headed the hospital board as well as being CEO of the auto company.

The 1930s had been a trying decade, one in which Ford Motor Company suffered walkouts, industrial unrest, and rising debt. In response, Ford Motor not only hired Black men but put them in higher-level and better-paid production jobs than did the other two, General Motors and Chrysler, of the Big Three automakers. By 1941, Ford Motor had employed 14,000 to 16,000 Black men, so many that they represented a full 50 percent of Detroit's male African American workforce.[13] Ford Motor Company's reality was not as hateful as Henry Ford's rhetoric, especially now that Edsel was in charge.

At Vanderbilt, Blalock's ploy was successful. Once he was assured by Brooks that he would receive the coveted promotion to full professor, he immediately declined the Ford offer. He explained to McClure, "As you know, I am the second man in the [Vanderbilt surgery] department [and] if I came to the Ford hospital at this time, I would be at best the third man in the department and would feel quite uncertain as to freedom in my experimental work."[14] Never had Blalock been asked to become the surgeon in chief. He certainly deserved his promotion at Vanderbilt and its accompanying pay raise, but not because he had turned down Ford's top position. Still, he kept the watch that Edsel Ford had given him.

The deception was never challenged. Everyone believed his inflated story, the narrative that Blalock gassed up like the Hindenburg, which was to meet disaster that same year. But unlike those blimp passengers, Blalock had a smooth landing. He was a man who lied to his colleagues and to Thomas, and he sustained this falsehood his entire life. As a result, books and articles wrongly state that Blalock was invited to become Ford's surgeon in chief. For example, Mark Ravitch wrote in the introduction to his two-volume compilation of Blalock's papers, "In 1937, he was invited to succeed Dr. Roy McClure," and as late as 2022, a book about Johns Hopkins Medicine repeated this audacious puffery.[15] The years went on and no one thought to question Blalock's version of his job offer. After all, he would later become a very influential man in surgery.

Here again, Blalock dissembled to Thomas, telling him that he had rejected the "chief of surgery" job because Ford hospital refused to hire Thomas on racial grounds. Thomas wrote, "As it turned out, Dr. Blalock turned down the offer because I was not acceptable to them."[16] Blalock's explanation agreed with what Olga had told her brother, so Thomas had no reason to doubt Blalock's word. Again, Thomas had no way to validate the truth; he had to rely on what Blalock told him. This mythos of Blalock as a progressive freethinker was memorialized by an esteemed chronicler of Johns Hopkins history, formerly its medical dean: as Thomas Turner, MD stated, "It was known that Blalock had previously declined a major surgical post at another institution because of the restrictive policy on the employment of Negroes."[17]

Blalock purposely deceived Thomas on this sensitive point of race discrimination. In fact, the very first time that McClure telephoned him to offer the associate surgeon position, Blalock told him right out that he wanted to employ his "colored" lab assistant. McClure immediately responded in writing: "You would be authorized to employ at our minimum wage a laboratory assistant whom you spoke of in our telephone conversation. While the conditions are not ideal for a lone colored boy, I believe that if he has tact there would be no difficulty whatever."[18]

Believing that the surgeon had turned down a prestigious job out of concern for him, Thomas was grateful, and he increased his loyalty to his double-dealing boss. (The worst of this deception for Thomas would have been that at Ford, even if he were only a minimum wage employee, he would have earned 50 percent more than Vanderbilt was paying him because of Ford's generous pay plans.)[19]

As that awful Depression decade of the thirties drew to a close, Thomas had numerous motives to keep things on an even keel at Vanderbilt. Also, with good reason, he was deeply worried about and maybe even angry at his oldest brother Harold, who was becoming a noted civil rights activist.

CHAPTER TEN

O Brother, Where Art Thou?

Vivien Thomas had an ingrained respect for his brother Harold's academic degrees and his decision to become a teacher at Pearl junior high school. However, when Vivien learned that Harold was inflamed over a risky legal court suit for teachers mandating equal pay regardless of race, Thomas was appalled. Harold, it seemed, wanted to get mixed up in the business of the NAACP, which Vivien felt would be foolhardy. He felt sick when Harold told him what he was involved with. He was dismayed, anxious, and fearful for Harold's future—and maybe even for his own.

Vivien Thomas did not believe in aggressive or organized approaches to solve hiring or pay problems; he thought it far better to be patient and work things out with as little publicity as possible. His way was to take things slower and avoid anything that smacked of radical change. "He was not a crusader," said a family member. "He was not the one to lead the movement."[1]

Harold confided that the NAACP had asked him to be its plaintiff representing Nashville's African American teachers in a lawsuit against the city schools. There and throughout the South, teachers were being paid different wages according to race; now, the national civil rights organization, founded in 1909, was seeking equal pay for all Black teachers who had the same credentials and length of experience as white teachers.

Harold had not volunteered; rather, the NAACP had chosen him, in his sixth year of teaching, because of his fine history and impressive degrees. It was the same approach taken fifteen years later, when it selected a woman with an impeccable reputation, Mrs. Rosa Parks of Alabama, to be a symbol of those who had enough of moving to the back of the bus.

Harold was an obvious choice to be its plaintiff: he had already earned a Collegiate Professional Certificate, which was the highest-level teaching certificate that one could receive from the state of Tennessee. He also had those two academic degrees from Fisk to his credit. Compare this to a good number of white teachers in Tennessee, who possessed A.B. degrees that were given after only two years of college. Moreover, Harold's master's degree was in biology, a specialized academic subject, rather than in education, which degree was considered not as rigorous. Another advantage was that Harold had divorced and his former wife, with their child, Valeria Thomas (later Valeria Thomas Spann), were distanced away in Indiana. There was little need to worry about their safety.

Despite Vivien's growing concern over his brother's intended lawsuit, on this fine early morning in Nashville in 1941, Vivien Thomas was, overall, content; he was working at his lab job the best and hardest he could, he was being a responsible husband and father, and he was serving God by improving the health of his fellow human beings. His second-class status at Vanderbilt, though, was always there at the back of his mind, nagging at him, no matter how hard he tried to silence its voice. However, his practical philosophy seemed imperturbable, and he wasn't going to rush Vanderbilt or its staff into treating him more equitably. And he still thought he owed his loyalty to Blalock.

On each workday, Thomas left his house and his young family to walk across town like any honest laborer or workman who carried his metal lunchbox and thermos of hot coffee. Only the jacket and tie that Thomas wore, and the leather briefcase that served to hide his sandwich and coffee from sight, identified him as an African American man who was someone a little bit different, a man who was concerned about serious issues.

Thomas thought about the day's work ahead and a passersby might have noticed that he even looked like an intellectual, his furrowing his forehead as he walked along in deep thought. Despite the noisy city streets, he could block out honking horns, screeching brakes, and the unpleasant stink of vehicles letting off their noxious gray exhaust. Thomas could concentrate on anything, anywhere, as if his mind were a scalpel cutting away at the superfluous material obscuring the answer to a problem. Approaching Vanderbilt, he was lost to others passing him in the street, so deeply was he thinking about the challenges awaiting him in the lab. Still, on this day, he thought of himself as an ordinary working man.

His brother Harold Thomas was quite a bit different, as everyone who knew them was aware. His goals were not necessarily wrong, Vivien believed, but maybe not as realistic as Vivien would have liked. For sure, Harold had outsized ambitions and thoughts, and welcomed the responsibility of bringing about change: change not just for himself but for other people, too. Harold enjoyed learning the ideas filtering down South from up in Harlem. People were saying that a Renaissance was going on in that Black community, with the showcasing of the talents of Black residents. There were throngs of educated and well-off white folks, too, going up to Harlem who were equally stimulated by this new thinking and novel perspectives.

Nearly 900 miles of hard driving separated Nashville from Manhattan, the headquarters of the NAACP. The geographic remoteness was slight compared to the difference in ideas between most of the Nashville Black citizens, even those who were constituents of Du Bois's Talented Tenth, and of the Black artistic and intellectual cadre in Harlem.

It had been ninety years since Walt Whitman had written the free-verse poetry that brought him fame, even though his breakaway vocabulary was sparse as he praised ordinary American workers, men and women alike, in his epic poem "Leaves of Grass."[2] Its well-known song included the poem "I Hear America Singing." Whitman celebrated hard-working Americans like the Thomas family. His words could almost make you believe he'd been watching William Thomas and his sons at work when he wrote that carpenters sing their songs as they work.

Now came along Harlem's Langston Hughes, who sang the praises of his own American people. Hughes had decided to tune Whitman's hymn to America to a minor key, and he declaimed at the beginning of his poem "I, Too" that he is the "darker brother" who eats in the kitchen but still "grows strong."[3]

It was a fertile time of rebirth and celebration for African Americans, and their history and their culture. Harold Thomas imagined a role for himself in this journey as a "New Negro," the phrase that he'd heard from Fisk professor Alain Locke, now an acclaimed Harlem Renaissance writer. Harold agreed that Black Americans needed to step up and realize their full potential rather than accept a stereotyped vision of themselves.[4] Vivien Thomas was far less sure that his brother should jump on this Northern accelerating engine. What if he were crushed by his ambitions?

As it ended up, both brothers' divergent prophecies for the future proved to be prescient.

This was the main issue: beginning in the thirties and accelerating in the forties, the NAACP's strategy was to tackle racial discrimination in employment bit by bit. The board members identified the most important issue in their quest for equal rights, which was education; everyone, Black or white, knew that schooling was the best way forward toward a more promising future. Just about all citizens, whatever their backgrounds and ethnicities, respected schoolteachers. Teachers were the ones who carried the shining lamp that would illuminate the coming time. Yet, throughout the South, Black teachers—public servants, all—were paid through a dual-salary schedule enforced by local governments and school boards, which meant they did and always would receive a smaller salary than their white counterparts. The NAACP realized that teachers, through their character and vocation, would make fine plaintiffs and that paying black and white teachers equally "was a 'benign' enough thrust for whites to accept."[5] After all, dual pay schedules based on race had been used long enough, the NAACP board thought, as "the cornerstone of the Southern system of caste education."[6]

O Brother, Where Art Thou?

Winning equal pay was also a symbolic goal. "When the Negro teachers in the South take their governments to court on a question of salary equalization, they prove themselves champions of the Negroes' cause and therefore worthy of the greater democracy of which we all aspire," noted the *Pittsburgh Courier*.[7] Education became the focal point of the NAACP's national campaign. One goal was to open access to universities that barred African American applicants eager to study law or other professions—cases that are remembered vividly in this day and time. Less celebrated and nearly forgotten were the struggles for equal pay for teachers.

After much thought and discussion by the NAACP board members, and many late-night meetings in the proverbial smoked-filled rooms which had necessarily followed a long day in court, the first teacher lawsuit for equal pay was filed in 1936.[8] The approach was far from radical. In fact, the NAACP's strategies were based on nearly conservative theories: not equal rights but equal Federal protections.[9] It would be a long and fatiguing battle, but the war would be won this way rather than by reaching for the amorphous and perhaps too distant goal of racial equality. Equal protection, as opposed to equality or even equity, could be easily defined because it was finite and measurable.

They strategically moved forward. The NAACP's unknown attorney by the name of Thurgood Marshall started to lay the groundwork for the equal pay campaign. Throughout what was dubbed "the solid South," the typical Black schoolteacher earned only 61 percent of white teachers' salaries.[10] Mr. Marshall's own mother was a Washington, DC teacher working on a dual pay system: it was said by the writer Juan Williams that Mr. Marshall "took it personally that his mother's work was valued less than a white teacher's."[11]

The NAACP began testing its litigation in those mid-Atlantic states—Maryland and Virginia—that leaned in a Southerly direction. And it won these cases, except that sometimes victory could backfire—and this constituted a good part of what made Vivien Thomas worry for Harold—as when a renegade school district would fire Black teachers rather than pay them equally. Or lower all white teachers' pay to equalize costs. The NAACP noted that several spiteful school districts tried to get around paying teachers equally through methods of "intimidation, chicanery, and trickery of almost every form imaginable." Still, the lawsuits were "wildly popular" with the organization's members[12] and membership spiked where the NAACP had brought suits.[13] In the years between 1939 and 1947, the NAACP would win twenty-seven of thirty-one of these cases.[14]

All this was fine and good for other people. Vivien Thomas blessed the NAACP's efforts and its results. He did not, however, want to see his brother stick out his neck and lead this effort in Nashville. No, sir, he did not.

Harold was profoundly disappointed by his brother's opposition, although not surprised. The men conflicted on nearly all levels, as friends and relatives remarked. Harold saw himself as growing the fruit; why, then, should he be satisfied to eat the rinds? Vivien, on the other hand, was trying hard to keep his own balance and maintain his dignity while supporting his family of four on his Vanderbilt poverty-level wages. He could accept the indignities for the sake of his family and because of his profound desire to conduct meaningful research. Harold, though, was defiant and disgusted by what he saw as his brother's willingness to settle for what was left over.

Despite Vivien's gloomy premonitions, on April 12, 1941, Harold E. Thomas, represented by local attorney Z. Alexander Looby and co-counsel Thurgood Marshall, filed suit along with the local teachers' organization against the president of the Nashville school board, Louis H. Hibbitts, to seek equalization of teacher salaries. The Metropolitan Nashville Teacher Association, which was integrated, stood with Thomas in *Thomas v. Hibbitts et al.*[15] The case was heard in a US federal court without a local jury; it was to be decided solely by Judge Elmer Davies. The judge had been appointed by President Franklin D. Roosevelt and therefore was assumed to be sympathetic to Thomas and to the goals of the NAACP. Of course, this particular filing with Davies's court was not coincidental; the organization had looked for districts where there were better chances of victory: Nashville was one. In fact, two years earlier, both the city council and the mayor had recommended complete parity in teacher salaries, but the school board refused to enact these equities. If it had, the Nashville trial could have been avoided.

Looby, Harold's principal lawyer, had an interesting and unusual background. He was born on Antigua Island in the Caribbean's West Indies and had, as a young man, actually worked on a whaling ship, a rarity by the 1900s. He went on to earn his undergraduate degree from Howard, his law degree from Columbia, and his doctorate in law from New York University. In addition to his practice, he also taught at Fisk. In the courtroom, Judge Davies made sure that Looby would be addressed as "Doctor," which irritated opposing counsel to no end.[16]

The NAACP did not have the money to pick up the entire cost of the lawsuit, so Looby held evening meetings to campaign for donations from Nashville's Black community. "The only ones who didn't go were those who were really scared to death or didn't give a damn," said one Nashvillian.[17]

The fact, as Harold Thomas, Looby, and Marshall presented to the court, was that there was a 20 to 25 percent salary difference in Nashville between Black and white teachers. Trying to circumvent the dual-pay schedule, minority teachers would spend their summers taking additional courses so that they might earn the maximum pay possible. As a result, "Negro teachers in Nashville are better prepared than white teachers."[18] Yet a beginning white teacher in Nashville's schools was paid $1440 while a beginning Black teacher would earn only $995.

Although it bothered Harold to admit it, some of Vivien's predictions were torturously proving true. Even at Pearl, the north star in the constellation of Nashville's minority schools, some teachers avoided Harold in the lunchroom or shunned him in the teachers' lounge. Very few went out of their way to indicate support.

Of course, the Black teachers were afraid of saying anything. Afraid of being fired, as they knew that what's what happened to Black teachers in other states who'd won equal pay. Afraid that their Black students would be assigned the least qualified white teachers, people who had no interest in the children's well-being and saw no future for them. They feared that these young people might not respect their white teachers and it would break down their self-confidence. Afraid that the students would ultimately comprehend that their new teachers had no expectations for them and that the students would follow suit—after all, why not prove their teachers' low expectations true?—and get into the worst kind of trouble. School officials would then have an excuse to administer the wrong kind of discipline, the harsh physical punishment of Black boys that was so well-known throughout the South. And, also, that those bonds between the schools and the Black community, so very precious, would be broken and would not be pieced back together.

The historian Sonya Ramsey points out that there were even fewer women teachers who would support Thomas.[19] Although teacher salaries were unequal based on race, Nashville was one of the school districts that did not additionally have a separate pay schedule based on sex, as was traditional throughout the entire nation. Particularly during the Depression, women teachers were paid less than men. Nashville's female teachers benefited from its sex-equitable policy and were especially threatened by the thought that Nashville might reconsider it to save money. As so many more Black women living in town had no choice but to work as domestics, the status of being a teacher afforded those women an elevated status that became part of their very own identity.[20] How lucky could these females be? After all, Nashville permitted married women to teach!

If many of Harold's colleagues saw his court case as a threat to them and their students, how would the worst of Nashville's white citizens behave toward Harold, with his buzz-cut hairstyle and his pleasantly round plump face, so unlike Vivien's lean face and longer hair? Those narrow-minded citizens perceived the unlikely Harold to be as big a threat as Samson was to the Philistines back in the biblical days. They saw his quest for equal pay for Black teachers as a destructive symbol of his tearing down their sanctioned temple of white supremacy.

Thomas had good reason to be fearful for his brother. In the late nineteenth and early twentieth centuries, more than 200 Black men had been lynched in Tennessee. Just a year earlier, a Black man in the western part of the state was lynched for working with the NAACP to register voters. Reavis Mitchell would remember hearing people talking about the Thomas case when he was a boy and how they had worried, "One of these days, old Harold's going to be found swaying from a tree limb."[21]

In the courtroom, there were numerous ways in which local officials tried to defend dual pay schedules. In Nashville, the local defendants were quite imaginative in their justifications: school board members said that lower pay for "colored" teachers was not due to *their* skin color but rather to the skin color of *the students* they taught. Therefore, anyone who taught "colored" students would be paid less. It just so happened that, in Nashville, all African American teachers were assigned to segregated schools of Black children while European American teachers were assigned to segregated schools of white children. The Black community of Nashville laughed themselves helpless when they heard about this argument.

The next claim by school superintendent Hibbitts was that there was an abundance of Black teachers who were more than willing to accept a lower salary.[22] However, the board failed to present any evidence to back this up, therefore, the court would not accept this argument, either. The defense pointed out that Black teachers paid lower taxes on average compared to the white population and therefore should receive fewer services and less pay from the city.[23]

Then, desperate for a way out, school district representatives told Judge Davies that "colored people" could live more cheaply than could whites. In fact, one expounded, a quart of milk is cheaper to buy for a minority teacher than for a white person. The judge inquired, "Where can a Negro teacher buy a bottle of milk cheaper than a white teacher?"[24] While trying to think of an answer, the city official gazed at the courtroom ceiling for quite a while before he allowed that he could not rightly remember any of the store names at that moment. Throughout the case, Nashville administrators also threatened that having equitable pay would result in minority schools having their already low funds cropped even closer to the ground.

Although the NAACP's Marshall would supervise more than 150 lawsuits that year, he still managed to step in as he deemed necessary for cross-examination. When the school superintendent claimed that

African American teachers "had a lowered standard of living and did not require as much pay as white teachers," Marshall asked him how many Black teachers' homes he had visited?[25] The man was forced to admit that, well, he had never been in any house but he still averred that many other people, both "colored" and white, had told him this was true.

Finally, on July 28, 1942, more than a year after the case had been filed, Judge Davies held for the plaintiff. Harold Thomas had won. The judge also moved that Nashville's violation of the Fourteenth Amendment needed to stop immediately, and he further gave Thomas "a declaratory judgment and an injunction" to make his point clear.[26] When the judge read the decision in Harold's favor, no matter whether his fellow teachers had supported him or not, a joyous shout of jubilee came forth from the room's Black observers. The teacher Sadie Madry remembered her reaction when she first saw her expanded paycheck in September. "I shouted," she said. "It was [the highest paycheck] I'd ever seen in my life." She added that for the first time, "We were being treated as first-class citizens."[27]

Harold was proud of his victory. As a news article declared, "[Harold] Thomas is said to have stood virtually alone in waging his suit."[28] Novella Bass, whose sister taught at Pearl, acknowledged the lack of support Harold Thomas received and gave him even more credit because he stepped up without fear. "Mr. Thomas had the God-given strength to serve as plaintiff. I am sure that others thought about [it], but nobody had dared touch that thing. He had to decide, 'If I lose my job, so be it.'"[29]

It was Harold alone—just as Vivien had predicted—who paid the price for drilling some cracks in the Solid South. He had become embittered by the actions of the school board and, more so, by fellow teachers. When the school administration transferred him out of Pearl, he left teaching.[30] He was sure that he could become a successful businessman in Nashville just like their brother, Maceo.

Harold's unexpected decision to abandon teaching made the news and was reported, along with his photo, in the *Nashville Globe,* well-placed on the front page above the fold.[31] Another paper wrote of Harold, "He

O Brother, Where Art Thou?

won out in the end, for all Negro teachers at the time and hundreds that followed him."[32]

Harold Thomas never taught again.

As for Looby, his full payback came later, in 1960, during the most dangerous year of the civil rights movement. It arrived in the form of a bomb consisting of twenty sticks of explosive dynamite, thrown into his Nashville house in the middle of the night.[33]

CHAPTER ELEVEN

MOVING ON UP?

Vivien and Clara never had given a thought to leaving their home in Nashville. In late 1940, though, Blalock was fielding an authentic promotion opportunity from Johns Hopkins University to become its chief of surgery at Johns Hopkins Hospital and chairman of the surgery department at the Hopkins School of Medicine. He wanted Thomas, of course, to go with him. The offer was as good as it got for Blalock, who still smarted from having had to leave Hopkins fifteen years earlier in shame. Now he was negotiating his contract terms with the university president himself.[1]

For nearly two years, Hopkins had been mired in its efforts to find an appropriate surgery chief to replace its acting head. Hopkins had only found two candidates of stature, and both had turned down the post. The futile search process became an embarrassment, indicating a slip in Hopkins's prestige and reputation.[2] The medical community had heard of its inability to fill a top spot and were idly chattering.

Finally, Blalock, whose name had been raised earlier in the process but not as a serious candidate, was given a second look. The search members discussed his pros and cons. His precarious health, including tuberculous and his sole remaining kidney, went against him. To his benefit was his substantial experience in experimental surgery and his impressive work at Vanderbilt on traumatic shock, as were his book, *Principles of*

Moving On Up?

Surgical Care: Shock and Other Problems, now in print, and the 143 papers he'd published by 1940.[3]

As the search continued, three names, including Blalock's, were thrown in for consideration. There was no clear-cut favorite and Blalock was selected only through a compromise, a point that is often forgotten.[4] When luck turned in his favor, he worked diligently and negotiated a beginning salary of $16,000 which was twice as much as he'd been making at Vanderbilt and was even more money than the president of Vanderbilt hospital made.[5] Blalock also gained a cushy retirement pension of 50 percent of his income earned in his last year before retirement. He received a generous deal—one that wasn't offered to the first two more desired candidates—that gave him more money, and more freedom and power within Hopkins, than the other department heads.

And he also received permission to bring with him from Vanderbilt five dogs and three staffers. The people he wanted to take with him were Frances Wolff Grebel, his ever-faithful secretary, along with George W. Duncan, MD whom Blalock immediately appointed as Hopkins's first chief resident, and his surgical laboratory technician, Vivien Thomas. He knew that Thomas would be the only Black man in the Hopkins lab, unlike at Vanderbilt. Given Hopkins's desperation to find a surgery chief, the institution seems to have been inclined to let Blalock have whatever he wanted. Besides, the typical laboratory worker is isolated—unseen and unpublicized—which would have gone a long way toward Hopkins's acceptance of this Black man.

Thomas was kept out of the loop on all this until December 1940, when Blalock was working out his deal. Before his contract was nailed down, Blalock took Thomas aside to tell him about the offer. "If I accept it," he said, "and I'm sure I will, I want you to go with me."[6] He further explained to him that the Hopkins position was something that "one does not turn down."[7]

Thomas decided not to share his news with Clara until Blalock received the contract terms he sought. When that moment finally came, Clara refused to offer an opinion about their move to Baltimore. Their one-sided conversations became moot when, in May 1941, surgery head Barney Brooks came in to give Thomas some news. He said that when

Dr. Blalock left, there would be "no place" for Thomas at Vanderbilt, something he communicated, Thomas felt, with relish.[8] It seemed that Brooks wanted to purge the hospital of Blalock's closest associates and, certainly, would not feel the loss of this particular Black lab staffer.

Brooks's words went a long way in convincing the Thomas family to follow Blalock, as did Vivien's concerns about living in Nashville during his brother Harold's lawsuit. If the job change meant leaving pleasant Nashville for industrial Baltimore, they assured each other that if they didn't like Baltimore, they would return to Nashville. In their absence, they would rent their charming house out rather than sell it. "Thomas hoped his relationship with Blalock would change up North," said a family friend, "not realizing that Baltimore was not like the North."[9] Of course, World War II was already underway in Europe and Thomas knew that the greatest contribution he could make to his country—if and when it joined the war—would be to continue his surgical experiments on shock research. Of course, doing the right thing to save lives would mean that he'd have to follow Blalock to Hopkins.

In June, Vanderbilt threw a joint farewell party celebrating both Blalock's departure for Hopkins and Tinsley Harrison's departure, on the very same day, to head surgery at Bowman-Gray medical college (now Wake Forest University). Later that month, Hopkins University threw Blalock and Mary a black-tie welcome party at the prestigious and segregated Maryland Club, which opened in 1872 and whose members were required to be white, Christian, and male. If you were one of Hopkins's few Jewish or female professors—Hopkins had no African American professionals in its employ—you were allowed into the club only for an official Hopkins function. In fact, the Hopkins dinner program for the evening carried a front page, pen-and-ink drawing of Blalock walking toward the Hopkins Medical campus Dome building while little dark-skinned children, obviously intended to portray Southern "pickaninnies," giggled and laughed among themselves.[10]

Blalock reported to work on the first day of July 1941 while his wife, Mary, kept busy settling into the family house they had just chosen in the swank Guilford neighborhood on Underwood Road. Mary was industriously interviewing applicants for household help. Some years earlier, a Hopkins physician had this house built for the large sum of $70,000. Apparently, there were ongoing squabbles between family members settling the estate: Blalock heard this from his realtor and used it to his advantage.[11] As he told Hopkins president Isaiah Bowman, "Our bid was $20,000 and rather much to my surprise, it looks as though this will be accepted."[12] He was delighted to lowball the estate and thought his charmed deal was an omen of his future at Hopkins.

Thomas, without Blalock's magic touch and family money, didn't have it so easy. He had not yet traveled to Baltimore to find lodgings for his family. Even his first visit to the city was difficult because Baltimore was officially segregated, and Blalock knew of no Black-owned hotel where Thomas would be allowed to register. Blalock had no choice but to invite Thomas to spend the night with his family.

However, Vivien, as the couple called him, wasn't surprised to find that he was placed in a bedroom on a different level of the house from where the Blalocks slept. With complete indifference to their guest, they explained that his quarters were intended for their future live-in help. The evening went comfortably. Mary ("Mrs. Blalock" to Thomas) retired early because "Dr. Blalock" wanted to talk to Thomas about the upcoming experiments at Hopkins. Before she headed up to bed, she mentioned, again, that the couple hadn't had time to hire any help. Thomas tried not to act surprised when Mrs. Blalock asked, as he remembered, if "I could cook and if I was going to prepare breakfast the next morning."[13] Although Thomas was a superb weekend chef with several delicious specialties in his arsenal, he was unprepared for her request and, perhaps, offended. He diplomatically told her that he knew how to cook—but only in an emergency. Mary laughed and said, that in that case, she'd make breakfast herself.[14]

CHAPTER TWELVE

"MARYLAND, MY MARYLAND"

Showing his good manners, Thomas started to clear the breakfast table the next morning, but Blalock stopped him, eager to start a tour of the Johns Hopkins University medical campus. From the lovely Guilford neighborhood, the surgeon drove a straight route south on Greenmount Avenue, and, as they drove, Thomas was shocked into silence as the neighborhoods became worse and more decayed. Then, as they turned left near the Hopkins campus, he could see the surrounding community was blighted, densely packed with rundown residential brownstone houses cut up into apartments for the city's minorities.

As Blalock parked the car, Thomas gazed at Hopkins's grim soot-covered buildings and couldn't help comparing them to the new clean structures at Vanderbilt University. The men walked toward the Dome building, built in the Queen Anne style with pressed red brick and terracotta ornamentations, which then and now is the icon of Hopkins's medical campus. Stepping inside, Thomas was taken with the statue of Christ (Consolator) in its atrium.[1] His hopeful mood changed fast when he entered its first hallway. He remembered, "To me, it seemed more a tunnel than a corridor,"[2] and he thought to himself, "So this is Hopkins, the great Johns Hopkins, of which I've been hearing as long as I can remember."[3] He thought the campus was far less attractive than that of either Fisk or Meharry.

"Maryland, My Maryland"

A few blocks from the Dome building, the two men entered the Hunterian surgery laboratory, which was to be Thomas's workplace and was named after the influential Scottish medical researcher, John Hunter, whose London house with its entrances on two different streets served as the model for the home of the fictional Dr. Jekyll and Mr. Hyde. Now the lab assistant comprehended why it was aptly nicknamed "the doghouse." He said, "Even though [Blalock] had more or less warned me, I was not quite prepared for either the age or odor of the laboratory building." It was "depressing" with an "almost revolting atmosphere."[4] Noticing his repugnance, Blalock told him that he could repaint the lab but only after scrubbing it down. Thomas silently thought that he would prefer to have used his own hands to tear down the building and construct a new one: "I would have gladly accepted the challenge."[5]

After the campus tour, Thomas left Blalock on campus while he went off to look at apartment rentals. In this industrial city, he'd realized that he probably could not find an equivalent dwelling to their Nashville house but was aghast at the expensive yet substandard housing open to them or any other African American family in Baltimore. The segregated apartments, he said, "could hardly be classified as fit for human habitation."[6] Levi Watkins, Hopkins's first Black surgery intern and later assistant dean for diversity, said of his friend Thomas's experiences, "What awaited Vivien at Hopkins was absolute segregation, absolute boundaries of who you are and where you will ever go."[7] A long-time resident would similarly comment, "Baltimore, at the time, was worse than Birmingham, Alabama. It was the largest small-town Southern city in the US"[8]

What the Thomases, and other people, didn't realize was that Baltimore was a peculiar city in a state with a unique history. Maryland lies directly south of the Mason and Dixon Line that had separated Southern slaveholding states from Northern free states. Currently considered a politically liberal state, Maryland's tradition of race discrimination is nonetheless ugly, especially in its largest city.

Eighty years before Thomas arrived in Baltimore, the pivotal 1860 presidential election had determined whether the nation would hold together or split under the threat of civil war. Maryland was then a burgeoning industrial area as well as laying claim to major tobacco plantations worked by enslaved Black people and owned by influential white men. In fact, the legendary Harriet Tubman had been enslaved by brutal owners on one such southeastern Maryland plantation.

In the 1860 presidential election, Abraham Lincoln received 40 percent of the popular votes nationwide but only a scant 2.5 percent from Marylanders. Instead, the state's voters supported the Southern Democrat candidate John C. Breckinridge, who had won the majority of the deep South vote and who later became the Confederacy's Secretary of War.

Baltimore showed its true Confederate gray a few months after Lincoln's inauguration. Pro-Confederacy advocates fought in the streets in the Civil War's first bloodshed, the Baltimore riot of 1861, that killed four soldiers from Union militia units and twelve civilians. Within a few weeks, the bloody street battle had led to Maryland being put under federal martial law, which meant that Maryland state legislators sympathetic to the South could be jailed. Only with these men removed could Lincoln be assured that the Maryland General Assembly would not vote to leave the Union. (The sentiment against Lincoln is reflected in the state song, "Maryland, My Maryland," with lyrics that call Lincoln a despot and a tyrant. The state did not abandon this song until 2021, six years after the killing of Freddie Gray by Baltimore police, and as yet no other state song has taken its place.)[9]

When the Thomases moved to Baltimore at the beginning of July 1941, the Maryland legislature still had not ratified the Fourteenth Amendment that granted citizenship, due process, and equal protection to Black citizens. Yes, it had been federal law since 1868, but that didn't mean that Maryland would vote in favor of it until 1959. The Maryland legislators also rejected the Fifteenth Amendment, which gave Black men the right to vote. It had been ratified in 1870, but the Maryland legislature did not vote in favor until 1973.

African Americans in Baltimore throughout the nineteenth and twentieth centuries were subjected to a level of race discrimination that no other American city practiced.[10] In 1899, the city began a "Negro removal" program when it evicted Black residents from their homes, churches and places of business and forced them to relocate in less desirable places.[11] In 1910, Baltimore had become the first city in the US to enforce housing segregation through law.[12] Fortunately, the segregation law was struck down as unconstitutional in 1917, not, as Edward Orser points out, because it was discriminatory but rather because it infringed on property rights.[13] It was not merely Baltimore's neighborhoods that were designated for white or Black families, as in other cities and towns. Baltimore brought racial segregation, block-by-block, down to the level of specific streets, specific blocks of streets, and specific sides of each street block. These intricate rules presented perplexing conundrums that were constantly being legislated by the city council with the intention of locking Black Baltimoreans in their second-class status, pointed out the Baltimore city planner Bernie Berkowitz.[14]

Euclid Avenue, for example, was open to Black residents on only certain blocks. In the 2300 block of Euclid, African Americans could live on the east side only. In the 2400 block of Euclid, the racial segregation might be reversed, with the west side of the avenue designated for African American citizens. The noted historian Louis S. Diggs, PhD grew up in Baltimore on Fulton Avenue's east side that was restricted to Black families; he would look over at the more spacious houses on Fulton's west side, designated for whites. He remembered the psychological distance between east and west Fulton, and between Black and white Fulton, saying of the white side, "It could have been the Moon."[15] Not until after the Thomases had moved to Baltimore did a courageous and affluent Black family dare purchase a house on the west side, prompting a few other well-off families to follow. Baltimore would dub this act "blockbusting," an ugly reference to war bombs that would decimate German cities overseas, one street at a time. In Baltimore, the presence of a Black family was considered as devastating to a neighborhood as a four-ton explosive.[16] Baltimore punished the Black Fulton Avenue blockbusters by ripping out the road's grassy landscaped median strip. Then it rezoned the avenue from residential to a major truck thoroughfare.

The same year that the Thomases arrived in Baltimore, the *Baltimore Sun* newspaper ran an editorial about the influx of Southern Blacks seeking jobs in the burgeoning war industry. Rather than lauding their patriotism and loyalty to a country that had treated them so badly, the *Sun* opined, "Keeping unneeded and unwanted Negroes out of Baltimore at a time like this is a national problem."[17]

CHAPTER THIRTEEN

Putting Up and Doing Without

When Clara Thomas joined her husband a short time later to tour Baltimore and looked at the costly segregated apartments they were allowed to rent, she was devastated and wanted to go back to Nashville as fast as she could. Given her customary belief in being her husband's helpmate, she lamented about the city, "It was something that I had to put up with. And I put up with it."[1]

The family initially had to take rooms in a rat-infested boarding house with a communal toilet. There were alleys nearby littered with garbage that remained home to dozens of rat colonies. At night, the neighborhood was even more depressing than in daytime. The sidewalks were illuminated only by a relic of the last century, the feeble yellow glow of gas streetlights. Thomas joked that city officials kept these flickering lights in the minority neighborhoods to promote the atmosphere of the macabre writings of Edgar Allan Poe, who had lived and died in the city.

Baltimore's segregation was reinforced by the poverty-level wages paid by local business and institutions to Black citizens. Salaries in the city were determined by race. Certain places of employment—most notably its two largest employers, Bethlehem Steel and Johns Hopkins University—were downright hostile to hiring Black workers and, if they did employ them, paid them less than a living wage.[2] Blalock had informed

Thomas that Hopkins would pay Thomas only $1,404 a year (currently, $29,000), take it or leave it, and he said that Hopkins had strict rules about salaries for employees who were not college graduates.[3] Although it was a higher salary by a few hundred dollars than at Vanderbilt, the cost of living in a Northern manufacturing city was far greater than in Nashville.

Now at work, Thomas spent his first week cleaning and painting the doghouse, trying to make it habitable. Only then was he ready to start his experiments but he soon found that "It took a while to get things rolling here."[4] He and the new surgery chief noted the "far inferior" equipment, instruments and supplies, compared to what they had at Vanderbilt.[5] Thomas drew up a supply list of necessary items and submitted it to the director of the lab, Edgar J. Poth, MD giving a full explanation why each was needed. Weeks later, a bewildered Thomas realized that he still couldn't begin the professor's assignments because nothing he had ordered had arrived. He could not even find basic needles and silk thread for suturing. Wary of directly confronting Poth, Thomas explained to Blalock why his research assignments had been delayed.

Blalock exploded when he heard that Poth was sitting on the supply order. He cussed, then yelled, "Who the hell does he think he is? I run this department."[6] He angrily pushed a handwritten note, addressed to Poth, over the desk: "Get anything Vivien asks for, for my work."[7] The supplies arrived, but Poth never acknowledged or spoke to Thomas again; the two men communicated only through writing.[8] And again, Thomas realized that he was an invisible man, to be completely ignored at will by whichever of the Hopkins staff refused to interact with a Black man. He had only the protection of Blalock, at Blalock's convenience.

Nor could Thomas help noticing that Hopkins's lab techs were white and were not particularly friendly. He noted, "This lack of hostility was only because I was there at the pleasure of one of the powers that be and that I had to be tolerated."[9] They knew he was "Blalock's man."[10] In fact, as he got ready for his first surgery, another lab worker realized that Thomas was getting ready to operate solo—without Blalock or anyone else—and the tech sarcastically said, "Oh, come on. Don't kid me."

Putting Up and Doing Without

Blalock, to his credit, had warned Thomas earlier that were no other "colored" lab workers at Hopkins.[11] The only people of African descent Hopkins would hire comprised "the mop and bucket squad,"[12] as Thomas referred to the housekeepers and janitors on the medical campus. Even then, Hopkins's separate wage scale for whites and Black workers in the exact same job classification was well-known.[13] Still, Thomas thought Blalock should have told him about the city's housing shortage for Blacks, which grew grave toward the end of 1941 after the attack on Pearl Harbor as more Southerners, both Black and white, moved up North for war jobs. The two men lived in entirely different worlds.[14]

Slowly, the coolness of his lab colleagues turned into respect. "There was no one in the laboratory who worked nearly as independently as I did."[15] He further explained, "I didn't have any real competition in my job, not even from the whites in the lab."[16] He added, "As technicians, they assisted but never carried out procedures on their own."[17] As time passed, Thomas was given more and more deference by his colleagues and he noticed, "I had become keenly aware of the situation I was in. I was sort of a curiosity, not only to whites but to the Negro community."[18]

As the only lab tech at Hopkins who was Black, Thomas was aware of his singular status. He'd only been at Hopkins for a few months when Blalock called him to bring some needed lab notes to the professor's office, which was a few blocks away. Thomas dashed from the lab carrying the papers, still wearing his long white lab coat—washed, bleached, and ironed by Clara. "As I met people along the corridor, some of them actually stopped in their tracks and watched me as I passed!!"[19] How could there be an African American employee who was not dressed in a one-piece janitor's blue boiler suit?

Although no one had complained to Blalock, the next time Thomas left the lab building, he removed his lab coat and walked over in his street clothes. This time, no one stopped dead in their tracks. Blalock asked him why he wasn't wearing his lab coat and he explained "how I had stopped traffic in the main corridor on my previous visit."[20] Blalock only laughed. A quick learner, Thomas had no desire to bring attention to himself. He noted that at Vanderbilt, as prejudiced as it was, "I had not previously been exposed [to] or experienced the Hopkins's atmosphere."[21]

While Vivien was at work, Clara kept herself busy at home scrimping pennies and stretching dollars. She would make her own and the children's clothes, including their snowsuits and the winter coats they now needed.[22] People at Hopkins also noticed that Thomas's lab coats were twinkling white and ironed to perfection. Although she was sympathetic to her husband's interest in medicine, she was understandably dissatisfied with her husband's ambiguous status and ill-paid job at Hopkins. Clara responded to the danger of her Baltimore neighborhood in her own way. Her daughter, Theodosia Thomas Dullea, explained, "Mother would not leave the house because she was afraid of the area."[23]

After some months, the family was able to find a better apartment rental that was affordable only because Thomas took a second job as the building's nighttime handyman. Although their housing had improved, one relative said, "At times, they would not have money for food."[24] The Thomases, though, shared an unspoken agreement: Vivien never brought his problems home.[25] Clara, in turn, did not irritate him by mentioning how much better off they would be if he worked as a master carpenter.

Across town, at the Blalock house, in its swank neighborhood, Mary wasn't seeing much of her husband during the week because of his long hours and increasingly heavy travel schedule. And when Blalock did return home, their two children (soon to become three, with another son born during the war) were asleep and often Blalock was too tired and too distracted to be the companion Mary needed. She knew no one in Baltimore and stayed at home most of the time.

Mary Blalock was a lovely social butterfly who was perhaps not the most well-grounded of women. As the prototype Southern belle, she had unrealistically assumed that her bright light would never dim. Her well-known sense of humor now served to irritate her husband, as many of her quips placed him as her target.

Family money, though, made possible a summer house rental on the Chesapeake Bay on Maryland's Eastern Shore. But Blalock would invite Hopkins surgeons and the students he valued to join the family for weekends, and the men would spend many hours playing tennis, fishing, golfing, and competing at the family ping-pong table. Mary was left to manage the children and get meals on the table for the many houseguests.

In early 1942, Thomas faced a hard choice. He was caught in a painful pay squeeze and remembered Blalock's promises, when they were at Vanderbilt, to raise Thomas's salary when he had his own department. Thomas matter-of-factly told Blalock that he needed to receive a living wage. His family could no longer manage on his salary. The surgery head demurred and suggested that if he needed more money, why didn't he put Clara out to work?

Thomas could not have been more offended if Blalock had insulted his mother. The Thomases were a traditional family, just as their own parents had been, and they did not believe that Clara Thomas should work outside their home. Thomas resented Blalock for, as he said, "interfering with my personal plans and affairs" and, furious, he rejoined that his daughters would not ever have to be "latch key children."[26] That Clara would have earned, as a Black woman with a high school diploma, only $0.35 an hour to clean houses was apparently of no concern to Blalock, whose own wife had hired a couple to live on their Guilford house and grounds. In fact, Mary had recently complained to her husband when their own servants left for better-paying war jobs.

Thomas would have been incensed to learn that Blalock, before leaving Nashville, had negotiated for Hopkins to give him $1,500 to cover his family's relocation expenses.[27] Thomas received no such help and had to shoulder the entire expense of his family's move, whereas the Hopkins check that underwrote Blalock's move was higher than Thomas's annual Hopkins salary.

Thomas simmered as he realized that he was not going to be treated any better at Hopkins than he had been at Vanderbilt: in fact, he was worse off. Originally, he'd thought that going to Hopkins would be terrific. As he said, "I thought it was great," and then he paused, blew out a breath of pipe smoke and added, "'til I got here."[28] His long work hours bent-backed over the surgery table and the significance and value of his experimental traumatic shock surgeries—the ones that helped Blalock be offered his surgery-in-chief position—counted for nothing when it came to his earning power.

However, Thomas made it clear to Blalock as they talked: he could not continue living in Baltimore on what Hopkins paid him. He said, "I left the office without waiting for a response. From his tone of voice and from what he had said, I felt that further discussion was useless."[29]

Blalock, despite telling his dean that Thomas "was the most valuable technician in the department," refused to increase Thomas's inconsequential salary with money from the surgery budget. Instead, he reached into the deep pockets of a generous and kind-hearted neurosurgeon, Walter Dandy, known for his generous and constant philanthropy.

In fact, Dandy had donated a substantial sum, $5,000,[30] to the surgery department in 1942 to supplement the pay of Thomas and others who were being hard hit by the expenses of wartime living.[31] After Thomas told Blalock that he urgently needed a raise, Blalock used a miniscule fraction of Dandy's gift to raise Thomas's salary by a princely $96.00 a year.[32] Thomas now earned exactly $1,500 and he never learned that Frances Wolff Grebel, Blalock's white secretary, was making about 20 percent more than he.[33] Thomas was caught like a mark in a confidence game operated by Blalock and the universities where he'd worked.

Even this nugatory boost made Blalock think he needed to justify it to his dean: "I have great fears of losing him unless this increase is granted. He has a wife and two children and is finding it difficult to live in Baltimore on his present salary. Vivien is a willing worker, and there are many days when he is at work in the lab for fourteen hours a day."[34]

One evening, Blalock made an unexpected stop at the Thomas household, now in a rented row house at the intersection of Caroline and Preston streets in East Baltimore, to talk shop. Clara's mood had been simmering red hot since the family's arrival in Baltimore. Mrs. Thomas was a Southern lady through and through, yet she could not keep herself from indicating to Blalock—in the most subtle and polite words that she could find—that he was not welcome to make another surprise evening visit.

Blalock had come by in person because the local Chesapeake and Potomac Telephone Company, a basic public utility, refused to install

Putting Up and Doing Without

private telephones in Black Baltimore neighborhoods. (A few red-lined neighborhoods were allowed to have a party line.) Finally, a frustrated Blalock intervened with C&P and demanded an exemption for a phone to be installed in the Thomas household.

Taking out his personalized 100 percent-cotton Johns Hopkins School of Medicine stationery, Blalock wrote to C&P, "Enclosed is an application for a telephone for my technician, Vivien Thomas. I have no way at the present time with getting in touch with Vivien Thomas except during regular hours when he is working here at the laboratory. It would be very helpful if this request for telephone would be granted."[35]

Even then, each time that the Thomases moved, C&P again would refuse them phone service. Blalock would need to intercede another time: "My technician, Vivian Thomas, has moved to 1113 Springfield Ave. and is having trouble getting a new telephone. It would be very helpful if his request for a telephone could be granted."[36] The Thomases had to wonder what they'd gotten themselves in to by moving to such a city.

CHAPTER FOURTEEN

HOPING TO DO GOOD

If Thomas had known little about Baltimore and its iron links to the Confederacy, initially he knew even less about the history of Johns Hopkins University. Being from Nashville, Thomas at first didn't realize that the university's name came from its Quaker founder. It's said of the Quakers that they set out to do good, and that they did very well, indeed. This was certainly true of the Quaker Marylander Johns Hopkins, who, with the largest trust ever given to higher education at the time, founded the university, its hospital, and its medical school in the late 1800s.

Johns Hopkins was born in 1795 into a devout family. (The unusual first name derived from his mother's family.) His grandparents had owned White Halls Plantation, a very large tract of land in southern Maryland, on which they initially farmed tobacco using enslaved labor and eventually substituted farm hands.[1] When Johns's father inherited White Halls, he put the couple's eleven children to work on the farm, which was not unusual. Young Johns, who was homeschooled, went into the fields at age twelve, when he might have appreciated having more time to play marbles or roll hoops.

Perhaps because he was denied formal education, as an adult Mr. Hopkins espoused its importance for all. Even more strongly did he promote abolitionism, racial and religious tolerance as well as equality for

Hoping to Do Good

women—all values he'd learned from his parents and the teachings of his religion on their isolated farm.[2]

At age seventeen, the tall and blue-eyed Johns Hopkins went into the more cosmopolitan Baltimore grocery business, eventually founding his own firm that grew to serve a number of mid-Atlantic states. Nevertheless, the greatest source of the wealth that allowed him to retire at age fifty-two originated from his exceedingly sound investments, especially his 1830 purchase of shares in the nation's first operating railroad, the Baltimore and Ohio. As talk of Southern secession grew louder in the early 1860s, Johns Hopkins astounded his fellow businessmen when they recognized that he was not merely an abolitionist in this Southern-leaning state but an outright Unionist (despite perhaps having owned slaves at some earlier point in his life).[3] Once the Civil War began, he allowed Union soldiers to travel free on B&O trains as they headed west toward Virginia and its new Union-friendly scion, West Virginia. The railroad became instrumental to the Northern cause and picked up steam when the war ended, making its stockholders wealthy men.

Mr. Hopkins lived into his late seventies but never married. When he died on Christmas morning 1873, with his dog by his side, he had accumulated a large estate of about seven million dollars. He was one of the nation's richest men. Referring to his egalitarian convictions, one of his obituaries described him as a "man who knew no race."[4] That he planned to donate nearly all his fortune had been well known. His gift was so considerable that even the New York City papers covered it, with the *Tribune* gravely admonishing his institutional heirs, "Make sure that his charity shall reach the object for which it was intended, which is the only adequate mark of respect which Baltimore can pay to the memory of her benefactor."[5]

The will of Mr. Johns Hopkins reflected his progressive philosophy.[6] First, as he had never married and had no children, he gave about a million dollars to more distant family members. The next six million dollars he gave to start four institutions: the Johns Hopkins University, the Johns Hopkins Hospital, the Johns Hopkins Medical School (by now, the medical school and hospital are unified), and a Johns Hopkins Colored Orphan Asylum. The university and the hospital had separate governing boards but nearly all the same members served on both, making them less independent than Mr. Hopkins might have wished.

Mr. Hopkins specifically stated that the hospital's mission was to "care first for the city's poor... without regard to race, sex or color" or "sectarian influence."[7] It also was to have space for a "limited number of persons who could pay."[8] Contrary to his clear instructions, the hospital was segregated by policy and practice nearly immediately after it opened.[9] It had "colored" wards, separate waiting rooms, and two blood banks—one for "colored blood" and one for "white blood." Some of the departments designated certain "colored days" when Black patients, who were always addressed by their first names, could enter the clinic. The hospital had separate morgues for Black people and white so that even the dead would not need to mix. Perhaps worse, by the turn of the twentieth century, only 20 percent of the Hopkins patients were indigent.[10]

Mr. Hopkins also made the hospital responsible for setting up and running the Johns Hopkins Colored Orphan Asylum and its accompanying school. The orphan home received the first two million dollars and opened in 1885. He had added a caveat in his will that if the orphanage did not spend all his two-million-dollar donation, the remnant should revert to Hopkins Hospital. Despite its huge endowment, the orphanage took in only twenty-four Black children.

The orphanage soon suffered from the Hopkins's hospital board members' extreme indifference and hostility to "colored" children. The establishment was quickly reversed into an all-female orphanage intended to train "colored" women as seamstresses, laundresses, or servants, contrary to Johns Hopkins's will.[11] After that, it segued into an orthopedic convalescent institution for "colored crippled" and "white crippled" children. The so-called orphanage was abandoned in the mid-1920s; the Hopkins hospital benefited from taking its remaining fortune. Baltimore's *Afro American* newspaper was horrified, and it wrote that "the entire Hopkins Trust has been perverted, and the wishes of the greatest of Maryland's philanthropists have been utterly disregarded and have been treated with scorn and contempt."[12]

For whatever reason, Mr. Hopkins had never stipulated in his will that the Johns Hopkins University's education institutions should accept

Hoping to Do Good

applicants who were Black, female, or Jewish. Because of this, its faculty and administrators soon reflected a deep Southern mindset and preferred to admit only students who were white, male, and Southern. With this limited student selection, by 1910, the Hopkins president admitted that the undergraduates "have the natural feelings of men from that part of the country" so that "admitting Negro students would be 'almost suicidal.'"[13]

Even in Hopkins's graduate programs, an applicant's race was prioritized over his achievements and the university was "particularly notorious for this."[14] As the Black scholar W. E. B. Du Bois had boldly stated in the late 1920s, "Race discrimination has been carried further in Johns Hopkins in Baltimore than in any other college in the country."[15] As a consequence, the first degree of any kind awarded by Hopkins to an African American student would not be until *after* World War II.[16]

The last of Mr. Hopkins's four institutions to open was the Hopkins School of Medicine. It had been delayed because the original financial gift suddenly fell short; B&O stocks were in free fall during the Panic of 1893. Hiring the distinguished physicians Hopkins medical school calls its Founding Four had to be postponed. However, the medical school could not have been opened with these four renowned doctors who brought the new hospital such prestige if it were not for the Financial Four: Mary Elizabeth Garrett (the businesswoman was the daughter of the B&O's railroad president), M. Carey Thomas, PhD, Mary Mackell Gwinn, and Elizabeth Tabor King, PhD, the Baltimore women who raised funds to make good its $500,000 shortfall. Garrett herself gifted more than $300,000.

The women required two things of the trustees. The first was that the medical school should admit only the nation's most highly educated applicants. Their elite standards prompted Osler to say to another one of the Founding Four, "Welch, we are fortunate to get in as professors; we would never have made it as students."[17] Alan Chesney, MD gave credit where it was due, stating that the women's "adoption of a high standard of admission not only helped to gain a commanding position for the new institution, but also did much to lift the general level of American medicine."[18]

The women's second condition was that female medical school applicants be admitted on the same basis as men. In an era when some women had growing expectations for equal rights and suffrage, entrance to medical school was a fiery issue. "In a surprising twist of fate, Johns Hopkins became ground zero and, initially, an unwilling partner in the late nineteenth century feminist battle for women's equality."[19] "Unwilling" is a fitting description. Carey Thomas said that "many of the trustees, and Gilman [the university's first president, Daniel Coit Gilman] seemed to prefer not to open the school at all if it meant that women were to be admitted."[20]

Black medical school applicants were not welcomed by the university either then or for nearly a century. Over the years, Hopkins University stood out in its unwillingness to admit Black students to medicine. By 1945, fifty-two of the nation's seventy-eight accredited medical schools, or 64 percent, had awarded medical degrees to African American students.[21] Only twenty-six schools, including Hopkins, barred Black applicants. Some Southern medical schools began to desegregate after World War II, but Johns Hopkins was not among them.[22] By 1960, it was one of only twelve medical schools in the entire country that did not admit African American applicants compared to eighty-six schools that did. Hopkins could no longer blame its failure on local sentiment: the University of Maryland medical school, also in Baltimore, had awarded its first medical degree to a Black student in 1955.

Not until 1967 did Hopkins finally award its first MD degree to an African American man, Robert Gamble. The Hopkins medical college's action occurred a mere 102 years after Confederate General Lee surrendered at Appomattox. Despite it being in the late 1960s, Gamble was "harassed and abused," said a fellow student. "There was tremendous racial hostility."[23] Gamble hung in, though, and graduated with his class in deference to his grandfather, who had been the sixth Black student to receive an MD degree from Yale University in the late 1800s.

For these reasons, and many more, the tension between African Americans and Hopkins runs deep and wide. It was sarcastically dubbed "the plantation" by many Black Baltimoreans and had a reputation for racism that made it particularly notorious among colleges and universities. Levi Watkins, a surgeon who became Hopkins's assistant dean for diversity at the medical campus, said that Hopkins's presence in East Baltimore "casts a billion-dollar shadow over its closest neighbors," mostly lower-income Black residents.[24]

Shortly after the death of Mr. Johns Hopkins, around 1870, the city's African American newspaper had stated that "Johns Hopkins will ever be regarded as a friend of the colored race in that we will teach our children to do honor for his memory."[25] Given the subsequent actions of the Johns Hopkins's boards, administrators, and professors, that prediction proved to be wishful thinking.

If Thomas's sister Olga had been a nurse in Baltimore rather than Detroit, she might have been able to warn her brother of Hopkins's reputation for unabashed racism and put him on guard. Most likely, Thomas would have come to Hopkins regardless. Once he arrived and recognized his unique position as the only Black professional on campus, he must have ascertained how critical a role he played in Blalock's career, and he said, "The only reason he brought me here was that it was to his advantage. I never kidded myself."[26]

Still, at the beginning of his employment at Hopkins, Vivien Thomas had respected its physicians and medical students and had admired and emulated their research talent, their dedication to patients and their capacity for hard work. If it weren't for the race discrimination that dominated the campus and dogged Thomas's salary and advancement, Hopkins would have been the perfect place for him to work.

CHAPTER FIFTEEN

IT'S WAR!

On the first Sunday of December 1941, as everyone slowed down to relax before the busy Christmas season, the peaceful day ended at 2:22 p.m. EST when the Associated Press radio announced the bombing of Pearl Harbor by the Japanese Imperial Navy Air Service. Seconds later, CBS News aired the news.[1] Within minutes, NBC ran the only live announcement of the sneak attack: "This is KTUH in Honolulu, Hawaii," said the terse correspondent. "We have witnessed the severe bombing of Pearl Harbor by enemy planes, undoubtedly Japanese. It is no joke. It is a real war."[2] Listening, you could hear his words being interrupted by the cacophony of exploding bombs.

Until then, it had been a typical day of rest. There was a New York Giants-Brooklyn Dodgers football game at the Polo Grounds and, at Chicago's Comiskey Park, the Chicago Bears were playing the Chicago Cardinals. Suddenly, at both arenas, fans heard a public announcement repeated every few minutes: "All servicemen immediately report to their units."[3] Worried, friend turned to friend, and stranger to stranger, wondering what this could mean.

Just two miles from the White House, the Washington Redskins[4] were playing the Philadelphia Eagles at Washington DC's Griffith Stadium and the spectators listened quizzically to the broader pages of individuals across the ranks that came one after another one after another as rapidly as machine gun fire: "Admiral W. H. P. Bland is asked to report to his

IT'S WAR!

office at once! Joseph Umglumph of the Federal Bureau of Investigation is requested to report to the FBI office at once! Capt. H. X. Fenn of the United States Army is asked to report to his office at once!"[5] Clearly, something was terribly wrong. Those at home, listening to the games on their A.M. radios, surely began calling out to their spouses, "Honey, you need to hear this!"

Shattered were the day's plans as families busily called each other, sent telegrams to friends and turned the radio up loud so it could be heard in every room in the house as frenzied news announcers alerted listeners. By evening, Americans knew that their world had changed. Routine was kicked aside for the exigencies of war. Blalock's phone was completely tied up: Washington's National Research Council office kept frenziedly calling him because he headed its Subcommittee on Shock. After all, he had published more than thirty papers on shock by this point, as well as his recent book.[6]

Everyone grappled with what the first steps should be.[7] Blalock's phone buzzed all afternoon and evening as he talked to either the Council staff or his committee members checked in with him and they agreed to meet with members of the military's Office of Scientific Research and Development. That night, Blalock began to write his first shock manual for the use of military physicians.

Shortly after, the Navy desperately called Blalock to Pearl Harbor, needing his advice on caring for the more than 2,400 burned and crushed sailors and pilots. When his military plane skidded to a stop on Oahu's airbase tarmac, sailors were still digging makeshift graves for the bodies that later would be reinterred in the national Punchbowl cemetery.[8] Blalock looked gray and weary after his long series of flights, especially because he feared flying. He'd barely stepped on land when a jeep pulled up to take him straightaway to the Navy hospital. A small part of it was damaged: an American ship's defensive fire had successfully hit a Japanese plane that spiraled down and exploded close to the building. Part of the hospital had to be evacuated, which explained the tents that mushroomed from the tropical green lawn.[9]

Fortunately, the Red Cross and Navy nurses had arrived and were working nonstop, each one carrying a pocketknife to defend herself in case of invasion. They had heard about the massive numbers of rapes of at least 20,000 girls and women committed by the Japanese Imperial Army when it invaded Nanking, China.[10]

Blalock briefly met the Army's Judge Advocate for the Hawaiian Islands, Thomas S. Green, to discuss the following day's activities.[11] Eager, though, to see the wounded, Blalock soon motored out into the harbor to board USS *Solace*, the Navy's newest mobile hospital ship. In his motorized boat, cutting through now tranquil water, Blalock must have seen the oozing "black tears" of oil seeping upward from the sunken USS *Arizona*.

Then, the surgeon for the Pacific Fleet met him on deck, gloomily telling him, "Burns, burns and more burns."[12] Seventy percent of *Solace's* patients were disfigured by first- or second-degree burns that covered up to 80 percent of their bodies. The sailors, to avoid being trapped in a sinking ship, had jumped into the water of the lagoon even though it was blazing with a layer of burning oil over its surface.[13]

The next day, the professor talked to the *Solace* surgeons and top medical personal about the treatment of shock caused by burns, as well as what he knew about medical responses to being crushed and suffering oxygen deprivation. The Navy still hoped to save the 1,200 sailors suffocating in the submerged USS *Arizona*, which, tragically, proved not to be possible. Metallic tapping noises continued day after day.[14] In this metal tomb, it took a full three weeks for the last man to suffocate to death.[15]

The physicians wanted to know how to improve their responses to shock as well as asking Blalock to identify the type of medical equipment that should be dispersed on all Navy ships. Of course, the first convoy of US ships had already left Pearl on December 8 without any supplementary supplies to hunt down the Japanese Pearl Harbor Striking Force.[16]

After Blalock returned home and shared his experiences with Thomas, the lab assistant reflected on his earliest burn studies at Vanderbilt in the 1930s, the ones in which he had become so badly nauseated by having to use a blow torch on anesthetized dogs. Thomas was satisfied, now, that his experimental surgeries meant that a greater number of Pearl sailors would survive because of his work. Then, Blalock informed Thomas that he himself would be constantly on the run, on the road and in the air, emphasizing how the lab assistant would need to work independently while

It's War!

Blalock was off campus. Indeed, the following year, Blalock seemed to be constantly setting off to give talks on shock at War Sessions meetings set up around the country by the National Research Council Committee on Transfusions. In these gatherings, he reiterated the effectiveness of blood plasma, which is far easier to transport than whole blood, which requires refrigeration.

Thomas knew that he was best serving his country by staying in the lab and aiding the military through his research. The draft, for all African American men, meant assignment to a menial job rather than meaningful work. Fortunately, the thirty-one-year-old Thomas would receive a II-A draft exemption in recognition of his research on traumatic shock. It was certain that Blalock would have been granted the same exemption; instead, his troublesome health history was enough for the military to judge him medically unfit for duty.

The US military's race discrimination was so overt that on December 7, of nearly two million servicemen and women, it could boast of exactly twelve African American officers.[17] This was noted by the historian Stephen E. Ambrose: "It is one of ironies of US history that while the nation fought its greatest war against the world's worst racist, it maintained a segregated army abroad and a total system of discrimination at home."[18]

Yet another example of how African Americans were treated came immediately, during the Pearl Harbor attack. Dorrie (Doris) Miller, an African American crewman who was cook third class on USS *West Virginia* at Pearl Harbor, had just finished serving breakfast and was collecting dirty laundry when his ship's battle station alarm shrieked. The former high school football player dropped his canvas bags and ran up to the deck, taking the stairs at double-step. Though he'd never been permitted to receive battle training, Miller fast figured out how to work the ship's starboard anti-aircraft gun after a few quick instructions from Ensign Victor Delano, who was firing up at the diving Japanese planes. Now Miller lifted the 84-pound Browning .50 caliber machine gun toward the sky and aimed at the incoming planes, expelling 110 rounds of ammunition at a time, to protect his ship from vicious bombs. At last, the enemy planes, their weapon bays empty, turned west to safety.

Miller fast pulled injured sailors from the water, "unquestioningly saving lives," the Navy reported.[19] As a result of his actions and a newly launched campaign by various African American organizations, he was awarded the Navy Cross, the service's second-highest honor for extraordinary heroism during battle.[20] Still, the Navy kept him on his same assignment as a kitchen worker and gave him no advancement. The *Pittsburgh Courier*, an esteemed African American newspaper, printed Miller's picture mopping the deck with the lede, "He Fought—Keeps Mop."[21] Such examples illustrated exactly why Thomas was content to stay out of the military and in the Hopkins lab where he could contribute far more to his country.

Within days, entry into World War II took a heavy toll on Hopkins's medical school and hospital. The military had called for total mobilization and, immediately, thirty-eight Hopkins physicians shipped out and another twenty-five were put on part-time status. Within eighteen months, a full ninety-two Hopkins physicians were absentee.[22] The situation added to Blalock's stress, taking time away from his lab work with Thomas, who also bore a significantly heavier workload.[23]

The young men and women in medical training at Hopkins had their education telescoped: although they worked even longer days and nights than their predecessors, they received a shortened curriculum. Their accelerated program meant that Thomas began teaching dog surgery methodology twice a week rather than the usual one time. Everyone was working at double speed. Thomas amped up shock experiments now that this work was immediately critical to the war effort. William Longmire described Thomas's work, giving him full credit: "Largely through the efforts of Vivien Thomas, the experimental work on shock was pushed forward."[24] Any thought of a getting a break for holidays or a summer vacation went up in a dark cloud of greasy black smoke when the first Japanese bomb hit Hawaii's airfield and harbor.

After the workforce depletion, Blalock was left with only a "small, relatively green" group of teaching surgeons who were not closely overseen by their chief, as he was absent so often.[25] He took even more care in selecting his interns and residents and came up with a distinguished group of young men, bringing in such notable future surgeons as Denton

It's War!

Cooley, William Longmire, and C. Rollins Hanlon, MD. In his wartime speaking and writing, Blalock emphasized the vital ounce of prevention in saving lives. He believed that the medic or physician should initiate treatment (using whole blood, plasma, salt, glucose solution, and/or oxygen) before shock set in. The preferred method on the battlefront was to use plasma, which was more easily administered than whole blood.

In wartime, the top priority was that Blalock needed to continue his shock experiments. Fortunately, he had just received a grant to accelerate it, not that any of its funding went into Thomas's pocket for his hours spent working overtime. In a downsized workforce, Thomas's unique ability to conduct surgery by himself, without an assistant, was critical.[26] Sometimes, both his fellow lab techs and surgical students would cluster around his table to watch him operate. He displayed his skill at devising and creating practical products that others had not thought of. As modest as Thomas was, the more he saw and heard about other people's lab work, the more he slowly became aware that he was different and perhaps more talented than most or even all experimental lab surgeons. He had never heard of a lab tech who worked as independently as he did nor one who could conduct his sophisticated operations, which included creating new medical instruments and materials. Little did Blalock realize how the war would cannibalize his own time in the lab. Little did Thomas realize that Blalock's war-related absences from the hospital would, eventually, bring Thomas into the limelight.

Thomas's lab was always productive as he continued research on a variety of environmental conditions that might influence shock: cold or hot temperatures, blood and blood substitutes, oxygen, circulatory failure, soft tissue wounds, and hemorrhage. When the war began, Blalock assigned both Thomas and George Duncan to more sophisticated research on crush injuries. As has been true throughout history, war advanced our knowledge of the best medical treatments. Civilians would be pulled out from the rubble of London's Blitz and appear healthy, only to go into shock shortly after, often with fatal results due to their crush injuries. Thomas described it: "People get buried alive . . . and would stay buried . . . until you took the pressure off them. Within minutes, their blood pressure would just bang-fall and they'd go into shock."[27] Blalock would author another fifteen articles on shock during the war. Two of the publications bore the name of George Duncan as coauthor with Blalock. There was never any authorship credit for the work Thomas completed, even for those studies which he created independently.

Despite Thomas's lack of personal attribution for his experiments, he was quietly proud of his work, knowing that it was saving lives. With fewer people in the lab and less oversight, he was able to carve out some office space for himself. He was allowed an assistant, Clara Belle Puryear, a trained chemist lab worker, and she helped him on some highly complex oxygen experiments. Thomas, with Puryear's assistance, organized four lengthy tables, each with thirteen variables, that demonstrated the effect of oxygen on graded hemorrhage, on extremity trauma, on tourniquets, and on burns. The tables Thomas produced constituted a full 60 percent of the article that Blalock published under his own name in 1944.[28]

The first time that Blalock had mentioned Thomas was in his 1940 book on shock when he wrote, "My excellent technician, Vivien Thomas, has been responsible for the execution of many of the experiments."[29] But now Thomas nearly jumped out of his chair as he reviewed his journal copy. There, on the last page, he saw that Blalock had written, "Clara Belle Puryear and Vivien Thomas rendered valuable technical aid."[30] This was his second published note of credit, although it did not count as a coauthorship. This second time around, Vivien must have wondered whether Puryear, a white woman, caused a halo effect that shone its reflected light on him, too.

The war years were ever-so-slowly changing his relationship with the professor. In Blalock's absence, Thomas acquired more decision-making authority in the lab and became its *de facto* chief. Now the surgical faculty learned more about the significance of Thomas's work and most acknowledged his ability to complete complex trials all while being an elegant surgeon. As J. Alex Haller, MD explained it, "It became clear to all of us that Thomas was the hand in Blalock's glove."[31]

Thomas was pleased that Blalock was tacitly acknowledging his capabilities and intellect, even though Blalock had not and would never express this straight out. It was typical of the men's mixed working relationship: rather than being able to speak honestly with each other, Blalock's narcissism and racial attitude wouldn't allow him to express gratitude to a lesser educated Black man while Thomas had to swallow his resultant anger to keep his job. The resentment and fury of both men, along with the unspoken presence of race, reduced Thomas to fight back indirectly through stubbornness and procrastination while keeping his mask of amiability. Thomas's exceptional resilience allowed him to stand up to Blalock, no matter how it was disguised. The two men, by now, had fallen into a type of passive-aggressive behavior that was frustrating to both. Their relationship was fracturing and would only continue to deteriorate.

In his own cool way, when Thomas was frustrated by Blalock's absence or lack of clear direction, he'd push back. Once, during the war, he stopped work on an experiment because Blalock seemed unable to give instructions on how he wanted it done. Thomas waited him out because he wanted to force Blalock to admit that he had no good ideas on how to proceed. Finally, Blalock gave him what he wanted: "Vivien, you do them however you want to. I just want them done."[32]

CHAPTER SIXTEEN

BLALOCK, THOMAS, AND CHARLES DREW, MD

On the home front, American citizens heard the shout-out, loud and clear, to give blood for wounded servicemen. The NRC shock committee had signed an agreement with the Red Cross to be the nation's conduit for blood donations and it already had commandeered brick and mortar storefronts in thirty-five cities to be blood donor centers and was operating sixty-three traveling mobile units. Along with Blalock's recent treatment for shock, the need for blood was critical to saving lives.

The Red Cross began education programs that urged citizens to give blood as often as was safe. You could see Red Cross posters pasted up everywhere. One was a sketch of an injured soldier lying on the ground with an explosion of fire directly behind him, while a kneeling medic infused him with plasma. The poster asked Americans, "He gave *his* blood. Will you give yours?"[1]

Lines snaked into Red Cross facilities across the country in the second week in December. Americans were furious at the sneak attack on Hawaii. Everyone wanted to help, especially after public service announcements explained why giving blood was vital to saving American lives. Nevertheless, after that huge first group of volunteers, blood donations came in and went out like the tide. When news would reach America of a battle won with relatively few injured men, few people would donate. If a dispatch told of a battle defeat with many American casualties, donors poured in. Some news, of course, was embargoed from the American people because the government did not want citizens aware of the extent of major military losses.[2] The first reports of casualties at Pearl Harbor totaled 350 people: the actual number of deaths was nearly ten times as high.

People who had never heard of plasma or blood types before were now learning. Blood has four important elements: the red blood cells carrying oxygen, white blood cells that combat disease, platelets that help wounds to clot, and plasma, a sticky protein salt-solution that is mostly water. Plasma is obtained from the liquid portion of blood, with its red and white blood platelets suspended. Blalock always emphasized that infusing plasma should be the first step in treating shock because it could be preserved significantly longer than could whole blood, and it carried fewer chances of transmitting disease. Also, it could be infused immediately, without needing to match blood types.

An African American physician, Charles Drew, MD, is known worldwide as "the father of the blood bank."[3] Only six years older than Vivien Thomas, Drew, whose father installed carpeting for a living, was accepted as a medical student in Canada at McGill University and, after graduation, earned a doctor of medical science from Columbia University. Drew took his expertise and developed a method to process and preserve blood plasma: the plasma was dehydrated in the US and shipped out so that, on the battlefield, it could be reconstituted with local water. So simple and yet so significant. Another of Drew's innovations was to establish mobile blood donation trucks, refrigerated to carry fresh blood as well as plasma.

Drew's brilliance led to his being named the assistant director of the first American Red Cross Blood Bank. In 1939, the American Medical Association had clarified that there is no difference between the blood of a person of African descent and that of someone of European descent.[4] Despite this known fact, the Red Cross excluded donations from African Americans for most of World War II; therefore, Drew, even as assistant director himself, was not allowed to donate blood. He left his Red Cross position in anger, protesting its methods as "unscientific and insulting to African Americans"[5] and, instead, became head of surgery at Howard University Hospital.

Dehydration of plasma offered an extremely efficient way to transport the miraculous elixir. Cardboard boxes filled with containers of powder were shipped overseas. Paratroopers landed with packages of dried plasma strapped on their bodies while South Italian donkeys and North African camels carried the jars on their backs. Navy aircraft dropped parachutes holding supplies of plasma over the Pacific islands, including Iwo Jima and Okinawa. The essential thing was to *get it to the men.*

Plasma was indispensable, a lifesaver. Ernie Pyle, the famous war correspondent, teletyped his story: "The doctors asked me at least a dozen times a day to write about plasma. They say that plasma is absolutely magical. They cite case after case where a wounded man was all but dead and within a few minutes after a plasma injection would be sitting up and talking."[6]

One wounded recipient described the sensation of being infused: "It was as though I was arising—being lifted right off the ground. The best thing I can compare it to is being out of breath, and all the sudden getting your breath back. Half an hour later I was up on my elbow, leaning over on my side, smoking a cigarette, and looking around the beach."[7]

During combat, soldiers could see plastic bags hanging from tree limbs with tubing snaking down to the wounded. On the beaches, medics would plunge a sailor's rifle into the sand with the barrel buried deep and the upright wood stock draped with a bag of precious plasma. Immediate intervention reduced the onset of shock and made it possible for a stretcher bearer to carry a soldier out of the battle area and into an operating theater.

Plasma cheated an otherwise certain death. Ninety out of every one hundred US men and women who had been injured in some way during the war survived their wounds. General George S. Patton, Jr. stated after Victory in Europe Day that "in the fighting in Germany just concluded, the death rate of casualties in the United States Army has been the lowest in all military history. While this situation was the result of many factors, it is safe to say that *outstanding among them was the ample and steady flow of whole blood and plasma.*"[8] (Emphasis added)

A few months after Patton spoke, when World War II ended after Victory over Japan Day on September 2, the US grieved for the 417,000 American servicemen and women dead and for the 2,000 civilians who also had been lost. Great Britain mourned its 383,000-military and its 4,000-civilian dead.[9]

The Third Reich, however, placed little importance on the necessity of plasma and blood in their forward medical units and the mortality rates for Hitler's soldiers shot up as high as its murderous V-2 rocket. The result was that its military suffered more than *five million* deaths with another two-and-a-half million civilian dead, including the bodies that were swept away in a riptide of lost blood and fluid.[10]

Generals and admirals—such men as Omar Bradley, George S. Patton, Dwight Eisenhower, Douglas MacArthur, Henry Arnold, Chester W. Nimitz, and William Halsey, Jr.—received due credit for winning World War II. One of them even became president of the United States.

For their role in keeping the injured alive and for saving countless lives, the list of war heroes should also include Alfred Blalock, Vivien Thomas, and Charles Drew.

CHAPTER SEVENTEEN

A Woman of Valor

The odds were strongly against Helen Taussig becoming a physician. Born one year earlier than Alfred Blalock, she had several congenital hurdles to overcome; she was partially deaf and apparently dyslexic. The biggest challenge, however, was that she was a female with intellect and ambition.

She had started her undergraduate studies at Radcliffe College, where her mother had trained as a botanist. Her father, the well-known and influential economist Frank William Taussig, PhD had chaired the US Tariff Commission and was an eminent professor at Harvard University, whose students included W. E. B. Du Bois. Worried that her father's fine reputation might stifle her own individuality, Taussig fled Cambridge for the West Coast and finished her undergraduate studies at the University of California in 1921.

Determined to become a physician like her grandfather, William Taussig, MD who had had an old-fashioned horse and buggy practice, she hoped to enroll in the medical school at Harvard University. Indeed, she met all qualifications—except for her sex, which excluded her from Harvard and most other medical schools. Harvard did allow her to take a special premed study program, although it required her to sit at a distance from the other students in the classrooms "so as not to contaminate the Harvard—male—students," she said.[1] When it was absolutely necessary for her to examine anatomical slides, the faculty insisted, for the sake of modesty, on sequestering her in an empty room away from the men.[2] In her desire to be a doctor, she put up with this silliness. After she completed her year of premed study at Harvard, she added a year of medical research at Boston University to her *curriculum vitae.*

Fortunately for her and for Hopkins, the Financial Four had made sure that a woman could be admitted to its medical school. The well-trained Taussig clearly was an excellent candidate for Hopkins, despite her clipped New England inflection that contrasted unfavorably (at least, in her professors' minds) with the drawl of her Southern teachers. She could also occasionally roar in a Nor'easter temperament that showed no resemblance to the demure mannerisms of their magnolia wives. In other words, some Hopkins men disliked her.

Nonetheless, her laser focus cut a swathe as she began her studies in Baltimore. After receiving her MD degree in 1927, Helen Taussig wanted to take an internship in internal medicine, but Hopkins forbade any more than one female in a specialty and internal medicine already had a woman.[3] Taussig ping-ponged to pediatrics and became an intern at Hopkins's Harriet Lane Home for Invalid Children, headed by Edwards A. Park, MD. (As with Mr. Hopkins, Park's unusual first name was his mother's birth surname.) Three years later, Park needed someone to supervise its pediatric cardiac surgery clinic and asked Taussig to apply to become its physician in charge. Although Hopkins, at the time, was reluctant to hire women, Park, fully aware of the university's prejudices, hired Taussig.[4]

It was a wise decision. She became renowned as a prescient diagnostician who compensated for her inability to hear through a stethoscope by sensing children's heartbeats through her magically perceptive fingertips. Congenital heart disorders became to be her specialty and, by the time Blalock arrived back at Hopkins, she was known as an up-and-coming authority. While she had been a pediatric intern, Taussig studied in Montreal with Maude Abbott, MD, the Canadian cardiology researcher, and the reigning expert on congenital heart abnormalities.[5] Taussig found Abbott wonderful, funny, and warm-hearted, despite her unjust treatment by most of her medical colleagues.[6]

While in Montreal, Taussig became fascinated by a congenital abnormality of the heart called Tetralogy of Fallot, or TOF. French physician

Étienne-Louis Arthur Fallot had been the first person to describe its four deadly characteristics in 1888.[7] These abnormalities resulted in babies who could not get enough oxygen in their blood.

However, it was Abbott who, in 1924, had coined the term still used for this congenital disorder, Tetralogy (a group of four) of Fallot (pronounced FAL-oh).[8] Newborns born with TOF faced certain death, maybe not today or tomorrow, or next month or even next year, but death would come before they reached adulthood. The TOF babies were born cyanotic, meaning that they were not receiving enough oxygen, which was a special concern to Taussig. Their skin typically had a noticeable odd blue tinge that derived from the oxygen-deprived blood circulating through their bodies, which is why they were dubbed "blue babies." When these infants or toddlers became extraordinarily fatigued, they were capable of suddenly and dramatically turning a darker indigo or purple shade all over their body.

By the time these babies turned a year old, their fingertips and toes would be clubbed and abnormally rounded. They were short of breath and could tire easily, which made them instinctively squat because that odd position increased the oxygenated blood flow to their lungs. (Taussig herself was the first to recognize squatting as a characteristic of cyanosis.[9]) Or they might lose consciousness for no apparent reason, sometimes for a full half hour. The only help that they could be given to extend their lives was to bring them back to the hospital and put them in incubators (isolettes) with incoming oxygen. It was a temporary measure that was not completely successful: at that time an oxygen tank could only increase oxygen in the incubator by about 8 percent. Worse, confinement in a hospital allowed for no acceptable quality of life. The behavior of these children terrified their parents, as did their knowledge that one of four blue babies died before they could celebrate a first birthday. Of those who lived a full year, few survived their childhood.

Each blue baby has the same four malformations that lead to oxygen-deprived circulation, although the severity differs from baby to baby. To begin with, the pulmonary (lung) artery, which enters the lungs from the heart, is too narrow. (Arteries are those muscular tubes that branch out from the heart and lungs.) The pulmonary artery's passage in a blue baby is so constricted that it cannot send a sufficient amount of blood into the lungs. The blood that doesn't get into the lungs obviously cannot pick up any of the lung's supply of oxygen. Adding to this problem for blue babies is that the cavity in their hearts (the right ventricle) is too large. It works harder and harder to push more blood into that cramped lung artery and the already oversized cavity may even enlarge in response.

As if these obstacles weren't problems enough, there were more. The muscle separating the two heart ventricles, called the right and left ventricles, has holes or openings that shouldn't occur: the muscle should be intact. These openings cause oxygen-deficient blood to travel the wrong way: not to the lungs to pick up oxygen but into the body tissues, which already are starved for oxygen. It turns out that the blue babies also were born with a misplaced large vessel, which, in a typical infant, carries blood to the body's tissues. In blue babies, though, this misplaced vessel is farther to the right than it should be, which means it is sending even greater amount of oxygen-starved blood through the body.

It may seem strange to us today, but as late as the forties, physicians thought the heart, and the area surrounding it, was inoperable. There'd virtually been no elective heart surgeries conducted by this point in time and the scant few that had been attempted were emergency responses to save adult lives as in, for example, a knife wound to the heart. The thought of operating on a tiny, sick blue baby was horrifying to most. In 1937, a surgeon had attempted to close, or ligate, the opening in a baby's vessel by tying the ducts' openings or holes shut, which was a "relatively rare congenital anomaly."[10] The first attempt failed, and the child died.

The following year, the young surgeon Robert Gross, MD, then the chief resident at Harvard University's medical school and working at Children's Hospital, wanted to close one artery leading to the heart (patent ductus arteriosus surgery). Unlike Blalock, Gross carried out his own experimental surgical research by operating on the dogs himself. He didn't have a Vivien Thomas to propel his work forward. In fact, Gross even held surgical rehearsals with other staff in case he had an opportunity to operate on a child. Despite all his preparatory work, he was thwarted by the hospital's chief surgeon, William E. Ladd, MD, who told him, "We don't touch the heart."[11]

Now, after having been specifically forbidden to try, Gross bided his time and waited until Ladd was out of town before he approached Ladd's acting chief surgeon. He got the man's go-ahead and was successful in performing the first closure of this type where the child survived.[12] Gross was only thirty-three years old, and he had taken an incredible risk.

Although a landmark, Gross's surgery was not the solution to the heart problems of blue babies. However, the intuitive Taussig realized that a basic mechanical technique—such as cutting, moving, and suturing an artery—might be used as a jumping-off point for mending the hearts of her blue babies. She hypothesized that, if closing an opening in a vessel was possible, there was no reason a surgeon couldn't operate to open a closed vessel. Then, the new vessel with its new opening could send a greater amount of oxygen-rich blood into the heart. If a surgeon could redirect the blood flow of a blue baby by opening a ductus into the heart, tying it and connecting it to a different blood vessel, the oxygenated blood could flow where it belonged—into the heart and not back into the body.

Taussig first pitched her idea to Gross, with whom she had worked during her post-baccalaureate studies in Cambridge. "If a surgeon can tie off an opening [ductus], why can't he build an open ductus that would help a cyanotic child?" she asked.[13] Her question was an astute diagnostic query that Gross dismissed out of hand. He had gained so many accolades for his closing a ductus (opening) that he explained that he did not see an immediate need to try the opposite technique on blue babies, who had four heart defects and not just one.

"I am not interested in opening ducts," he responded. "Only in closing them."[14]

Taussig reminisced, "I think he thought it was one of the craziest ideas he'd heard in a long time."[15] Gross is recognized as a great surgeon, but his refusal to follow up on Taussig's idea was a decision he'd come to regret. He lost a chance to claim credit for a medical revolution called heart surgery.

Taussig remained undeterred. Though Gross had turned her down, she was still convinced that her blue babies could be helped by some type of surgical procedure designed to augment oxygen-saturated blood flow. She couldn't shake the idea of opening an artery to change the direction of blood flow. Creating a new arterial opening or duct, she surmised, would give significant relief even to a baby with severe cyanosis because it would increase oxygen throughout its body. She was aware that Blalock, at Edwards Park's suggestion, was developing, with Thomas, an experimental operation to relieve the constriction of the aorta. In fact, Blalock had insisted on sharing credit and made Park the coauthor of the resulting article, published in 1944, although Thomas's contributions were not mentioned.[16]

Not letting Gross discourage her, Taussig approached Blalock in late fall 1943, and decided that the best way to pique his interest was to flatter him, a technique many other women have used. She said, "I stand in awe of your surgical skills, but the really great day will come when you build the ductus for a cyanotic child, not when you tie off a ductus."[17]

Blalock replied, "When that day comes, this [earlier surgery] will look like child's play."[18] She then requested a meeting to discuss the possibility of a special blue baby surgery that might help these oxygen-deprived babies. Blalock set up a time and told Thomas to be there.

In that first and only meeting of the three, Taussig kept her blue baby description simple and elegant. She spoke of some type of mechanical "plumbing" surgery, as she put it, that would reconnect the heart's great vessels to each other. Thomas remembered the detailed thoughts and ideas she brought to their first meeting and the precision with which she highlighted the numerous problems involved with these hearts. With Taussig's background, her experience, and her intelligence, she concisely stated that the answer for her blue babies was a case of changing the pipes around. In its simplicity lay its genius. However, she had no specific ideas on which "pipes" should be switched.

Bringing the blue baby surgery problem to these men turned out to be partly serendipitous because of their past work at Vanderbilt where, in the late thirties, Thomas and Sanford Leeds had tried to increase blood pressure for an experiment in an ill-fated attempt to raise blood pressure. In the failed experiment, they had attached the heart artery, or aorta, to the lungs (pulmonary artery) to circumvent the heart's original plumbing. However, in the course of the surgery, Thomas had used a technique whereby he had opened an unclosed vessel and then sewed it somewhere else by using a suturing technique called anastomosis, which removes the vessel from where it was connected and joins it somewhere else in the body.[19] However, neither man thought about using this procedure for a different purpose at the time.

There was never a eureka moment when Thomas and Blalock met eyes and silently yet triumphantly communicated that they knew what to do. In fact, they both were at a loss for how to treat blue babies and, with the ongoing war, Thomas knew he could not rely on Blalock's presence in the lab to assist him. The responsibility now lay on his shoulders. Fortunately, Thomas's prepared mind and his surgical experiences would lead him to success. In the meantime, though, he saw only a complex and perplexing problem that he was told to solve. He believed that Taussig had presented him with an idea, brilliant in its simplicity, but he knew that finding the right answer to correcting four separate malfunctions of the heart—in an infant, no less—would be extremely challenging, even for him.

He remembered an earlier conversation with Blalock when he'd asked the doctor why he couldn't assign easier projects. Blalock's answer? "All the easy things have been done."[20]

CHAPTER EIGHTEEN

Thomas Decodes the Blue Babies

Now, after Taussig left the lab, Blalock tasked Thomas with planning the experimental lab research that would create a surgery to help blue babies. This included creating any new instruments or surgical apparatus that Thomas might need, as well as figuring out any particular surgical techniques required to pioneer the revolutionary surgery envisioned by Taussig. He wasn't entirely confidant that he could pull it off. Yet he could only imagine the misery of parents who knew their baby would die; he needed to come up with a solution as fast as he could. To make matters worse, Blalock stressed that Thomas was to conduct his work alone, due to the wartime staff shortage. Even lab techs and medical students would only be available for assistance on his new project when absolutely necessary. For his own part, Blalock said he would make himself available weekly to consult and advise Thomas.

Thomas liked a challenge more than anything. But he couldn't fathom when he'd find the time to ponder, let alone execute, research on Taussig's and Blalock's ideas. His work on shock in the aftermath of crush-related injuries was not to be suspended, Blalock said, and the professor commanded him to work on both problems of crush injuries and the blue babies, as difficult as that would be. Fortunately, Thomas had started work on the crush syndrome with George Duncan when they were at

Vanderbilt. At least Duncan's presence working on shock would remove some pressure off Thomas so he could have more time to concentrate on the blue baby conundrum.

In their meeting, Taussig had emphasized that she'd collected a great many preserved TOF hearts from the babies and children whom she had already lost. Thomas's first step was to walk over to the pathology lab to examine her extensive collection of blue baby hearts and analyze their anatomical abnormalities. He was confounded as he studied these miniature hearts that were as small as a walnut and had arteries and veins no thicker than the slimmest of wires.

The four defects in these TOF babies presented Thomas with a congeries of problems. He spent hours and days in the pathology lab studying the specimens. "I'd never seen or examined a defective heart and what I actually saw defies verbal description," he said.[1] And, as there was no literature on operative procedures for TOF babies, his own research could not take, as he put it, "an armchair strategy."[2] Thomas's first task was a difficult one that no one had ever tried: he had to recreate a TOF heart in the lab dogs. "In order to be able to treat any ailment or disease, whether it be medical or surgical, in the lab, we try first to produce the syndrome as a model and then try various methods of treatment," he explained.[3]

Within weeks, he reported back to Blalock and told him that trying to replicate each of the four heart defects would take years and years, and therefore would be too ambitious a goal. Thomas told him that, instead, he'd try to recreate cyanosis in his lab dogs by reproducing only one rather than all four of the TOF heart's congenital abnormalities. He wasn't sure that creating just one defect in dogs would cause their oxygen deprivation to become as severe as in the blue babies, but he had to give it a try.

Tackling pulmonary stenosis in the lungs of the lab dogs was his first choice, he told the professor. It would require Thomas to narrow the pulmonary artery of a healthy dog to stop it from sending a healthy supply of blood from the heart to the lungs for reoxygenation. To imitate the blue babies, Thomas needed to ensure that the dogs had so little oxygenated blood flowing through its body that they would turn cyanotic.

Unfortunately, Blalock's promise of weekly consulting turned out to be empty, through no fault of his. He was pressed to educate military doctors about shock, ever urgent given the war, and get in as much teaching at Hopkins as he could manage. The professor did not have adequate time to advise him on the experiments and, even when he was on campus, it was difficult for him to squeeze in meetings or lab visits. Although this failure frustrated Thomas, he realized that Blalock's complete reliance on his performance was a great compliment, even if the professor never raised the possibility of paying Thomas for his extra work hours. It wasn't unusual for the lab tech to put in fourteen-hour workdays.

There may have been another reason for Blalock's willingness to allow Thomas such freedom. Despite his rank as surgery chief, he acknowledged to a few friends that he was not a great surgeon.[4] He was better known for his theoretical work and ideas than for his surgical skills. As a result, he became a limpet in the operating room, dependent on the advice of others. Even Blalock's acolytes, and he had many, would not compliment his surgical skills.[5] Denton Cooley, who became a renowned heart surgeon, said, "He was sort of average, a deliberate surgeon, who was somewhat insecure in many respects." If Blalock ran into a problem, he choked in emergencies; he'd become tense and frustrated and would start to whine.[6]

While more isolated than ever from Blalock—their offices weren't even in near proximity in Baltimore as they had been in Nashville—Thomas proceeded with his hands-on approach to figuring out how things functioned or, in this case, did not work the way you'd expect. Starting from scratch was his natural creative style and it differentiated him from surgeons who relied on published medical research for their surgical approaches. Thomas's sophisticated understanding of mechanics, added to his technical skills and his self-taught knowledge of physiology, made him the perfect person to create an operative procedure to fix and improve blue baby hearts.

His days were filled with experimental trial and errors. Blalock's already cool demeanor toward Taussig indicated to Thomas that he should avoid meeting with her to brainstorm. He feared that Blalock—who did not work well with women, especially one with Taussig's strong personality—would automatically reject any of her ideas. Thomas "had no further contact or communication with her until the project was completed."[7] Certainly, there was no one else in the hospital as well versed as he was. As a consequence, Thomas was on his own.

Hopkins may have benefited from his long hours, but his family did not. Clara and the girls were rarely awake when he came home, and only Clara would be up and out of bed when he set out for the office before dawn. Working six or often seven days a week, at times he feared that he might need to check himself into the hospital for exhaustion. He used his house primarily to shower and sleep. Most days, he didn't have time to eat at home, other than to drink a quick morning cup of strong black coffee with his wife. He always brought her the first cup and would hear her say, "Thanks, Bunch," which was her usual shorthand for "Honeybunch."[8]

Things were not as copacetic at the Blalock household. The surgeon's absences put even more stress on Mary Blalock, who was struggling alone to raise two adolescents, William, thirteen years old, and Mary, twelve. Then, she unexpectedly found she was pregnant again and gave birth to in 1943 to their third child, Alfred Dandy Blalock, who was called Dandy and, later, Dan. When Al Blalock was able to get home, he expected, not unreasonably, to find a calm and well-managed house, which was no longer a given. The couple they'd hired to care for the house and yard had deserted them, using Mary's expression, for better-paying and less menial war industry jobs, working to build ships in Roanoke, Virginia. Things on Underwood Drive were really falling apart.

Mary was showing signs of depression and her mood worsened during the war years. The couple's old friends back in Nashville had hoped that her marriage to Blalock would help him curb his own drinking but rather it gave her permission to increase her drinking. In their fourteen years of marriage, Mary had gone from being an admired, witty and fun-loving young woman to a lonely wife, isolated in a new city. She was seeking relief in alcohol. What had started as an evening cocktail with her husband had now become an early morning ritual. The less happy she was, the more she drank.

Everyone in the surgery department realized that the Blalock marriage wobbled.

Blalock finally called his mother-in-law, Mrs. O'Bryan, for help and "Mrs. O.," as he called her, moved in with them, providing a little companionship to her daughter while standing in for the children and attending their needs. Still, family relations deteriorated. When Blalock's own mother had a birthday, there was no one to remind him and he sent her many notes of apology over the years for forgetting to call or send her a gift, sometimes excusing himself by telling her, "There wasn't anything good enough for you."[9]

The scant attention that he paid to his Baltimore family was, perhaps, sublimated by his focus on his medical students. His students enjoyed and benefited from the attention Blalock spent on them. Of course, he only accepted white men, including one candidate who attached a photograph of his beautiful wife, having been told of Blalock's eye for women. Rowena Spencer, MD was the one exception to his all-male students. She paid a price for her acceptance, however, and tolerated the allegedly playful spankings she received from Blalock and her male colleagues, both on campus and off.[10]

At this early stage of his blue baby work, Thomas had to focus on the basic supplies and equipment he'd need for an operation that had never been attempted, and on a fragile small heart, at that. Even before he figured out how to surgically change these babies' hearts, he needed to create and manufacture, on his own, new operating instruments. There were so many things to figure out before he even got close to lifting a scalpel.

One issue was that the hearts of dogs do not have the same fixed physical barrier (called a septum) between the two halves of their heart the way that humans do but rather have only a fragile membrane separating the two heart sections. Then, if a dog's chest were opened on only one side, both lungs would collapse rather than just one, as would happen to the lungs of a person.[11] He would need to keep the second lung of his lab dog open by using positive pressure, which equalizes the air in the lungs with the surrounding environment and keeps a lung from collapsing while it also administers anesthesia. A costly intratracheal catheter (a tube inserted in the windpipe) could do the job, but the Hopkins lab did not own one. Nor did the hospital on a wartime budget see the need to purchase it for him.

Thomas turned to Thomas Satterfield, a senior lab technician who had become his right-hand man. Satterfield's primary task was to administer positive pressure oxygen and anesthesia to a dog during surgery by manually and rhythmically compressing the dog's trachea (windpipe). The problem was that Thomas would need to perform hundreds of these surgeries before he could gather a satisfactory number of experimental outcomes and Satterfield, justifiably, feared that his arms and hands would wear out before then.[12] A different solution was called for. Rather than attempt to persuade Blalock to purchase the proper catheter amid wartime austerity or to pressure Satterfield to work manually at the strenuous pace, Thomas concluded that he would need to make his own artificial breathing apparatus if he were to succeed in making the dogs cyanotic.

William O. Jones, the medical school's skillful machinist, was the person Thomas approached. With Jones's capable assistance, he devised a basic motor-driven valve that automatically inflated a dog's lungs with air and anesthesia, and then deflated the lungs. It sounds simple but, in reality, it was a very complicated procedure because a machine small enough to accommodate surgery on underweight newborns had never been manufactured. Its construction required making a very small inflatable cuff that would seal the trachea from the endotracheal tube outside the windpipe.[13]

Because he'd observed how the little hearts were "surrounded by abnormal dilated blood vessels," he'd have to create his own miniature suturing needles for the tiny babies' vessels.[14] The only manufactured needles that were available would damage these precious little veins, so he bought the smallest needles commercially sold and sharpened them down with a metal emery board. Now they were so diminutive that he had to attach a spring clothespin to be able to hold onto each needle. Their eyes were so small that he couldn't thread them with regular suture material and had to separate the silk threads to make them extra thin to fit into the needle's eye. Once he'd completed that task, he had to pick up a magnifying glass to thread the needle.

He ascertained that a standard "bulldog" clamp, used to close small blood vessels during surgery, would not work for these vessels. Thomas first chose to modify an Allis forceps to block off the large aorta, but it was cumbersome. Searching through a lab cabinet, he found a long intestinal clamp but feared its length would irredeemably damage the aorta. He ran the instrument over to the talented Jones in the machine shop and asked him to cut it down to a four-inch length, to alter its guide pins for better alignment, and to add slots to make its size flexible. The instrument was created and built by Thomas to stabilize arteries, but it is identified in medical circles as the Blalock Clamp.

Having conceived and created all the operative tools that he needed, Vivien next focused on artificially shrinking the width of the dog's pulmonary artery to create cyanosis. Some type of material was needed to narrow the artery by wrapping around it. Blalock suggested using linen to set off the cyanosis cycle, but his idea failed: the heavy linen ligature did not come close to narrowing the artery and, worse, cut into the vessel, as Thomas learned when he autopsied his dogs.

Then Thomas tried using umbilical tape, which was wider than the linen he'd used, to restrict the artery, assuming that tape would be less likely to cut into the vessel. He was wrong; the umbilical tape sliced into the artery and his dogs died from extensive internal bleeding. Next, he tried using a sheet of connective tissue (fascia) from an ox to narrow the artery: failure, again. He was more frustrated and tired than he'd ever been before. Although the dogs were turning slightly cyanotic, their oxygen deprivation was minimal. However, Thomas needed to increase the percentage of unoxygenated blood in the dogs in order to bring their blood closer to the level of unoxygenated blood in the blue babies.

Finally, Thomas managed to grab Blalock to tell him that his attempt to create pulmonary stenosis was not entirely successful. During their long conversation, Thomas's suggested a completely different route to create a cyanotic dog; he wanted to try creating the third TOF defect, a hole or opening in the heart (ductus arteriosus). He would not make an actual opening, but he might be able to create cyanosis by allowing unoxygenated venous blood to bypass the lungs and to return to the heart, in a right-to-left shunt. The procedure is called a pulmonary arteriovenous fistula, which means that there is an atypical vein that connects to the artery in the lung.[15] Thomas used a less important vein from the dog's limb to join its heart and lung.

To test whether he'd successfully created cyanosis, he instructed his lab tech, Clara Belle Puryear, to take the dogs' blood chemical measurements. Mind you, at that time there were no ways of conducting instant blood count determinations through electronic instruments. Thomas, at first, and then Puryear had to conduct these counts by hand: for oxygen content, for sufficiency of the arterial blood and for hemoglobin (that allows red blood cells to transport both oxygen and carbon dioxide), and for hematocrit (the percentage of red blood cells).[16] It seemed to take forever and was painstakingly tedious. He then needed to compare the dogs' level of cyanosis to the level of the TOF babies, which had been calculated earlier by Taussig.

To his great joy, he realized that he had finally succeeded in reproducing the effects of two of the TOF heart defects by lessening the blood flow into the lungs and by mixing oxygenated and unoxygenated blood. The dogs were cyanotic: their skin was blue, they lacked energy, their blood was thick and plum-colored, and they could not exercise. The oxygen in their blood was 25 percent lower than before his last try. The figures proved that the dogs were less severely cyanotic than the babies, but the measurements demonstrated an oxygen deficiency that was finally similar to theirs. Best of all, he'd replicated cyanotic dogs that survived and remained healthy, except for their shortage of oxygen.[17]

More than a year had passed before he'd reached this stage. The dogs were given time to heal before the last step in his experimental research because Thomas was never callous about his dogs. Throughout his entire career, he insisted that all the lab workers handle them well and call them by names rather than just their identifying numbers. To keep the dogs safe and free of pain, Thomas used aseptic surgical techniques and administered a mixture of morphine sulfate and atropine sulfate.

At this point, he had to relieve the dogs' cyanosis by allowing them a way to gain oxygen-rich blood in their body tissues. In other words, the only thing left was to figure out how to cure them or at least ameliorate

Thomas Decodes the Blue Babies

their symptoms by using whatever surgical technique that could bring more oxygen to the blood. The technique he would invent for the dogs would eventually be used on blue babies to let them live normal lives.

His last step was to create an artificial ductus arteriosus by cutting the dog's aorta in two places and then excising a short portion of the tube-like vessel that carries blood and fluid. It would not be the exact surgery that Thomas had created at Vanderbilt in 1938 to create high blood pressure, but it was very similar. At Blalock's suggestion, Thomas produced a lung's arteriovenous fistulae that shunted the low oxygen blood in the right side of the baby's heart over to its left side. Then he cut the vessels and everted them by turning the very ends slightly inside out and then he sewed the subclavian artery to the pulmonary artery. Thomas had devised a way to switch blood flow to the lungs and increase the mix of arterial and venous blood flowing into the dog's general circulation. This method of surgical connection is called a side-to-end anastomosis (specifically an anastomosis of the subclavian artery to the pulmonary artery). The shunt he created is named the Blalock-Taussig shunt and is used currently to treat at least four other heart and lung conditions.

The first dog of several hundred that lived through both procedures, the one that caused cyanosis and then the one that alleviated it, was named Anna. She was a small, off-white mixed breed with an unusually sweet disposition. Her singular status convinced Thomas to retire her from undergoing any more research surgeries; subsequently, she enjoyed her favored position roaming around the lab and lived a long life. In 1952, a Baltimore animal association had an artist paint her portrait for Hopkins, and the framed image still hangs on the wall of the hospital's pediatric ward.

Thomas, after more than a year of unceasing experimentation, finally found "what pipe to put where" to promote greater blood oxygenation.[18] He prayed that it would work as well for the blue babies as it had for the lab dogs.

CHAPTER NINETEEN

A BLACK MAN, A BLUE BABY, AND THE DAWN OF HEART SURGERY

The phone's shrill ring in the Thomas household at nearly 9:00 p.m. on the night of Tuesday, November 28, 1944, alerted Vivien. He grabbed the receiver, sure that the only person calling at that hour would be the professor. What Thomas had not anticipated was Blalock's solemn voice telling him to prepare first thing in the morning for a special surgery. As Thomas listened, he was shaken by the importance of the event: his blue baby operation was to be put to the test.

As Helen Taussig had feared, one of her most seriously ill blue baby patients, fifteen-month-old Eileen Saxon, was rapidly deteriorating and close to death, slipping away. The wee infant had been readmitted to the hospital a full six months ago and had never been able to be discharged. She'd spent the entire time in an incubator, relying on a tank to supply her with extra oxygen, but it wasn't enough. She was barely alive, gasping for air, her color turning from blue to deep purple. This precious baby's last chance at life was the experimental operation that Thomas had devised but only had tested on dogs. There was no alternative: as Eileen's mother said, "We had no choice."[1] It was either a new surgery for her infant daughter or certain death. Surgery would be Blalock's desperate effort to save her. Taussig was insistent on it; although Blalock strongly disliked being told what to do, particularly by a woman, he had to admit that she was correct. He, bravely, would take responsibility for the surgery.

The problem for the professor, Thomas knew, was that Blalock had never performed this surgery before: in fact, his total experience with the techniques and instruments Thomas had created constituted serving as Thomas's assistant while the lab tech demonstrated the operation to him only once, a few days earlier. This was quite a sight for everyone to see—Thomas, a younger Black lab assistant, calling out directions to Blalock, the older white head of surgery. Now Blalock would try it on a fragile nine-pound, fifteen-month-old critically ill baby.

Before Blalock put the phone down, Taussig, at his side, sternly told him to go home and get some sleep. She would stay with her patient, waiting out the night with Eileen's mother in the ward at the Harriet Lane Home for Invalid Children. In 1944, hospital visiting hours were strictly enforced, even for parents of a dying child. Anything else violated house rules and was considered inappropriate mollycoddling. That the baby's mother was allowed to stay demonstrated both the severity of the infant's illness and the extent of Taussig's kindness.

Blalock and Thomas slept fitfully that night. Before daybreak, Thomas, as always, walked to the Hopkins medical campus. Blalock lived farther away in his fashionable neighborhood and, this morning, he was so nervous that he asked his wife to chauffeur him. Mary dropped him at the front of the medical campus's iconic Dome building. As the tense Blalock entered it and walked past the statue of Christus (Consolator) with its outheld arms, the Carrara marble figure placed to welcome patients and provide hope, he stopped to rub its big toe, a Hopkins tradition said to bring good luck.

Blalock wanted to check on his undersized surgery patient. He walked a few blocks to the Harriet Lane Home to examine Eileen, discuss her case with Taussig, and then speak to Eileen's mother. Afterward, he returned to the old Halsted building to receive a last-minute briefing from Thomas.

When Thomas had arrived, he headed straight away to Elizabeth Sherwood's office. Sherwood was nicknamed "the King" due to her power in supervising the hospital's surgery theaters and, although she had known nothing about this last-minute surgery, she understood its importance. She walked Thomas over to review the standard surgical instruments that would be available in the theater. Thomas knew that they wouldn't suffice for the minuscule Eileen, so he jogged back to the dog lab and grabbed the custom-made needles, sutures, and clamps that he had designed for the operation and then met with Blalock. When their conversation ended, Thomas returned to his lab.

By 9:00 a.m., the medical team was gathered in the scrub room annexed to Halstead room 706, an operating theater. The men and women scrubbing in were an exceptionally talented group. First, there was Taussig, her conservative hairstyle looking immaculate despite her having spent the night fitfully sleeping in a chair. She had scrubbed but was present to observe the operation only. The other people at the table included Hopkins chief surgical resident William Longmire, thirty-one years old, who was Blalock's first assistant. Thomas always said that Longmire was the best surgeon he had ever known. Denton Cooley, a twenty-four-year-old intern, joined the team; Thomas thought that Cooley was the second-best surgeon of his generation. Cooley was tall and athletic with a patrician nose and intense blue eyes. And, of course, Alfred Blalock, chief of surgery, was the lead man at the table.

They were all waiting for the baby to arrive. She had been in her crib on floor four of the Harriet Lane Home and was now being moved into the old and temperamental elevator that took her downstairs. From there, she was wheeled through a hospital corridor into Halstead and then up another elevator to floor seven. Taussig approached the baby lying on the gurney, gently lifted her frail patient up, and carefully placed her on the operating table.[2]

The atmosphere was sober and tense. Most of the hospital staff found it hard to believe that anyone would contemplate operating on a pathetically ill baby, who looked shrunken and emaciated. Even the younger men, Longmire[3] and Cooley,[4] were astounded by Blalock's decision to proceed with the surgery, with Longmire thinking, "My God, this man isn't going to operate on this patient."[5]

In fact, the hospital's anesthesiology chief, Austin Lamont, had refused to participate because he was sure the baby would die. Instead, a young anesthesiologist, self-described as the "low man on the totem pole," Merel Harmel, was assigned this responsibility and he joined the small team.[6] Harmel had nervously changed from his blue blazer and ascot into scrubs, and felt greatly relieved when he saw that Olive Berger, RN the devoted and experienced nurse anesthetist, was present and ready to begin open-drop ether on the baby. They were joined by Charlotte Mitchell, RN, the scrub nurse.

Thomas was absent because he was trying to distract himself, puttering around in his dog lab. Puryear, his chemistry technician, informed him that she was walking over to watch the new surgery and asked if he wanted to join her. "I might make Dr. Blalock nervous," he responded. Then he added, "Or even worse, he might make me nervous."[7] After she left, he continued to keep himself busy, picking up one report after another to review, but couldn't keep his mind focused on anything. Instead, he kept checking either his wall clock or his watch as the minutes ticked on.

He jumped when his phone rang. With Blalock in the operating theater, who could it be? When he answered, he recognized the voice of his chemistry tech. Puryear had been in the upper level of Room 706, waiting for the surgery to begin, when Blalock saw her and shouted, "Miss Puryear, I guess you'd better go call Vivien."[8] She dashed out to call and told Vivien that Dr. Blalock wanted him to report to Room 706, *stat*.

When Blalock had walked into the operating theatre a few minutes earlier, he had been dismayed that Thomas was not there, scrubbed and waiting. He had assumed that his senior surgical lab worker would know, somehow, that Blalock would want him right next to him during the surgery. Thomas, though, had never anticipated being a member of the operating team; in the past, he'd been limited to the research phase in the dog lab. Only a few times earlier had he walked into the viewing area of an operating room to observe Blalock at work.

As Thomas dashed across campus, looking grim and oblivious to any odd looks he might have received, he silently and briefly prayed for Eileen. The modest man felt awed by the results of his two years' work: his experiments, his inventions of unique surgical instruments, and his creation of innovative surgical procedures. He may not have been able to become a physician, but he was fully aware that his repeated effort to duplicate in lab dogs the heart defects that were killing blue babies was a stunning achievement. In doing so, he had invented a way to basically reverse these congenital problems through an "extracardiac" (directly outside the heart) operation.[9] The country's best surgeons had deemed any surgery on the heart to be impossible and refused to even try. Now the old insecurities driven into him must have whispered to him: "Who are you to attempt this when better educated men than you would not?" and, worse, "What if this baby dies because of some error that you didn't foresee?"

As he was hurrying, Eileen was being brought into the operating theater for a last chance at life. Thomas, breathless now, raced into the second-story gallery above the operating theater. Blalock spotted him above and immediately called out, "Vivien, you better come down here."[10] The spectators looked confused. Who was this man?

The whole scene must have seemed unimaginable. Here was the vaunted Hopkins surgery chief needing the advice of his Black lab tech. Reflecting on the oddity of the situation, Alan Woods, MD commented, "Blalock is the only surgeon I know who trained his own coach."[11]

Blalock had asked for a step stool that he had placed slightly behind him and to his side. Reentering the room after scrubbing and putting on a fresh white coat, Thomas heard Blalock tell him to stand on the stool so that he would be able to see everything. The surgeon was deeply afraid that he might commit a surgical error that could be fatal and, if so, he needed his lab assistant to warn him. Thomas gently assured the surgeon, "If you don't get ahead of yourself, and break it down into smaller and smaller steps as you work, it can be done."[12] When Thomas, more than six feet tall, stepped on the stool, he loomed over Blalock and everyone else. Then, when he first looked down, he was shocked that Eileen was "so small, weighing nine pounds, that it was difficult to ascertain whether a patient was beneath the sterile drapes."[13]

Taussig and Harmel stood at the head of the table. Blalock stood in the middle of the left side with Longmire facing him on the right side. Blalock started his cut-down, or incision, on Eileen's side, close to her fourth rib. Typically, red blood spurts out from an incision. Eileen's blood, instead, flowed out thickly and slowly, and was blue-black in color. Although this was not a complete surprise to the medical team, it disconcerted them because it was so unusual. She bled much less than expected, possibly because the great vessels of her heart were so tiny that Thomas called them "almost capillary in size."[14] In fact, his smallest dog had heart vessels that were twice as large as hers. Eileen's heart was miniature, and she obviously struggled to continue breathing.

The operating team must have also been slightly disconcerted when Thomas acted as a virtual cosurgeon. Thomas began guiding Blalock through the surgery, step by step, tactfully offering his suggestions and answering Blalock's questions. "Vivien, is the transverse incision long enough?" Blalock worried. Thomas responded, "Yes, if not too long." The queries continued: "Was this subclavian artery dissected far enough out?" and "Should the continuous suture be interrupted at this point?"[15]

As prompted by his lab assistant, Blalock placed one of the unique clamps created by Thomas in Eileen's left subclavian artery to stop her bleeding. Now he could incise the artery, so he cut into it. Next, Blalock put two more clamps on the left pulmonary artery, then placed a strip of umbilical tape under it to block the blood flow and paused to ensure that Eileen could tolerate the blockage, or occlusion.

Blalock cut a very small opening, a transverse incision, in the second artery. Thomas knew that they had reached the point of no return because after this second incision, they had to proceed with the experimental surgery until its end.[16] Blalock picked up one of Thomas's minuscule threaded needles and began to suture the two vessels together. They were so tiny, "no bigger than a matchstick," that the sutures had to be sewn as close together as possible.[17] Blalock, ever so gently, pulled his stitches tight. Then he sewed the stay sutures, which kept the other sutures in place.

The placement of sutures in the posterior line, which was inside the blood vessel itself rather than outside it, commanded the surgeon's full attention. Sewing just one suture in the wrong direction could be disastrous. Thomas, with an eagle eye, watched Blalock as he connected the end of the shortened subclavian artery with delicate silk sutures to the side of the pulmonary artery. Thomas interrupted when Blalock started suturing the wrong way, which he did on several occasions, by saying quietly but forcefully, "The other direction!"[18]

At one point, Harmel, the anesthesiologist, turned slightly toward Taussig to whisper in her ear that the baby was doing worse, that they could lose her at any time. When Taussig blinked at this frightening news, but remained standing impassive and unspeaking, he further murmured, "[It] upsets Dr. Blalock when we tell him that."

Taussig whispered back, "Then let's not tell him."[19]

After more than two hours, Blalock finished connecting the left subclavian artery to the left pulmonary artery. He also introduced an antibiotic in the incision that would help prevent infection. The connection, or anastomosis, between the two arteries was complete.

Taussig, except for her whispered command to the young Harmel, had been silent all this time. She had watched and hoped that this surgery would mean that all her blue babies, present and future, would have a chance to live. The entire operating team held its collective breath. What would happen when Blalock detached all the clamps from the arteries?

Blalock removed each clamp, one by one, slowly and deliberately. He cautiously paused after the clamp came out to examine each area to ensure that there was practically no bleeding. Everything in the surgery had gone exactly as Thomas had envisioned. Blalock needed only to close Eileen's chest. She was alive and breathing. She did not immediately turn pink, as the story is often told by dramatists, but her color had improved, and she appeared somewhat healthier. In the recovery room, Eileen's mother caught her first glimpse: "When I was allowed to see Eileen for the first time, it was like a miracle. I was beside myself with happiness."

Helen Taussig slept on a cot next to Eileen for several nights until she felt assured that Eileen would survive her surgery. The infant had to be put into intensive care immediately after the operation and her recovery was slower than hoped. Still, two months later, Eileen went home.[20]

Blalock had been able to perform the world's first blue baby surgery because of Thomas's research, his operative techniques, his improvised instruments, and specially designed supplies, as well as Thomas's whispered suggestions, directions, and answers to the surgeon's queries. Blalock also owed a large debt to Taussig because he would have never thought of operating without her original idea and her explanation that laid out the problem. Also, he was obliged to his first resident, Longmire, who throughout the operation gave words of encouragement to the anxious chief of surgery.

In the larger world outside the hospital, it had been six months since D-Day and the Allied landings at Normandy. By November 1944, the Allied nations were quickly advancing through France and Belgium, faster than the Germans had anticipated. Within a few weeks, the Third Reich would launch a major counter-offensive campaign, the Battle of the Bulge, with US forces bearing their greatest number of single battle casualties of the war, with 19,000 killed. Though the carnage of war was ever present, on this day in late November 1944 the staff at John Hopkins were not focused on it. Jubilant that they were able to save the life of a blue baby, and mindful of the tens of thousands of other children in the future who would live, it was time for celebration.

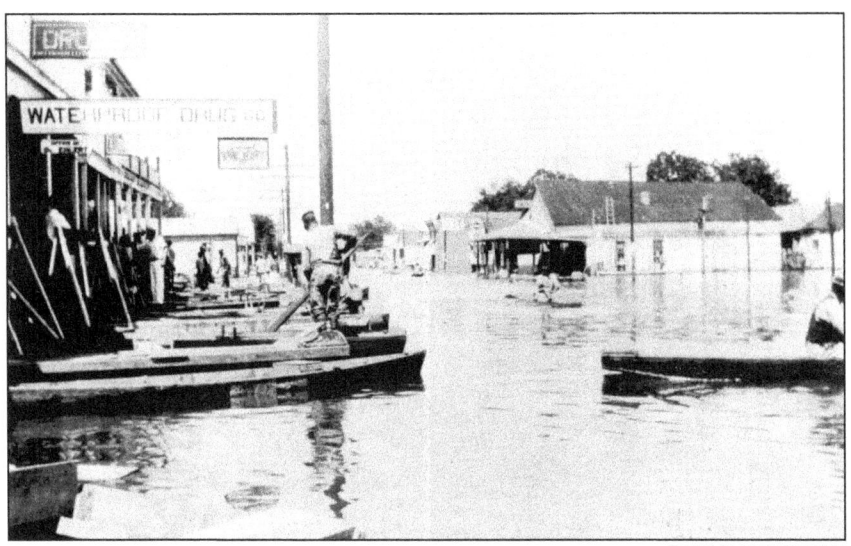

BETTY JO HAZLIP HARRIS

To avoid the springtime Mississippi River floods, the Thomas family leave Lake Providence, Louisiana, in favor of Nashville, Tennessee, when Vivien Thomas was two years old. They were safely in Nashville when this photo of a Mississippi River flood was taken in 1927.

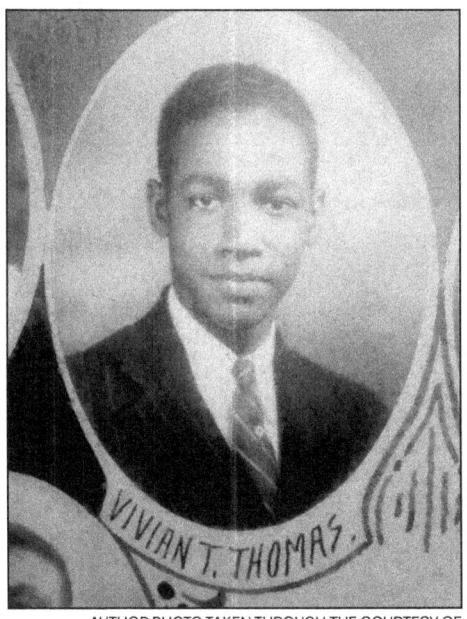

AUTHOR PHOTO TAKEN THROUGH THE COURTESY OF
MELVIN BLACK, PEARL HIGH SCHOOL ALUMNI ASSOCIATION

Vivien Thomas graduates from Nashville's outstanding Pearl High School in 1929. Yes, his first name is spelled incorrectly.

143

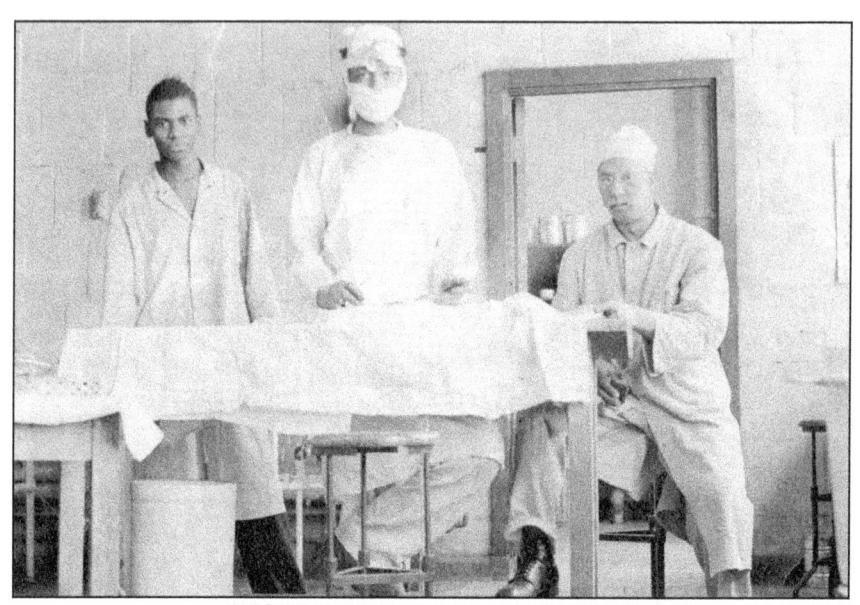

THE CHESNEY ARCHIVES OF JOHNS HOPKINS MEDICINE, NURSING AND PUBLIC HEALTH

Vivien Thomas (middle) is hired by Dr. Alfred Blalock as a surgery lab technician at Vanderbilt University. Vanderbilt's Black lab techs didn't know that the university was hiring them as lab techs but assigning them job titles of assistant janitor or janitor. In this 1940 photo, Samuel Waters is on the right and Andrew Manlove, the younger brother of Thomas's best friend, is on the left.

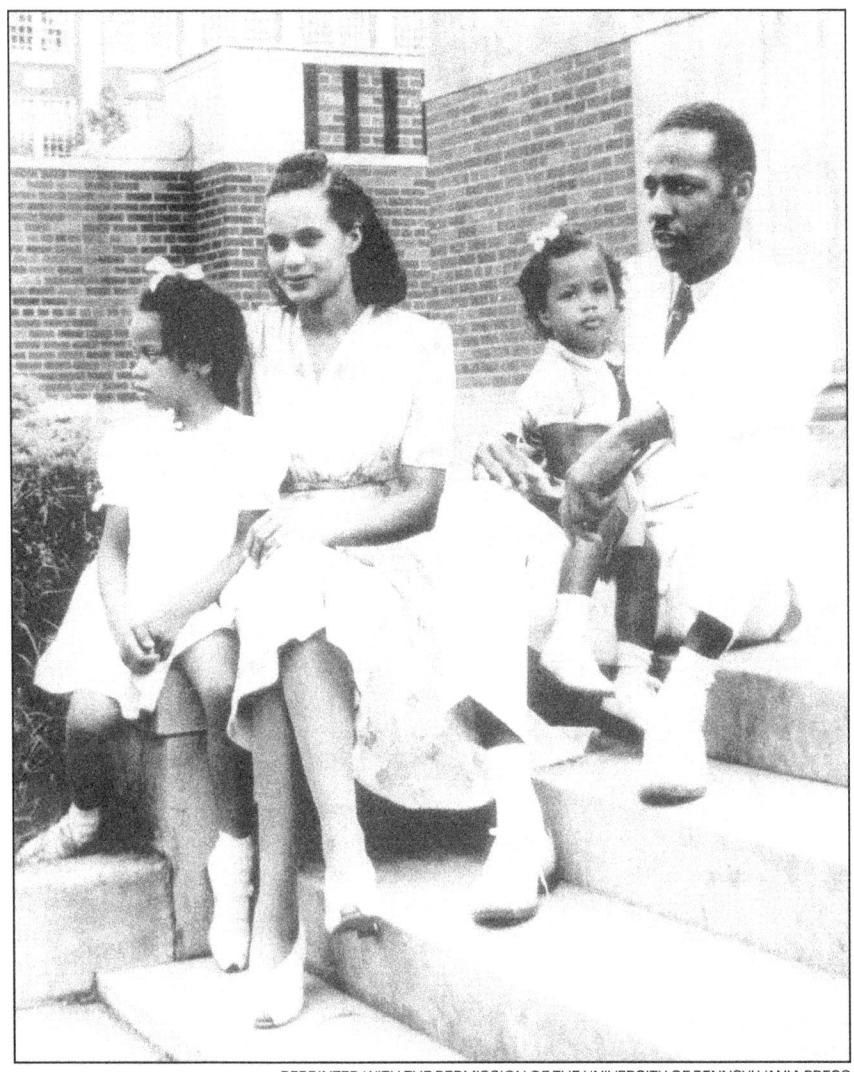

Vivien Thomas, age twenty-three, marries Clara Flanders, age twenty, in 1932. They have two daughters: Olga, born in 1934, and Theodosia, born in 1938. This photo was taken in 1941, just before the family left for Baltimore.

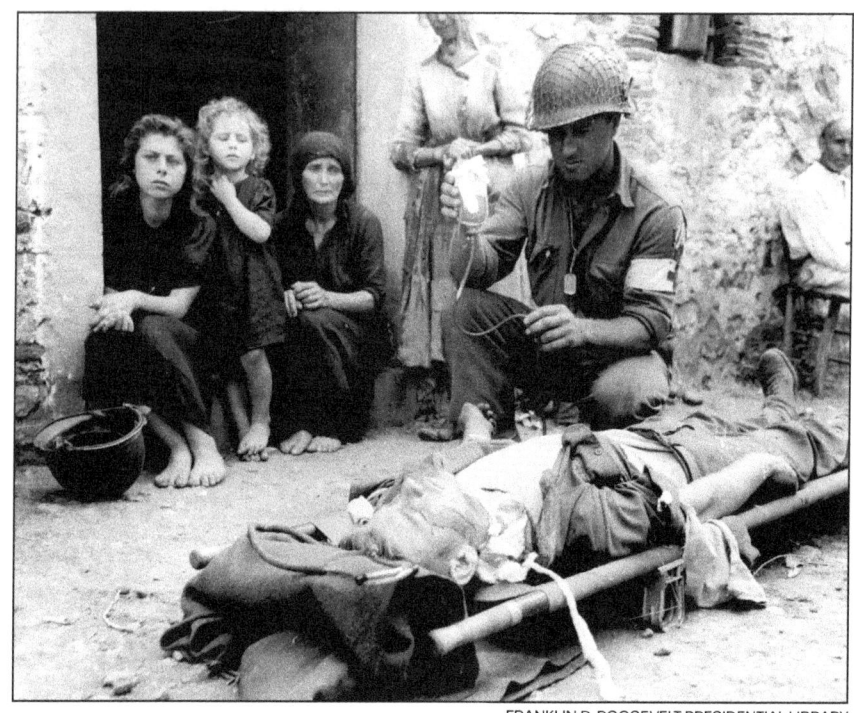

FRANKLIN D. ROOSEVELT PRESIDENTIAL LIBRARY

Countless lives were saved during World War II through the treatment of traumatic shock with plasma and other fluids, conceptualized by Blalock and verified by the experimental surgeries of Thomas from 1930 onward.

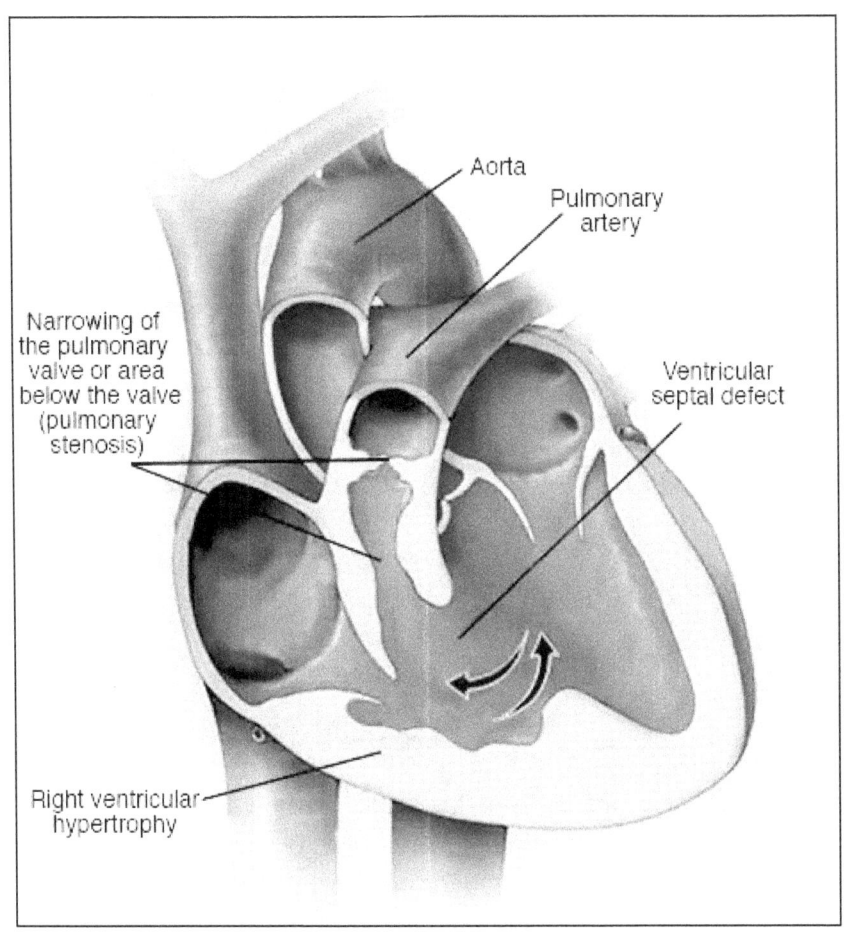

USED WITH PERMISSION OF MAYO FOUNDATION FOR MEDICAL EDUCATION AND RESEARCH, ALL RIGHTS RESERVED

A blue baby born with Tetralogy of Fallot has a significant shortage of oxygenated blood circulating through its body. This image of a blue baby's heart shows its four defects: a hole in the heart (called ventricular septal defect), a narrow pulmonary valve (called pulmonary stenosis), a misplaced aorta, and a thickened lower right chamber wall (called ventricular hypertrophy).

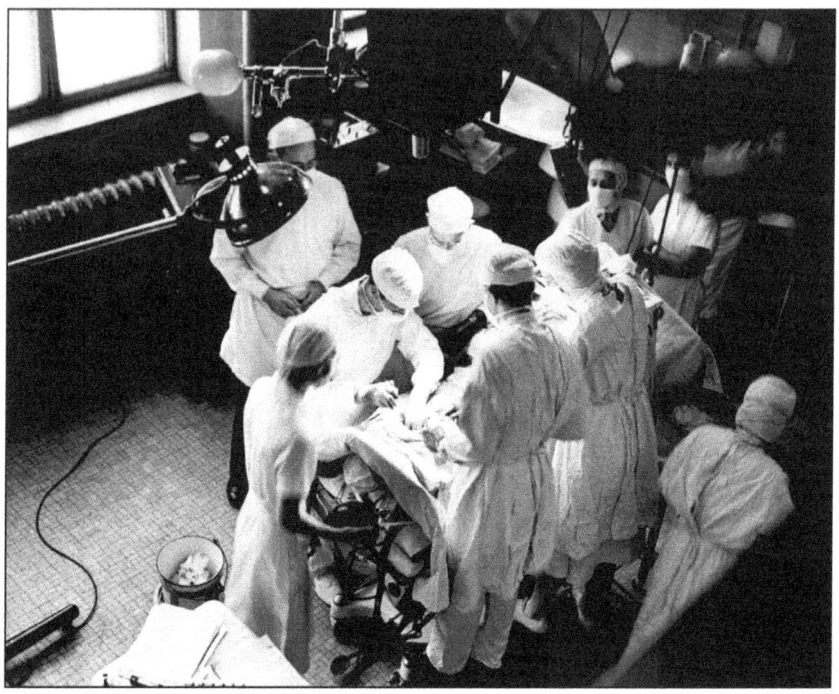

THE CHESNEY ARCHIVES OF JOHNS HOPKINS MEDICINE, NURSING AND PUBLIC HEALTH

In late 1944, at Johns Hopkins Medicine, the first blue baby surgery took place, stunning the world with its originality and impressing everyone with the risk-taking of Alfred Blalock. This 1947 photo shows Vivien Thomas, who created the operation, standing behind Blalock so that he can coach the Hopkins chief of surgery through the operation. Thomas, the only Black person in the photo, was never identified by Hopkins Medicine and the step stool on which he always stood, at Blalock's request, was removed before the picture was taken. This surgery is called the Blalock-Taussig shunt.

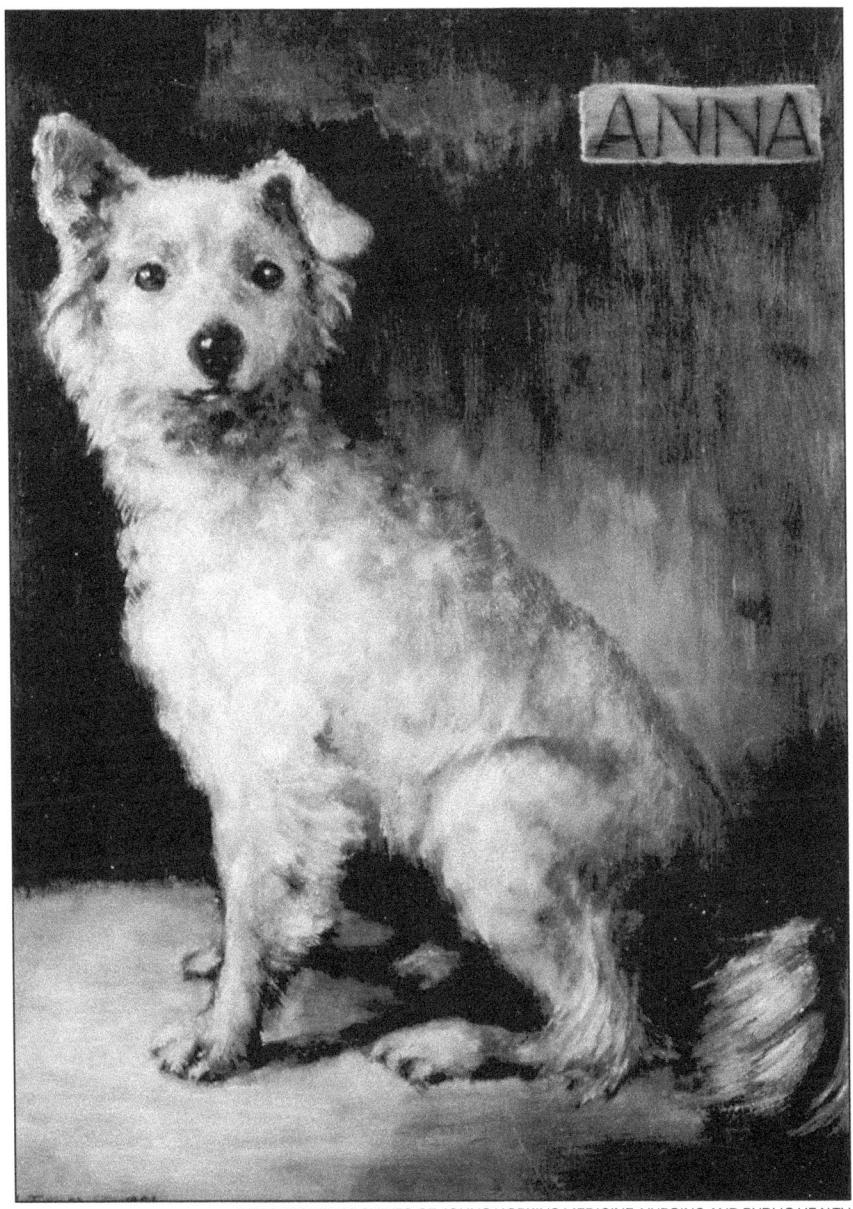

THE CHESNEY ARCHIVES OF JOHNS HOPKINS MEDICINE, NURSING AND PUBLIC HEALTH

An oil painting of Anna, the first dog to survive both experimental blue baby surgeries: the first to make her oxygen deficient and the second to ensure that her level of oxygen is improved. She was Vivien Thomas's favorite dog due to her sweet personality. An animal rights group in Baltimore commissioned this painting and presented it to Hopkins, where it hangs in the Children's Center.

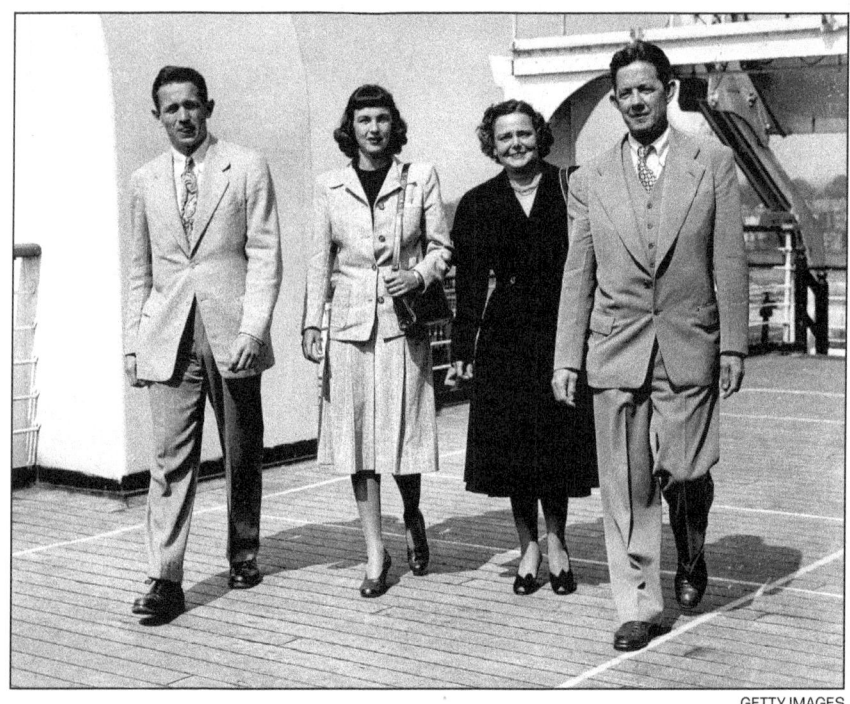

Arriving in Southampton, England, in 1947 to demonstrate the blue baby surgery. To the far right is Alfred Blalock with his wife, Mary Blalock, on his left. On the far left is Henry Bahnson with his wife, Louise Bahnson, to his right. So much fuss was made over the surgery that Hopkins referred to this as "the Royal Tour." Vivien Thomas stayed in Baltimore.

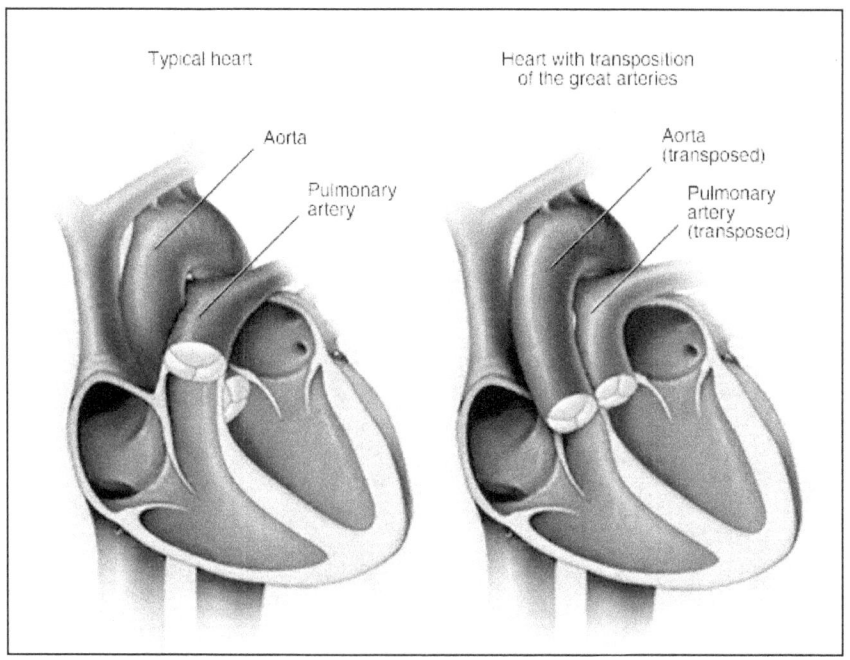

USED WITH PERMISSION OF MAYO FOUNDATION FOR MEDICAL EDUCATION AND RESEARCH, ALL RIGHTS RESERVED

In 1948, the second critical cardiac surgery that Vivien Thomas creates is for the Transposition of the Great Arteries (TGA). These babies, like the blue babies (TOF) lack a normal amount of circulating oxygen in their blood, but it is caused by a different set of cardiac defects. A typical heart is on the left, and on the right is the heart of a TGA baby born with its main arteries (the aorta and the pulmonary artery) switched or transposed. Thomas's surgical experiments give physicians a method creating an atrial septal defect (ASD), or a hole in the septum) that allows enough oxygenated blood into the infant's blood circulation to keep them alive and active. The surgery is called the Blalock-Hanlon procedure.

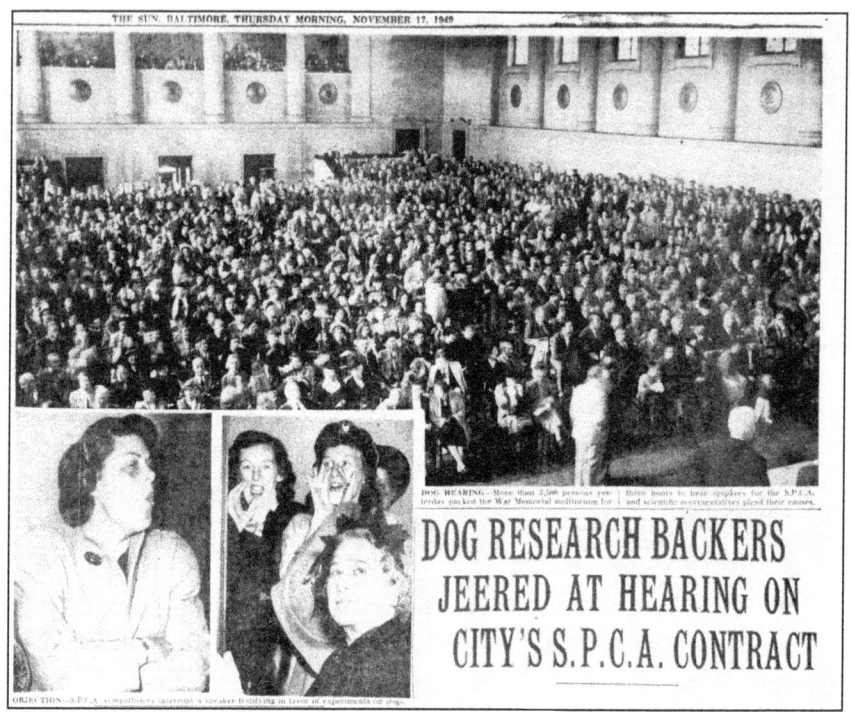

The use of animals in medical research was becoming a highly contentious issue. In 1949, Baltimore holds a public hearing on the issue with 3,500 attendees. The overheated hearing makes the front page of Baltimore's newspapers.

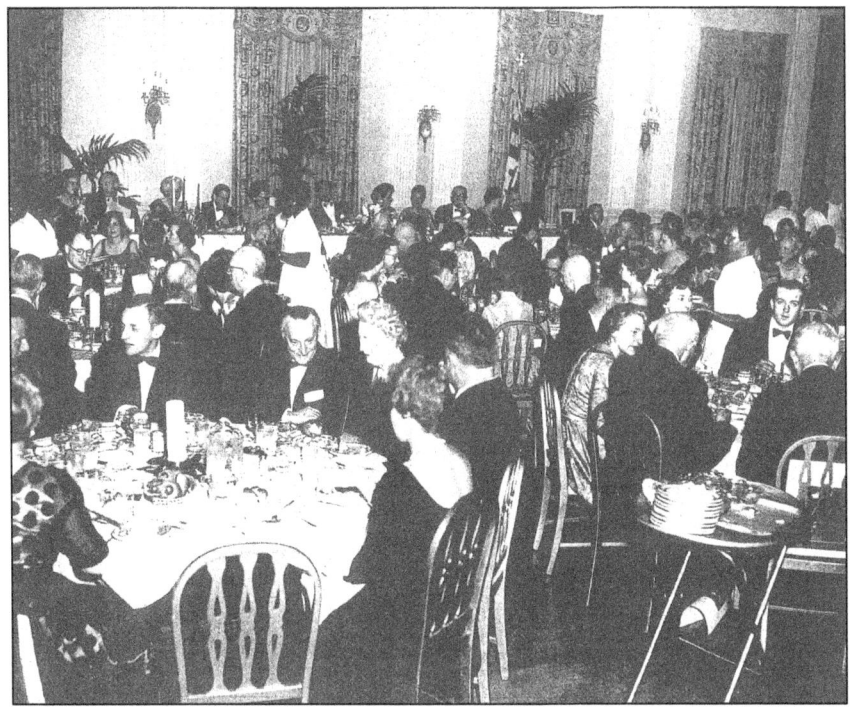

DUKE UNIVERSITY MEDICAL CENTER ARCHIVES

In 1960, a commemoration party for Alfred Blalock's achievements is held at Baltimore's Southern Hotel. Although more than 400 people are invited, Clara and Vivien Thomas were excluded by Blalock because he doesn't believe that whites should eat with Blacks: it's "simply something that isn't done," Blalock says.

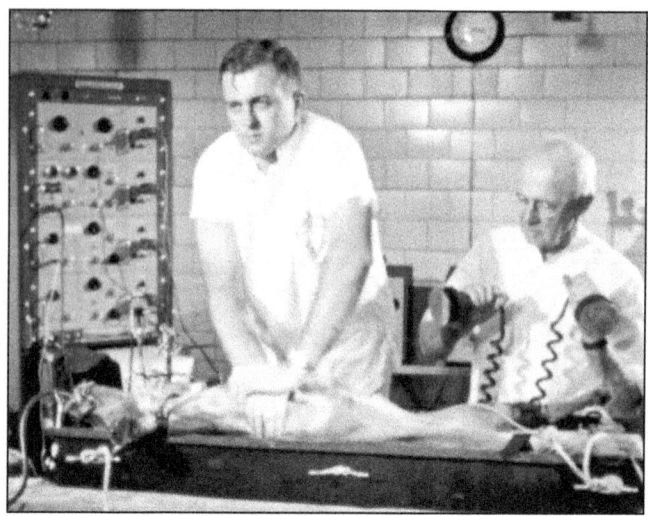

THE CHESNEY ARCHIVES OF JOHNS HOPKINS MEDICINE, NURSING AND PUBLIC HEALTH

Vivien Thomas makes important contributions to the development of CPR. Seen here is G. Guy Knickerbocker demonstrating external cardiac message on a dog, with William B. Kouwenhoven, their team leader.

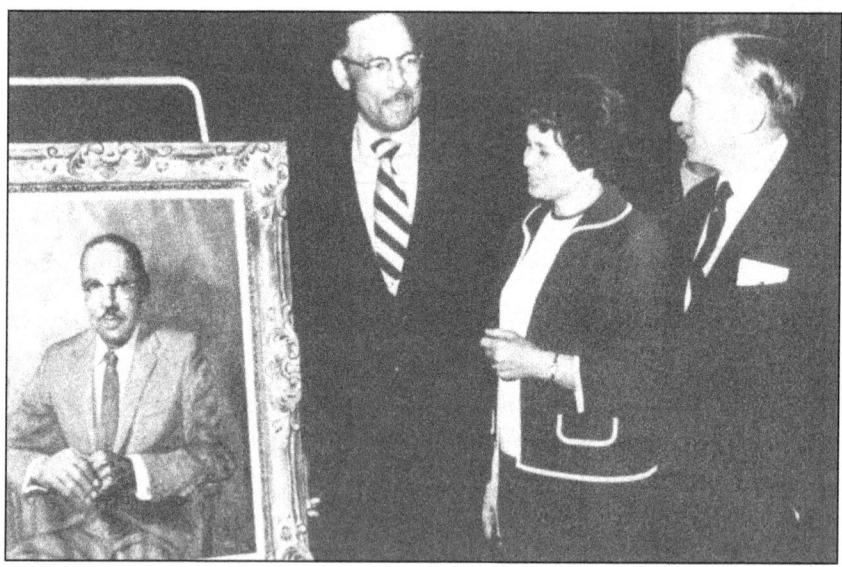

THE AFRO AMERICAN NEWSPAPERS, BALTIMORE AFRO AMERICAN

A collection is taken up in 1969 by Hopkins surgeons for a portrait of Vivien Thomas. Once painted, it sits in Thomas's closet for two years before Hopkins agreed to hang it in 1971. Vivien Thomas is on the left and Clara Thomas is to his right. To the far right is C. Rollins Hanlon.

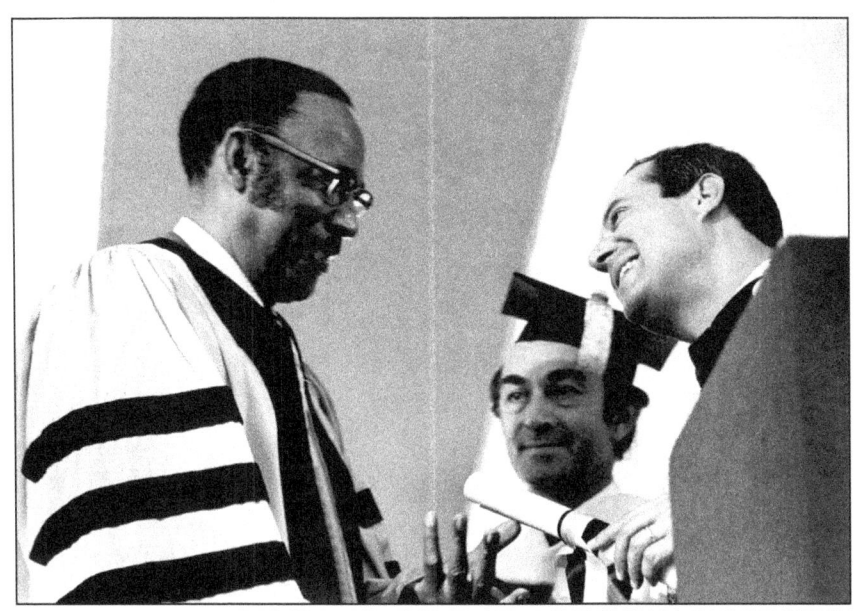

THE CHESNEY ARCHIVES OF JOHNS HOPKINS MEDICINE, NURSING AND PUBLIC HEALTH

When Hopkins learns that the University of Maryland is interested in awarding Vivien Thomas an honorary DSc (doctor of science) degree, it quickly votes to give him an honorary LLD (doctor of laws) in 1976. Thomas is on the far left and to his right are Harvey Woolfe, Hopkins's provost, and Steven Muller, president of Johns Hopkins University.

GWENDOLYN MANLOVE CLARKE

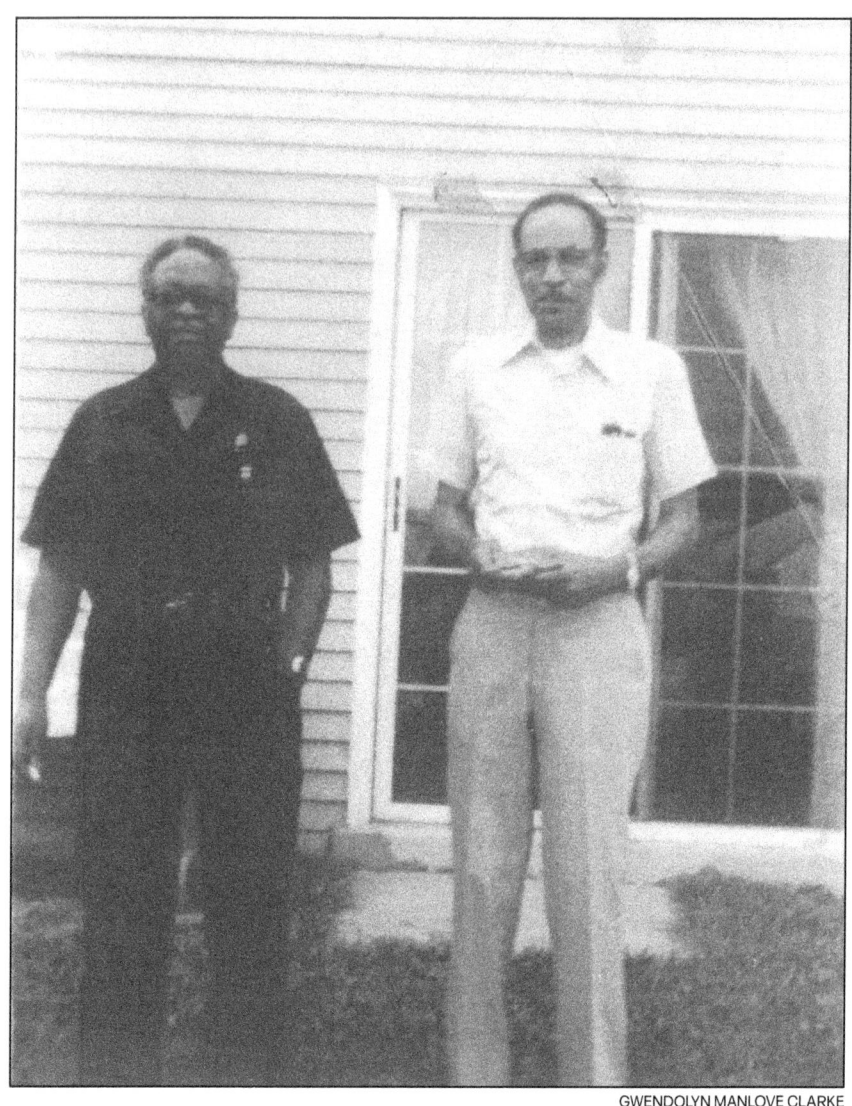

Vivien Thomas, on right, remained lifetime friends with Charles Manlove, on left, who had introduced him to Alfred Blalock at Vanderbilt University in 1930. This photo was taken in 1981, when Thomas was seventy-six years old.

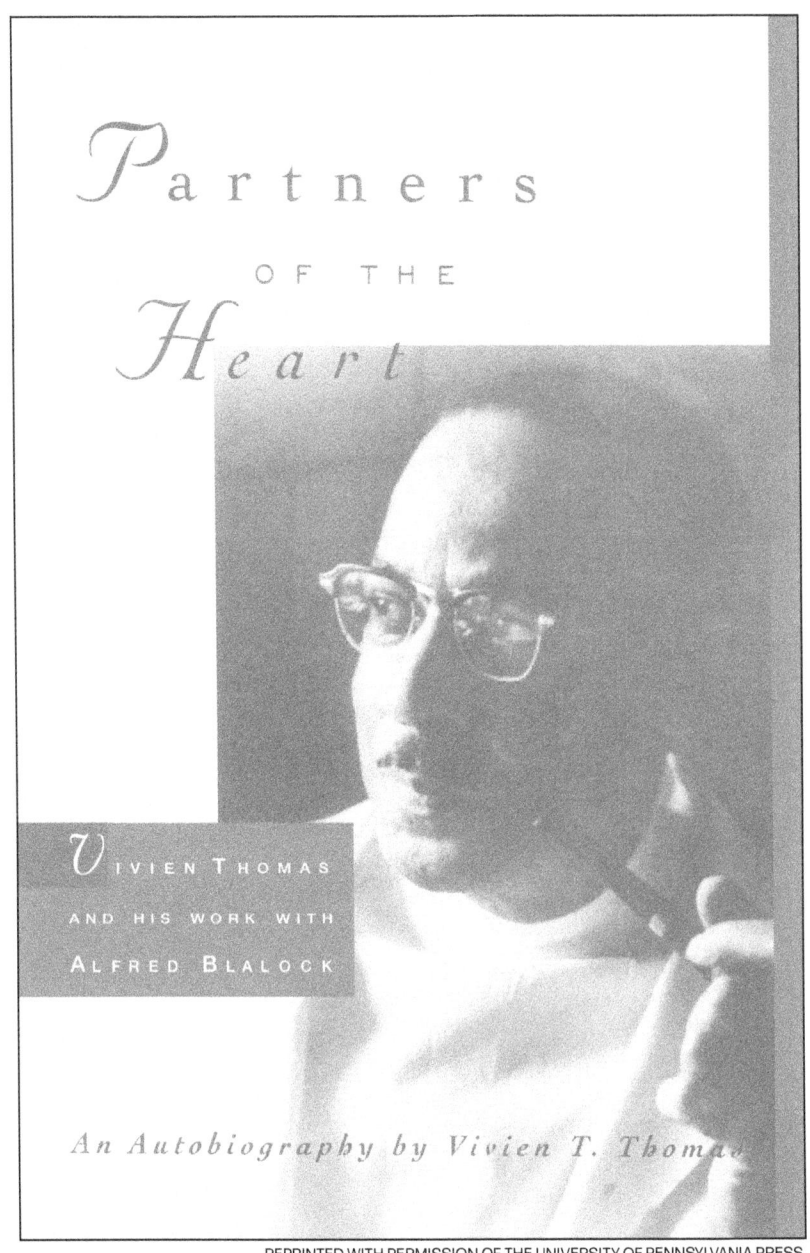

In 1985, Vivien Thomas has his book, *Pioneering Research in Surgical Shock and Cardiovascular Surgery: Vivien Thomas and His Work with Alfred Blalock*, published by the University of Pennsylvania Press. It is now named *Partners of the Heart*, after the title of a PBS documentary on Thomas. Thomas dies a week before the book is published.

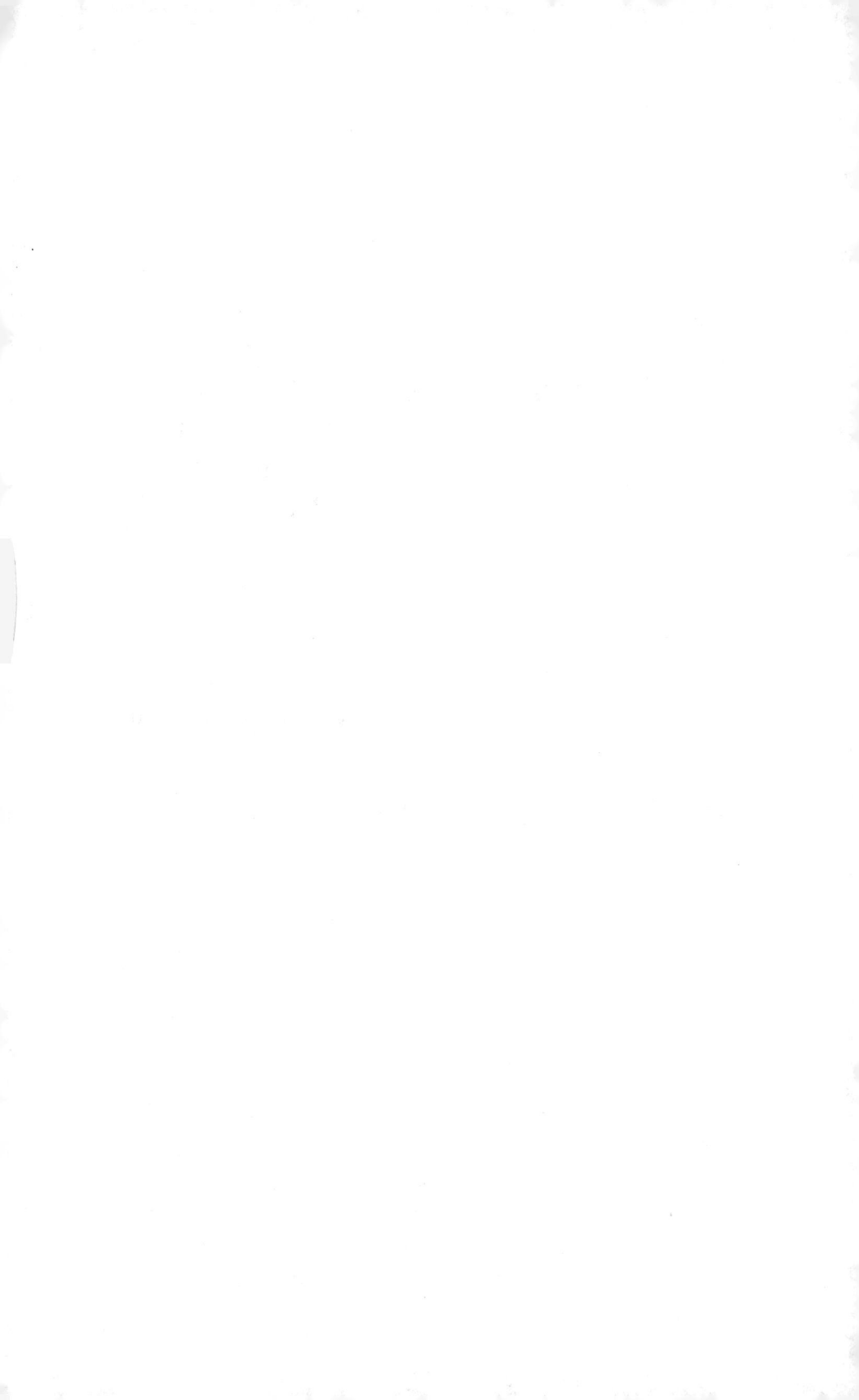

CHAPTER TWENTY

A VACATION, AT LAST

In 1946, following the end of the war, Clara and Vivien's mood lightened and they decided to take their first vacation in more than five years.[1] It was high time for a trip to Nashville and also to Macon, Georgia, where Clara had been raised. The couple wanted their girls to reconnect with family, and they also wanted their kin to see how the girls, one in junior high school and the other in elementary school, were turning into young ladies.

Olga, who was eleven years old, and Theodosia, the younger sister at seven years, were especially excited and high-spirited. Clara kept a wary eye on them while Vivien watched their delighted reaction to their *first vacation ever*—at least, within their memories. Before the long trip, though, this strict father let them know that any complaints or arguments would not be tolerated. Clara, anticipating hot and grimy hours ahead in the car, allowed the girls to wear cool cotton outfits, although she would have made sure that her daughters looked pressed and sharp.

With Thomas behind the wheel once they'd set out of Baltimore, Clara would have reviewed their state maps and the *Green Book*, an annual publication written out of necessity for Black motorists in the South.[2] The *Green Book* listed the motels, rest stops, and coffee shops where African American travelers were allowed service. In the hostile Jim Crow South, it was an indispensable tool.

Other than stopping for gas, the Thomases planned to drive straight through to Nashville to avoid as much unpleasantness as possible. Clara took her turn at the wheel while her husband slept, which always made the family a little nervous because she was a speed demon. Clara had been taught to drive by her brothers, whose concept of driver's ed was to push down on the accelerator, hard, with one of their feet on top of hers.[3] Speeding was a matter of course to Clara and they made the trip to Nashville in a long day and a night.

Clara, home manager that she was, would have parceled out her carefully packed meals and snacks that would sustain them until Nashville. Why worry about finding a restaurant that would serve them or spend good money when food from home tasted better? After a full meal and miles on the road, the children found themselves lulled to sleep by the wheels' thumpity-thump rhythm on the pavement. When the girls slept, Vivien and Clara had a little time together for quiet conversation. Although they rarely showed their emotions, they were as excited as the girls about returning.

Once they finally pulled up to Thomas's mother's house in Nashville, word quickly spread of their arrival. Friends and family stopped by day and night to visit and reconnect, often with syrupy summer-fruit pie. The couple's friends would exclaim over how much the girls had grown in four short years, just as elders have done generation after generation.

While everyone chattered and exchanged stories, Thomas was, as usual, reticent when asked about his job. Back in Baltimore, he'd learned not to mention that he was working at Hopkins to friends and neighbors because they ragged him about the racist institution. Nor would he ever admit the level of his accomplishments because everyone, not even knowing the skyscraping level of work he was fulfilling, was quick to accuse him of being foolish by working for Hopkins: "Hopkins is making money as a result of the work you've done—they have the money to pay you!" said one.[4]

The neighbors wanted to know how Clara could afford to stay home when his salary was so abysmal. Vivien deflected them by complimenting his wife and her careful budgeting. He felt that he had to keep everything about his achievements to himself, which added to his loneliness.

A Vacation, at Last

All anyone knew was that he worked in a medical lab with dogs, and they could guess that the job didn't pay much. He would never let his friends, siblings, or children know that those headline stories were based on his own work. His younger daughter remembered, "He didn't tell us anything—not me or my sister."[5] So Thomas beat on alone, for his family and its future.

During the Nashville visit, nearly every evening, the Thomas family was invited to dinner at someone's house. Treated to trademark Southern hospitality, there would be so much home-cooked food—such items as biscuits *and* cornbread, green beans (cooked with a nice fatty piece of salted pork), butter beans with a little sweet Vidalia onion, maybe a yellow and red tomato salad, and a delicious-smelling roast, carved at the table with its juices running down its side—that they never went hungry. After, there was dessert: coconut cake so light it could fly, tart cherry pie, and maybe even dark chocolate pudding as rich as Rockefeller. The ever-present percolator sat bubbling, ready for someone who needed something to cut the sweetness of dessert.

The Thomas children and the other kids at the table would eventually get fidgety and be excused to go play. The adults could chat at the dining room table or, depending on the weather, go out onto a back porch. There were plenty of high spirits as well as the nostalgic sights and sounds of children laughing. As darkness fell, the birds got softer and the insects grew louder, and a calm descended on all. Nothing could compare to the satisfaction found in a good dinner with old friends.

Once the coffee's caffeine had kicked in, folks would try to convince the Thomases to stay in Nashville. "Vivien, the housing market has exploded! Everyone is building new houses. Why, you can't find a carpenter who doesn't have a dozen employers begging for his skills," exclaimed one.[6]

"And the pay! Sweet Jesus," said another. A third interjected, "You can make $3,500 to $4,500 a year [currently between $46,000 and $59,000] just by putting in eight hours of work every day!"[7] Only Vivien and Clara knew that his Hopkins salary still remained set at $1,500.

The conversation immediately changed direction by implicit agreement whenever a child stepped over to the table to ask permission to do one thing or another. Adult decisions were for parents to make, and how a man made his living or where he chose to raise his family were not topics discussed with children. When the elders settled on a choice, the young ones would be told.[8]

On these tranquil evenings, Thomas got to thinking. He was still earning the same salary as when he had received a ninety-six dollar increase at the beginning of 1942, paid for by Walter Dandy. In the past four years, he'd been offered no bonuses, no cost-of-living increases, and no adjustment for the higher pay that Baltimore's industrial Black war workers had enjoyed. Yet his successful blue baby operative techniques were bringing thousands more patients to Hopkins and had given the hospital a much-needed boost in reputation.

There was another concern that nagged at Thomas. His firstborn, Olga, would start college in six years. Thomas ached for his daughters to have the opportunity that had blown past him like a dust storm in 1930, taking the last of his boyhood with it. There was only one obstacle in his way, and that was his paltry income. He vowed to put this right, thinking, "I want to give them a better chance than I had."[9]

The only route to higher pay was through his boss, and Blalock was uninterested in promoting Thomas. He was only concerned about the welfare of his many protégés, whose background reflected his predilection for Southern students. When they'd arrived in Baltimore from Vanderbilt, Blalock boasted, "I'm going to bring in some good old Southern boys to turn it [the residency program] around."[10]

Some thought that his strongest interest lay in the progress of his most promising surgery students. Those who trained with Blalock held distinct advantages because he chose nearly all his students from prosperous, well-connected families. He also was known to give his best doctors second-author credit on papers he wrote based on any research they completed. He made sure that "full recognition was accorded everyone who had made even a minor contribution."[11] Everyone who was a white physician, that is.

His lab assistant, although also Southern, was a cageling bird, one that Blalock did not want to set free. Despite how Blalock jump-started his students' careers, Thomas often remarked that Blalock "never encouraged me to attempt to continue my education."[12]

Still, Thomas decided to give it one last shot. After the war, plenty of former soldiers, including older men, returned to college now that the GI Bill had made it affordable. Thomas thought that this was the time for him, too. No one would stare and wonder why a thirty-six-year-old man was sitting in the classroom. Thomas, of course, could not take advantage of the GI Bill due to his military exemption and, even if he were eligible, very few African American veterans were able to gain its privileges because it was locally administered and did not carry any anti-discrimination rules.

Predominantly white colleges took some Black students, but only a few of those who'd applied. The historically Black colleges like Fisk were overwhelmed with applicants and, of the 100,000 Black veterans who applied for admission to historically Black colleges and universities, there was space for only 20,000.[13] (The GI Bill also provided funds for a veteran who wanted to own a house to be put firmly into the middle-class, but a minuscule percentage of Black veterans, under the GI Bill, could benefit: only one hundred of 140,000 assisted veterans were Black.)[14]

When Thomas looked in to entering undergraduate studies at Maryland's Morgan College (now Morgan State University), a historically Black institution, the college insisted that Thomas take a full class load for four years, regardless of his knowledge and experience, when he was qualified to teach some of his mandatory science coursework. Thomas informed Blalock of this dilemma, and the professor remained aloof and provided absolutely no support, for example, by documenting Thomas's splendid research skills or his knowledge of science and math. Without this, the college refused to waive any undergraduate course work. Nor was Blalock willing to reduce Thomas's long work hours or allow him the flexibility necessary for him to attend classes.

While Thomas was navigating the choppy waters of academe, he received no helping hand from any surgeon whomever at Hopkins. Many of them knew of Thomas's abortive attempt to return to school and some even sympathized with his goal, but they—including those men who claimed to have been friends with him—asked him nothing, said nothing, offered nothing, and did nothing. No one, from Blalock down, even made a phone call on his behalf. Perhaps they shrugged him off, thinking that this is the way life was for a Black man. The daughter of his best friend, Charles Manlove, remembered, "He knew that he was going to have to let the dream of college go. And that hurt, that was very crushing."[15]

Thomas's dream of becoming a physician, which he held on to for two decades past his high school graduation, dissolved as if it had belonged to a man he had known in another life. He would never be a doctor, and he concluded that this had wrecked his life. But he would be darned if Blalock would stop his daughters from getting the schooling that he wanted for them.

To make ends meet and maybe set a little money aside, Thomas was supplementing his salary by bartending at the parties given by Blalock and other Hopkins surgeons. He noted of Blalock, "He was aware, of course, that I was moonlighting for additional income for house parties given by the professional staff, his parties included."[16] Sometimes, Clara would work at these parties, too, catering the food and helping to serve. This way, she could get out of the house and make some much-needed cash.[17] Clara was more of an extrovert than her husband and was curious about the people in Vivien's life. If serving them was her only opportunity to meet them, she would take it. The couple certainly wasn't being invited as guests to any party given by Hopkins surgeons.

Most of the invitees were the same men with whom Thomas worked during the day, many of whom he was training or had trained. Naively, some guests thought Thomas felt on par with the invited guests. Alex Haller, a strong supporter and admirer of Thomas explained, "It was not awkward for Vivien to serve me drinks. We would talk shop about the lab. It was more like Vivien was a host of the get-togethers."[18] He insisted that Vivien was treated "just like a colleague," yet it seemed doubtful that Thomas would have viewed his situation in the same way.[19] As one surgeon recalled, with some embarrassment, "We called him Vivien and he called us 'Doctor.'"[20] Another admired Thomas for his grace while bartending, "It was humiliating to him, but you would never detect it.[21]

All these thoughts were swirling around his head when he learned of the well-paying carpentry opportunities in Nashville. His mood turned from being relaxed to being frustrated and anxious. One lazy morning after breakfast, as soon as it was polite, Clara and Vivien decided that it would be nice to drive out to look at their old house, the one they'd been renting out. After a short ride, Thomas braked to a stop, shifted gear into park and, for caution's sake, yanked the safety brake up. The couple looked across the broad green lawn leading to their front stoop and sighed in nostalgia. The lovely neighborhood, the comfortable house, and the relaxed pace of life was so different from the urban streets of Baltimore.

Of course, they gazed at each other and said what was in their hearts, "Why not move back home?"[22] It was an idea they couldn't shake.

CHAPTER TWENTY-ONE

CLASH OF THE TITANS: BLALOCK VS. TAUSSIG

During the first two blue baby surgeries, before anyone outside the Hopkins hospital knew about the incredible surgical advance taking place there, a sign outside the operating room had identified the surgeries as the "Taussig-Blalock" operations.[1] That would soon change.

Running parallel to this great accomplishment was Blalock's deep vein of narcissism, which he mined for his sole benefit. He did not want Helen Taussig's name listed before his despite her idea "that proved correct both physiologically and clinically,"[2] as Thomas said. In fact, he didn't want her name to be included at all. He jealously tried to block any blue baby credit from Taussig and "insisted on dropping Dr. Taussig's name from future surgical blue baby postings."[3] Blalock's denial of credit to Taussig seems particularly small because Taussig moved from being "depressed at having to stand by" while her blue babies died, one after another, but then, after the successful surgery, "acted as if a great burden had been lifted from her shoulders."[4]

His actions enraged Edwards Park, Taussig's longtime supporter and the head of the children's clinic. He stormed over to confront Blalock and they had a shouting match that was overheard by other staff. Austin Lamont said the incident displayed Blalock's "petty and ungenerous spirit."[5] Olive Berger was shocked by the tempest and said she had never seen Dr. Park so angry at anyone.[6] Of course, everyone who overheard the argument repeated the delicious details to others; in a hospital, gossip spreads even faster than a virus. Perhaps Blalock had thought that Taussig's status as a low-ranked female instructor would mean that he could seize all acclaim for the blue baby surgery. Fortunately for the pediatrician, Park's intervention and clout was at least as great as the surgeon's and Blalock failed at his attempt to erase her name. After that, what had been their quiet dislike of each other exploded into "a thinly suppressed hostility."[7]

Despite their mutual aversion, Taussig and Blalock knew they had to continue working together if they were to gain any acknowledgment for their innovative surgery outside of Hopkins. They couldn't publish a paper that was based on the results of only one surgery. In February 1945, Taussig identified two more possibilities for surgery: a twelve-year-old girl and a six-year-old boy, both of whom were older and more stable than little Eileen had been. The third surgery, Taussig reported, was the first time they'd seen a dramatic color change, when they boy turned from blue to pink.[8] The success of these last two surgeries helped salve the sadness felt by all at the death of Eileen Saxon on New Year's Day, 1945.

Finally, after the first three surgeries were successfully completed, Blalock and Taussig's article was published in the *Journal of the American Medical Association* in May 1945. It was titled "The Surgical Treatment of Malformations of the Heart in Which There Is Pulmonary Stenosis or Pulmonary Atresia."[9] Recognizing the momentousness of the story, the medical reporter for the Associated Press newswire clattered out a nearly unbelievable piece about a miraculous heart surgery freshly devised by a pair of American doctors in Baltimore. The journalist marked the story so that five bells clanged when it came through the teletype machine, indicating it was urgent, worthy of immediate attention. (A rare ten-bell alarm would be used later, on August sixth of that year, to announce the news of an atomic bomb dropped on Hiroshima.) The AP announcement kicked off a story that ricocheted throughout the world, and it held its own while competing with the press attention being given to the aftermath of the Victory over Europe Day announcement signifying the end of the World War II in Europe. After the war ended, Thomas would receive a certificate "for contributing to the successful persecution of the Second World War" from the US Office on Scientific Research and Development for his shock research, but he was not acknowledged by Hopkins in any way.

Editors jumped at the story about a rare heart surgery that could let sick children live because it hit their readers' hearts and minds. *LIFE* magazine would run a five-page feature with eleven photographs[10] and *TIME* magazine announced the operation's success on its "Medicine" page.[11]

Richard Bing, MD, who was hired by Blalock to open the first ever cardiac catheterization lab, was on his way to start his new job at Hopkins via a small ferry that shuttled between New Jersey and Baltimore. He said, "I had a premonition of what was to come when, on the drive from New York to Baltimore, we went across the Chesapeake Bay on the ferry. I encountered at least six TOF patients on the short boat ride."[12]

The blue baby research and surgery had put Hopkins back on the map: its first-class reputation had suffered for several decades and had lost its shine. Now, Hopkins's star was rising again. Thomas noted, "The influx and deluge of patients that came into the hospital was something this hospital has never seen before and I do not think it will ever see again. It caught the hospital unprepared."[13]

A woman who'd worked at Harriet Lane described the chaos. "Every few days an exhausted young mother would get off the bus at the Monument Street after a long trip hastily arranged by her sympathetic townspeople. Nobody expected her. She brought no medical records," and had no place to stay in a crowded wartime city.[14] One mother from Appalachia actually hitchedhiked all the way to Baltimore, carrying her child in her arms.

There'd been so much commotion over the blue baby success that the hospital became choked with parents and infants. Finally, a waiting list of babies was created and the surgery department acknowledged that there was up to a three-year delay. However, in 1946, a child could be bumped to the top of the waiting list if his distraught parents could afford to pay $500 cash rather than the standard surgery fee of $100.[15] By 1948, the price of jumping the queue had risen to $1,000 cash.[16] Conducting two surgeries a day, Blalock sometimes waved his personal fee.[17] Often, raising money was a local effort. Parents asked for donations from friends and neighbors, church and synagogue members, fire and police officers, and any retail shop willing to put out a cash box. When time pressure was dire, youngsters traveled to Hopkins on chartered Army transport planes and trains, and on Navy bombers.[18]

The news swept through the country's medical schools, too. At Vanderbilt, one undergraduate remembered the school's dramatic announcement of a successful surgery on a blue baby's heart. "There was a sort of awe, then a quiet, and then there was this emotional upheaval and outstanding applause," he said of the reaction.[19] It was a sign that the fog concealing both cardiac surgery and surgery on infants was dissipating. The implications were great for men like Blalock who weren't timid about puncturing medical wisdom or challenging the establishment. No one had thought the heart could be touched and so physicians called this surgery "an epochal event,"[20] and declared that "all questions about operating on the heart had been challenged and vanquished."[21] It was a very big deal for Johns Hopkins, indeed.

Thomas wasn't sure that he could carry a bigger workload, but he did. Meeting each day as a new challenge, he spent his mornings in the operating room with Blalock, walking him through the surgery at least another hundred times until the surgeon felt fully comfortable with it. Anticipating a spike in patient load, he knew he could not keep up with the demand if he continued using his hand-devised surgical instruments and materials. Taking the initiative, he contacted J. A. Deknatel & Son, a suture company, to inquire about the possibility of their manufacturing fine-size braided silk pre-attached to an eyeless, or swagged, needle. Then he met with a representative of Murray Baumgartner, a local surgical supply house, and described the special non-crushing vascular clamp (the Blalock Clamp) that he wanted it to manufacture.

Although the issue of joint contribution by Blalock and Taussig had been resolved, Vivien Thomas remained totally uncredited for his work for many decades. The first sign of his anonymity can be seen in the original 1945 Blalock-Taussig article, which contains no mention whatsoever of him. He was ignored in the public affairs releases from Hopkins that credited Blalock with nearly every aspect of this innovation, including the creation of new medical instruments invented by Thomas and the more than 200 experimental dog surgeries Thomas had performed. He was, as W. E. B. Du Bois, termed it, shrouded by a "Veil" that kept him from being seen by white people.[22]

There were no photos taken of the earliest surgeries because no one was assured of the consequences. Then, in 1947, Vivien Thomas appears fleetingly in a blue baby surgery still-shot photo taken from Hopkins's first black-and-white televised closed-circuit film of the procedure.[23] He is respectfully situated in the background, several feet away from Blalock, looking completely impassive, hands crossed and idle, watching Blalock work. His face is partly blocked by a floor spotlight that makes it impossible to determine his race. He is only partly scrubbed, wearing a white scrub coat, a surgical mask, and a scrub hat on his head. His hands are bare, without the rubber gloves everyone else is wearing. The pants and shoes are his own street clothes, and the customary step stool had been removed before the posed image was shot.

Certainly, Hopkins never mentioned Vivien Thomas's name in their press releases and identified only the white people in the operating theater. Neither did the press ask Hopkins any questions about this unnamed man. The prejudice of his university forced him to go "incognegro," using the wry term others have coined. He was just another invisible Black man.

CHAPTER TWENTY-TWO

THE BLUE BABY TOUR

By 1947, major international hospitals were vying for Blalock and Taussig to leave Baltimore to lecture and to perform a series of blue baby operations abroad. The doctors decided to go to London, Paris, and Stockholm. The day before they embarked for England, Blalock's tobacco habit had him running around Baltimore, buying up all the Viceroy packets he could find. He was, by now, a two-pack-a-day man and smoked at least forty cigarettes by bedtime. He had always been a little vain and was embarrassed by the look of his fingertips, stained orange-yellow by nicotine. Soon he would purchase a cigarette holder to prevent his discoloration from becoming more noticeable. He correctly assumed that, in Europe, he could find his necessary six to eight bottles of Coca-Cola that he drank daily.

A characteristic blip of Blalock's pride initially stymied his entrance into the United Kingdom. To clear customs in Southampton, England—the group had journeyed on the transatlantic ship RMS *Mauretania* because Blalock disliked flying—Blalock had carefully prepared letters, written on Johns Hopkins stationery, that explained why Hopkins staff would be working in the UK. The officials duly permitted people holding these letters into the country. It had never occurred to Blalock that he might need some type of formal acknowledgment from Hopkins for himself that would explain his own activities in England, and he was held in customs for quite a few hours before being released.

Once that was cleared up, Taussig and Blalock went first to London to lecture on the blue baby condition and its palliative operation to large crowds of doctors. Everywhere they spoke, physicians jumped to their feet and thanked them with standing ovations. At London's Royal College of Surgeons, they had to give the same lecture twice to accommodate the huge overflow crowd. For dramatic effect, they had brought with them a two-year-old Baltimore girl with a TOF heart modified by Blalock; at the conclusion of the lecture, they'd throw a spotlight on her. It was "a Madonna-like tableau, a perfect climax to an impressive lecture on an epoch-making contribution."[1]

"They operated all over Europe with accolades up and down the continent," said Haller.[2] The European physicians were filled with awe, but Blalock and Taussig eventually became exhausted from the attention given them. They were garnering so much idolatrous publicity that soon Hopkins staff were joking about the "Royal Tour."[3]

Nonetheless, the operations were especially draining for Blalock because there were so many surgeons watching his every move. Blalock had anticipated fatigue and had asked Denton Cooley, who was already in Europe participating in a tennis match, to join him as his substitute surgeon. Captivated by the matches, Cooley declined the opportunity in favor of the tournament. He would come to regret this decision, saying he missed "the greatest professional opportunity of my life."[4] Instead, Blalock's surgical resident, Henry Bahnson, MD, picked up the slack when he tired from churning out healthy pink babies. Before too long, Blalock turned the operations over to Bahnson entirely.

Overseas, both Blalock and Taussig were smothered with honors. In France, they received its premier decoration, the *Legion d'honneur*. In every country they visited, they were given laurels, many that included substantial financial awards ranging from $1,000 to $25,000. By contrast, in the US it was Blalock, then fifty-six years old, who received the lion's share of recognition. He, for example, was immediately inducted into the National Academy of Sciences while Helen Taussig was made to wait another twenty-five years, until 1973, for membership. She was named an assistant professor in 1946 by Hopkins but was not promoted to a full professor until 1959. "It hurt," she acknowledged. "A man would have had the promotion long before I got mine."[5]

Cash gifts also poured into the surgery department. Although the money was generally to be spent at the discretion of Blalock, a few donors suggested that their gifts might be given to underpaid staff. If anyone ever received this money, it wasn't Vivien Thomas. Some of it was used for such items as a portrait of Alfred Blalock to be given to the American College of Surgery, which cost $1,000, and the trips overseas that cost up to $1,500 to speak at conferences, and for two dinners for surgery staff that each cost about $550.[6] However, Thomas received absolutely no form of recognition from Hopkins for the blue baby surgery: no salary increases, no cash award, not even a letter of commendation.

With these awards and their accompanying news coverage, an enormous amount of disruptive attention crashed down on Hopkins. Thomas noted, "If Johns Hopkins had a public affairs office, it was completely ineffective."[7] Taussig and Blalock had no control over the press or the frequent articles that appeared on their work. There was the hopeful story "Operation May Save 'Blue Baby,'" and the emphatic "French Blue Baby Held Cured," and the peace-loving "German Boy Has Surgery in US," and the cautious "Ex-Blue Baby Back to School." And there was also the sentimental Brooklyn story, "Gift of Health Fills the Stocking of Boy Who Was Doomed to Die." There were a few sad stories, too. "Detroit Child Loses 4-Year Fight for Life" detailed how "little Patricia Connor died seventeen days before she was to undergo an operation" at Hopkins because local citizens had been too slow in raising the needed hospital fee.[8]

That the two physicians had been civil to each other in Europe did not keep them from resuming their sniping after they returned to Baltimore. In retrospect, their disputes seem comical. Because the two now refused to speak to each other—except when they were in the public eye—they communicated via endless correspondence. A letter from Taussig, which Blalock read in dismay, royally announced that she should be first author on all their joint articles or they should publish separately.

Continuing the feud, Blalock replied, "The more recent and insulting letter makes it necessary for me to write to you in a very unpleasant manner." He further explained, "I intentionally placed your name first, providing you do not return to your former habit of placing your name in parentheses throughout the paper and in all those places in which you refer to what you call your own original work. If you do this, and if you insist, as you did in connection with our first joint paper, that all reference to my work be deleted, then there will be disagreement."[9]

Yet Blalock was himself unreasonable and squawked to Taussig that she didn't give him enough credit in her talks. Her subtle but sardonic response was guaranteed to irritate him. "Again, my most humble apologies if there was anyone in the audience who thought that I did not give you full credit, but I am quite sure that most people are 300 percent convinced of the brilliance of your work."[10]

Blalock eventually proposed to open a pediatric cardiac service within surgery so he could be independent of Taussig and her students, many of whom who were female. Clara Belle Puryear recalled Blalock lamenting that Taussig wouldn't give him any peace. The organizational change never happened. Longmire implies that Taussig, "the patron saint" as he dubbed her, would not allow any part of pediatrics to fall under the surgery department.[11] Of course, Edwards Park supported her.

The following year, more argumentative letters flew between their offices. Which department should pay for the necessary blue baby long-distance calls, pediatrics or surgery? Letters went back and forth until these two capable, well-educated, and emotionally immature adults finally compromised: if the blue baby patient who warranted out-of-area phone calls did not have an operation, pediatrics would pick up the long-distance costs. If the child did go to surgery, surgery paid. One more item settled but at the expense of those who had to reckon with the onerous billing statements.

Soon after this teapot tempest, Blalock called Denton Cooley into his office. "Denton," he said, "you seem to have a reputation around the hospital of getting along well with the women."

Cooley, who was tall, extraordinarily handsome and a natural athlete, thought it best to answer noncommittally. "Do I, sir?"

"Yes, that is the rumor. You know, Denton, I am going to make you my cardiac resident. I know it is a little premature for you, but I want you to do one thing for me."

Cooley looked quizzical, so Blalock explained, "I want you to get all those damn women out of my hair."

Cooley responded, "I will try, Dr. Blalock."[12]

CHAPTER TWENTY-THREE

THE EVERLASTING SALARY ISSUE

A few months after that Nashville vacation, Thomas made up his mind. He headed directly into Blalock's office and declared, "I'm leaving." Thomas was thirty-six years old, and he had decided that his devotion to surgical research must take second place to his duty to his family and, particularly, to his daughters' college education. He also was angry that his Hopkins salary did not provide "enough money to salt away for the future."[1]

Thomas explained to his stunned supervisor that, with the post-war building boom, he estimated that he could make "anywhere from two to four times what I'm making here" by returning to carpentry.[2] He reminded Blalock that he'd had no pay increase in four years and, at that, his income of $1,500 was shockingly low for anyone, particularly a man of his accomplishments. It was also far, far less than that of Black male industrial workers in defense factories whose salaries, during the war, had risen by 61 percent.[3] In fact, had Thomas worked as a janitor in Baltimore for the federal government in 1946, even without having a high school diploma, his pay would have been substantially higher.[4] Instead, the Hopkins wages paid Thomas, despite the importance of his surgical shock research and his creation of the blue baby surgery, placed his family in an income category *below* the poverty line for a Baltimore family of four.[5]

Thomas had barely spoken his first words of resignation when Blalock began sputtering in surprise and horror. Thomas explained that his family could return to Nashville, where he would earn a lot more money and live in a far better neighborhood than in Baltimore. Thomas always referred to his Nashville place, which had no mortgage, as his "go to hell house. That is to say, you could tell the boss to go to hell, you still had a roof over your head."[6] Blalock was flabbergasted; his knowledge of Thomas's personal life was so scant that he had no idea that the family had kept their Nashville house. Now Thomas confronted him about his statement at Vanderbilt, when he had said that he would pay higher staff salaries if he were a department chief.[7]

Blalock now acted as if he had been betrayed in some way and began his characteristic whine. "Well, Vivien, you're making more money now than anyone here without a degree."[8] Thomas did not know if what Blalock said was true, but he knew Blalock was caught off guard, shocked, even. Thomas cleverly used Blalock's statement to his advantage, explaining that what Blalock had just said was precisely the reason Thomas needed to leave Hopkins and its miserable salary to put his girls through college. He pointed out that on his meager earnings, he couldn't afford to send his daughters to Maryland's Morgan State College, which charged only about forty dollars each semester.

It quickly became clear that compared to the two prior salary disagreements between the two men, this one was the ugliest. Blalock offered another option. If Thomas needed more money, he could take on a *third* job as a sales rep for medical supply companies. Lab tech, bartender, and sales representative. Blalock assured him that Hopkins would buy only from Thomas and would stop its purchasing from the companies' other sales reps. Again, Blalock had identified another way for Thomas to earn money without having to take a penny from the surgery budget. Thomas objected immediately. He knew that the Hopkins commissions amounted to a large proportion of the sales reps' income, and he rejoined that to take other men's jobs from them would be "unconscionable." He would not do this.[9]

In response, Blalock started in on him, lecturing that many of the men he'd be working with in construction wouldn't even have a high school diploma whereas, at Hopkins, Thomas could work with the brightest and best-educated surgeons. Vivien would not be persuaded. He was firm that he was quitting. He made this clear, "I'm not even asking for more money here."[10]

Thomas resigned, offering to stay three more months before leaving. Blalock was so enraged that he could barely speak.

A month later, Blalock called Thomas to offer him a raise so minuscule that Thomas asked if he were joshing. More time passed before Blalock offered a higher salary, but one which did not come close to matching the $3,500 to $4,500 a carpenter could make in bustling Nashville. Thomas turned him down out of hand. Blalock now mocked him, purportedly humorously, telling the talented dog surgeon with extraordinary surgical skills that, after fifteen years away from carpentry, he probably could not hammer a nail straight. He also charged Thomas with trying to force him to violate Hopkins's personnel and pay regulations. An offended Thomas reminded him he hadn't asked for a penny, much less trying to break Hopkins regulations.[11] Thomas walked out.

Of course, Thomas had never been told that his research on blue babies had been partially supported by funds provided by the Robert Garrett Foundation, whose trustees were related to Mary Elizabeth Garrett, the generous woman who was primarily responsible for the medical school.[12] Part of the foundation's generous donation could have been used to supplement his miserly salary if only Blalock had chosen to do so.[13]

Even worse, no one had cared to quantify at any time Thomas's contribution to the financial windfall that the blue baby surgery brought to Hopkins. In 1945, the year that Blalock and Taussig had published the groundbreaking blue baby surgery article detailing the first three operations, the surgery department had taken in $15,223 in private patient fees.[14] That wasn't much. From 1947 through 1952, the annual surgery income from private patient remuneration had risen to between $134,000 and $151,000, close to ten times the money as before.[15] In 1947 to 1948, surgery took in so much money that the surgery department fees equaled

The Everlasting Salary Issue

patient fees from all other Hopkins hospital departments combined.[16] Thomas certainly warranted a livable salary for the money he helped bring to Hopkins. Who could argue with his influence on Hopkins's stratospheric jump in income?

The day before Christmas in 1946, Blalock called Thomas to his office in late afternoon—Hopkins was nearly deserted, most people had already left to celebrate Christmas Eve—and told him that Thomas would receive a small $300 salary increase in January and then a larger one six months later, in July, to raise his salary to $2,500 (currently close to $34,000). Blalock said that Hopkins had agreed to create a new personnel category to increase his wages.[17] Blalock added that this offer was good only through that day. It didn't matter how long Blalock had stalled: now he said that Thomas's decision had to be made immediately, on Christmas Eve.

Thomas was amazed at what he thought was a generous offer, yet he knew that the new salary was still significantly less than a good carpenter could earn in Nashville, or what he could have made as a full time medical supply sales rep in Baltimore. Yet the raise offered Thomas the opportunity of staying in research, which was his passion and the closest he could ever get to his dream of being a physician. Even if no one outside Hopkins would ever know of his spectacular achievements, Thomas derived his own inner satisfaction from his accomplishments. He feared that he might suffocate if he could not continue working in medicine. Thomas considered the salary adjustment to be in-house recognition of the fact that, as he modestly said, he was somewhat of an asset.[18]

Unsure of how to respond and feeling coerced by Blalock's impending deadline, Thomas told Blalock that he wanted a Coke from the soda machine and used this as a respite to ponder the offer. As he swigged down the cold drink in the hallway, he thought on it for a spell and then headed for the nearby public phone.

He called Clara and recounted Blalock's offer. She was quiet, and then she responded in her typical fashion, telling him that it was his choice to make, not hers. Her words reflected the family's values; as Thomas explained, "I had always assumed full responsibility for the welfare of my family."[19]

Now the pressure was back on Thomas. The minutes were passing; in fact, it had already turned dark and the building was quiet. He vacillated for another thirty minutes, then returned to Blalock and told him he'd take the salary and keep his job at Hopkins.

Not willing to let well enough alone, an injured-sounding Blalock snapped back at the thirty-six-year-old man that if Thomas made any other salary "demands"—presumably for the rest of Thomas's life—he'd be out of a job.[20] Blalock also dropped the news that the salary adjustment was promised for eighteen months only and then it might revert to his 1942 salary.

Thomas's cheeks turned hot and again he tensed, telling Blalock that he should have given him these conditions when he first made his offer. With all the calm he could muster, Thomas added, "One thing I would like you to get straight is that I have not made any demands on anyone, not you or the university."[21] With a determined voice, Thomas declared that he would stay at Hopkins only for the eighteen months of the higher salary guarantee. If his salary were then cut, he would give Blalock only a thirty-day notice before leaving, not the three months he had proffered in November. He silently swore that he would never humiliate himself again in front of Blalock by asking for a raise.[22]

Blalock always played his cards close to his vest, maneuvering to keep control of any situation. He ended the conversation about salary, as Thomas described it, "with the smile of a victor."[23] Then the professor gratuitously added, "Maybe we can get some work done now."[24] Thomas turned his back and, as he walked out, he retorted that he had been working the whole time.

"Merry Christmas!" Blalock called out to him.

Thomas, a churchgoer, and the most courteous of Southern gentlemen, did not respond. Instead, he went home and reflected, "He must have had a Merry Christmas, but I wasn't sure I had made the right decision."[25]

CHAPTER TWENTY-FOUR

Hopkins's Greatest Surgeon?

Now that Thomas had agreed to stay on at Hopkins, the demands on his schedule accelerated. His duties became so time-consuming and fraught with pressure that he often joked that he needed a long hospital stay to recover from his deep exhaustion and long hours. Late into the night, five days a week, he'd still be on campus in a deserted lab because Blalock insisted that only he calculate the just-in-time blood tests to determine the oxygen concentration measurement required before morning surgery. The surgery chief couldn't have made his wishes clearer. "I want *your* figures," he said.[1] The calculations Thomas completed by himself; no sophisticated laboratory device to determine blood values yet existed. Thomas was returning home so late at night that he saw his daughters for a short time on the weekends. After all, the professor needed the critical oxygen results to be waiting when he arrived in the early mornings.

In addition to Thomas's never-ending blood work in the lab and his indispensable surgery advice in the operating room, he also counseled blue baby parents. He did this on his own: no one asked him to. Thomas firmly believed that parents would feel less anxious if they understood what the operation entailed. A psychologist whose daughter was a blue baby said, "I remember Thomas as this very kindly, gentle, soothing man.

He described the procedure step by step. He told me exactly what to expect and he made it un-scary. He really did. He created a profound impact and, of course, as an adult psychologist, I know he was way ahead of his time in terms of how to prepare children for something like this."[2]

Thomas was also working with Richard Bing in cardiac studies. One day, Bing was to conduct a cardiac catheterization (a diagnostic test involving a catheter or flexible tube that had to be inserted in the heart) on a child. This would be the very first cardiac catheterization done at Hopkins and both he and Thomas were jittery. As Thomas said, and as Bing has confirmed, "The patient, a four- or five-year-old boy, had been sedated. When we were ready to begin, Dr. Bing suggested I do the cut-down [first incision] saying that I, not he, was a surgeon."[3]

No wonder Thomas grew weary.

Who was the superior surgeon? Was it Alfred Blalock or Vivien Thomas? Hopkins surgeons recognized Thomas's natural talent at the operating table. In fact, in the late 1940s and through the 1950s, when less-experienced Hopkins surgeons began performing these surgeries, they'd call Thomas at his lab to run over to assist them.

Despite his fame as the savior of blue babies, Blalock was an average surgeon, as reflected earlier by his failure to be admitted by Hopkins to its surgical residency program in the 1920s. He knew it and others recognized this shortcoming, too. Blalock had even admitted his lack of smooth technique to Thomas, who remembered, "Only months after coming to Hopkins, before we really had just gotten down to work in the laboratory, he stated in conversation with me that some of the men on the resident staff 'could operate circles' around him."[4]

By now, the clear superiority of Thomas's elegant work was frustrating to Thomas when he painfully watched the surgeon's awkwardness. Sometimes, he said, he wanted to say to his surgery chief, "Move over and let me do that."[5] Blalock also knew that this "fabulous assistant," as Denton Cooley described Thomas, had superior skills.[6] His long and elegant fingers, with his cool ability to stay unruffled, made him a fast and precise surgeon. He was a natural. In fact, Cooley said that Thomas in the late 1940s was the best surgeon in the US.[7] The *Johns Hopkins Magazine* itself

HOPKINS'S GREATEST SURGEON?

referred to Thomas as "the man who may have been Hopkins's greatest surgeon."[8]

More telling than Alfred Blalock's unexceptional surgical skills was that he lacked the emotional maturity that any surgeon, much less the chief of surgery, is expected to demonstrate in the operating room. In contrast to Thomas's patience and level-headedness, Blalock's disturbing emotional mood swings were well remembered by his students and staff. Memoir after memoir recounted Blalock's nervousness and resulting insecurities.

"Emotionally, he was juvenile and had great difficulties mastering himself," said Richard Te Lind, MD.[9] Another surgeon, Henry Bahnson, normally a great fan of Blalock, said, "His number one characteristic was his complaining and his whining. He did not realize that he had a job to do."[10] He called Blalock's "scenes in the operating room occasionally unbearable."[11] When Blalock became frustrated during surgery, he would stamp his feet like a small child. One time, the professor suddenly noticed that the members of his operating team were all inexperienced, having never worked on blue babies before. Ignoring the presence of Vivien Thomas next to his shoulder, Blalock shouted, "Is there anyone here that's ever seen this operation besides me?"[12]

Thomas, possibly for a bit of fun or possibly out of irritation, wrote out a list headed "Famous Blalock O.R. Sayings" that included Blalock's frequently heard complaints, "If you can't help me don't hinder me," and "Can't somebody do something to help me?" and, when something went wrong, "Same operation—we been doing every day for the past six months."[13] When a nurse fainted from heat, Blalock waited until she regained consciousness and then turned to sarcasm, "I'm sorry, I wish I could do that sometime."[14]

Another great difference between the two men was that Thomas had the imagination and dexterity to make anything, whether it was a new surgery clamp or a lamp for his house.[15] His mechanical ability was amazing, sculpting lovely wooden toys for his girls and helping Clara cut heavy fabric and hang it, too, for their living room drapes.[16] Koco Eaton, MD, a young relation of Thomas's who later became a Hopkins surgeon, will never forget spotting Thomas at home, in his backyard, flipping hamburgers with a medical instrument that he'd modified to be the best hamburger turner in the country.[17]

Blalock was Thomas's opposite when it came to mechanical ability and constantly relied on others to assist him with the tasks of daily living. His faithful secretary, Mrs. Grebel, told Leeds, who reported in turn, "He could never do anything. He couldn't open a window. He couldn't turn on the heat. He couldn't adjust the thermostat. He was completely helpless, and she would have to do everything."[18] Of course, part of Blalock's ineptness was purposeful so that he could make others take care of the ordinary chores of daily life and leave him more time to work.

Yet no one can doubt that Alfred Blalock had many notable attributes. He was incomparably top rate at spotting new talent in his students and employees: hiring Thomas was an early example. A good number of his picks went on to head surgery departments at major university hospitals. By the early forties, he had brought to Hopkins such notable future surgeons as William Longmire, Hank Bahnson, David Sabiston, Walter Merrill, C. Rollins Hanlon, and Denton Cooley, who would ultimately conduct 120,000 open-heart surgeries and was viewed as "one of the deities" of cardiac surgeons.[19]

Still, Blalock's stated preference was to choose "good old Southern boys" as Hopkins students, but he also inspired them to do their best, mentoring them and serving as a father figure to some.[20] Walter Merrill, who became chief of staff at Vanderbilt University, found him to be an inspiring and caring teacher and thought that Blalock's "real joy in life" came in working with residents.[21] Blalock continued to look after his students' professional welfare well after they'd left Hopkins and, in turn, many revered him because he was instrumental in making their careers. This behavior, of course, contrasted sharply to his treatment of Thomas, whose goals he never recognized.

However, Blalock was ambitious to a fault and smoothly politic.[22] When Blalock wanted something, he was an astute bargainer, capable of aggressively pursuing his goal. For example, he had been frustrated over what he saw as his relatively low salary since he came to Hopkins in 1941. He saw an opportunity to improve his income in late 1945 when Columbia

University's Physicians and Surgeons medical school approached him to be its surgery chair. When he told Thomas about "their" possible move to New York City, Thomas succinctly retorted that if his family was to move, he would need a salary that permitted him to live in Long Island.[23]

What Blalock could not admit was that he was content to stay just where he was and viewed Columbia's offer as an opportunity to raise his pay at Hopkins, just as he had done at Vanderbilt by leveraging a proffered position at Henry Ford Hospital. Despite his true motives, he wrote Columbia's Dean Willard C. Rappleye, MD, "The more I think of it, the more I am convinced that the thing for me to do is to join you in New York."[24] Then he listed nine changes that he wanted Columbia to make, including raising its salary offer from $30,000 to $36,000 writing, "I might add that they [Hopkins] have offered to raise my salary quite appreciably here if I remain."[25] When Columbia committed to paper, Blalock verbally accepted it but then brought the proffer back to Baltimore.

Leeds remembered, "Dr. Blalock manipulated things—this was Dr. Blalock as a politician, and his character as a politician—he manipulated things and waved this Columbia appointment and threatened to leave and go up to New York, until he got his raise." And Hopkins did raise his pay to $25,000, a 56 percent increase.[26]

Warfield Firor, a Hopkins surgery faculty member, bumped into some P&S surgeons at the Southern Surgical Association meeting. He asked them what had happened to the Blalock proffer. The Columbia doctors denounced Blalock: "He came, looked over our position, and accepted it. Five days later, President Bowman of Johns Hopkins had increased his salary. He [Blalock] resigned [from P&S]." Consequently, Firor said, "The P&S people were very, very upset."[27]

To keep Blalock in Baltimore, Walter Dandy had reached into his wallet, once again, and offered the surgery department a large sum of money to augment Blalock's salary. However, Dandy died unexpectedly before this money was transferred and he'd never updated his will with this bequest. He had a large estate which he divided nearly equally among charities, his children, and his wife, Sadie.

Between her inheritance of only one-quarter of the estate and the taxes due, his widow felt she could not spare the money to increase Blalock's salary. She waited for Blalock to release her from this obligation, but she never heard a word from him. Finally, Mrs. Dandy felt obliged to write Blalock a letter explaining her altered financial status as a widow and her inability to contribute money to Blalock.[28] She must have been humiliated at having to openly explain her finances, but she knew Hopkins was fully capable of paying for his raise.

Blalock, however, with his higher income ensured, was now seeking the crown jewel of recognition and status. He coveted the Nobel medal something fierce and pleaded with his colleagues every year to nominate him for his traumatic shock research, which they did, thirty times in all.[29] The Nobel, though, remained out of his grasp and he was never elected a laureate. That was a great disappointment to him.

Blalock had cynically treated the Columbia offer as just one of his deals, a negotiating strategy for a raise. On the other hand, Thomas assumed that a move to New York might be an opportunity for him. The ever-practical man would rarely allow himself to think "What if?" because it would be far too painful. A shadow must have passed over him, though, when he realized that Columbia would have paid him a higher salary and would be significantly less racially biased than the segregated Hopkins. Any thoughts he might have had of a higher income, a better work environment, and a more pleasant living style for his family were dashed by Blalock's decision to stay at Hopkins, in which Thomas—again—had no say.

CHAPTER TWENTY-FIVE

THEFT AND DECEPTION

The constant blue baby work was wearing Thomas down. After having spent more than a year advising Blalock through more than one hundred blue baby surgeries, Thomas was eager to return to his lab full time and start some new experiments. He was fed up, tired of standing in the operating theater behind the professor. His boredom made his mind wander and then he'd be lost in thought. One time he was wool gathering and failed to catch Blalock's sewing a suture incorrectly. He quickly whispered, "Professor, the suture is going in the wrong direction." Blalock blew up. "Vivien!" the surgeon querulously reprimanded him. "You watch and don't let me put them in wrong!"[1]

Surgeons and physicians from all over the world were coming to Hopkins. The already crowded observation gallery of the operating room was jammed.[2] As Thomas climbed that step stool, already placed to Blalock's side, he must have felt awkward standing there on top, sticking out high up for everyone to see. Still, he was content, knowing that this international audience could see him, a Black man, assisting Hopkins's number one surgeon. The visitors had to acknowledge that he was providing vital assistance to Hopkins's chief of surgery. Yes, his brother Harold was the lead plaintiff who won an important civil rights case that equalized pay for Black and white teachers in Nashville, but Thomas knew that his own work was important; he saw himself as a Black man who could demonstrate to these international physicians what African Americans could accomplish. Maybe his quiet example could alter some people's expectations.

Sometimes, following the surgery, Blalock would bring his most esteemed guests back to the dog lab, and he'd take care to introduce these brilliant pediatricians and surgeons to Thomas, who would go home that night, excited to tell Clara (but only Clara) about whatever big shots he'd met that day. For the rest of his life, Vivien cherished the memories of chatting with the medical greats, including Russell Brock, who was knighted as Lord Brock of Wimbledon a few years later for his surgical accomplishments.

Johns Hopkins Hospital had grabbed the world's attention with the blue baby surgery. While it had successfully concealed Vivien Thomas's role as the operation's creator and surgery coach, it allowed Blalock to fly as high as its iconic Dome. Enjoying his financial awards and jump in status, in 1946, Blalock's ambition led him to tackle another congenital heart problem of newborns, called Transposition of the Great Arteries (TGA). These babies are born with misplaced aorta and pulmonary arteries. The aorta should be connected to the left ventricle but instead it is connected to the right, while the pulmonary artery, which should be connected to the right ventricle, is attached to the left. As a result, their oxygen-deprived blood does not travel to the lungs to pick up additional oxygen, but rather is recirculated throughout the body. Additionally, the oxygenated blood, which should circulate through the body, returns to the lungs.[3]

Consequently, newborns with TGA and those with TOF (blue babies) are both cyanotic, without enough oxygen in their circulating blood. Their skin will have a bluish tinge. In that sense, TGA newborns also could be described as "blue babies." Although a greater number of babies are born with TOF defects (one in 2,500 births) than TGA defects (one in 3,400 births),[4] the TGA babies have a dramatically shorter lifespan and most die in their first six months.[5] Blalock believed that Thomas, who had ameliorated the problems of TOF babies, might also be able to

THEFT AND DECEPTION

enhance oxygenated blood flow in TGA babies to let them live beyond infancy.

Often, babies with TGA have such additional defects as a hole in their hearts' septum (the wall that divides the heart). If there is a hole between the upper chambers of the heart, it is called an atrial septum defect or ASD. If the opening is in the lower chambers of the heart, it is called a ventricular septal defect or VSD. (This is the type of opening that TOF blue babies also exhibit.) Oddly, an opening in the heart's septum is functional in the TGA cyanotic newborns: the gap allows blood to mix, which causes a greater amount of oxygen-rich blood to circulate throughout the oxygen-starved body.

At their first meeting, Thomas and Blalock kicked the idea of this new operation up, down, and around. First, Blalock would talk. Then, as Thomas said, "I'd say what I thought about it. What we were going to do. How should we approach it?"[6]

Blalock and Thomas agreed that Taussig's description of changing the pipes around might be the answer for the TGA newborns, just as it had for the TOF blue babies.

Back in his lab, Thomas began puzzling it out. With typical modesty and, as yet relatively little rancor over his lack of recognition, he had been positive that he would never have a chance to work on any surgery as important or acclaimed as the TOF blue baby operation. What he could not forecast was that he would soon be the creator of another path-finding pediatric cardiac surgery that would lead to a palliative fix for newborns with TGA.

Working with Blalock's suggested methodology, Thomas's initial set of experimental surgeries were aimed at connecting the right pulmonary vein to the nearby right atrium. Discouraged when his first set of experiments failed, he slightly altered his methodology for his second group of surgeries by cutting an oval-shaped incision rather than a straight-line incision and leaving a longer vein. That didn't succeed, either.[7]

Thomas realized that he'd improve his odds with an alternative surgical solution. He talked it over with Blalock, who assured Thomas that he could conjure a means that would bring more oxygen to these sick infants. Still, Blalock hoped to produce a constructive idea and, with this in mind, he would stop by the lab to watch Thomas operate. Unfortunately, the surgery chief came up empty and, again, turned the issue back to his lab assistant.

Starting over, Thomas returned to reexamine the heart specimens of deceased TGA babies. This time, he noticed the atrial septum adjoining the upper right border of the heart was surprisingly thin, and he envisioned that he could surgically remove part of the atrial septum to create an artificial opening in the heart wall, allowing more oxygenated blood to mix to keep the babies alive. In essence, he wanted to create an atrial septum defect. He was hampered, though, by the instruments at hand because none of them let him gain the access to the septum he needed.[8]

With the medical student Rowena Spencer as his assistant, he went rummaging through dusty boxes of old medical instruments, devices that had not been used for years. Thomas's quick eye caught an odd-looking thing with curved cutting jaws and a long-handled shaft. After studying the shaft with its rounded metal blades, he thought that it just might work. As often happens to creative people like Thomas who also had extensive experience, he saw further possibilities: the instrument's rounded shape would allow him to get closer to the heart's atrial septum. First he completed his usual mechanical modifications to improve the curved instrument, which included placing an everyday rubber band around the scissors' shaft to keep them in place.[9]

He used this mysterious contraption for the third series of operations. With this jury-rigged curved instrument, he set out to cut incisions in the heart's wall. Once he'd isolated part of the septum, he saw that he needed a larger surface to make these cuts. Accordingly, he tugged the septal wall with thumb forceps and successfully exposed more of the surface.[10] With his clamps in place, he precisely excised the atrial septum, removing a substantial piece of tissue. Finally, he finished by sewing the "edge of the right atrial incision" to the "edges of the pulmonary vein with the continuous mattress suture."[11] He carefully everted "the edges of the vein" and the atrial wall.[12] After Thomas closed the dog's pericardium with silk sutures, he told Tom Satterfield, who'd assisted him with the dog's anesthesia, that the operation had gone well. Indeed, it had, for the dog survived and was awake and well within thirty minutes.

Still, Thomas remained cautious. Nearly twenty years of experience had taught him that it was possible to leave a seemingly healthy dog in the surgery lab at night, only to return the next morning to find it cold and stiff. This time, when he entered the lab the next morning with his heart beating fast, he quickly looked over toward the cages. The dog was still healthy and healing beautifully.[13]

Giddy with delight, he and Spencer kept his operation hush-hush until he was absolutely sure it was correct. To prove that his surgical technique was valid and reliable, he rushed into completing a half-dozen dog surgeries. He could barely muzzle his joy at this surgical triumph, but wanted so much to surprise Blalock that, once again, he suppressed his emotions.[14]

He patiently waited for one of Blalock's before-lunch lab visits. When the professor finally walked in, Thomas bubbled with excitement about his new surgery, talking so quickly that he wasn't making make much sense. So he grabbed his red and blue pencils and sketched a diagram that demonstrated how the dogs' blood could now mix to gain more oxygen.[15] Blalock cut him off with, "Let's autopsy one."[16] Thomas scurried back to the autopsy room and asked Satterfield to sacrifice one of the dogs, and then he brought its heart and lungs to Blalock.

The professor grabbed some scissors and forceps and opened the heart. Blalock had seen congenital atrium septal defects before, but now he was looking at one that was artificially created by his lab tech. He concentrated, focusing on the heart for about five minutes as he tried to see Thomas's incisions and sutures. By now, Thomas was worrying about the length of time Blalock was taking and he nervously waited for Blalock to speak.

Apparently, the surgery chief couldn't spot the tiny sutures because they were so gracefully sewn. He finally stopped looking and stared, instead, at a fixed spot in the room as he used his fingertips to feel the location of the sutures. His fingers moved slowly, millimeter by millimeter, as he touched the incredible evenness of the healed edges. It appeared as if the septal defect had been formed by nature rather than by a human being: the healed edges of the sutures seemed impossibly smooth. Blalock became quiet for a moment. Then he queried, "Vivien, are you sure you did this?"[17]

Thomas didn't take umbrage but reassured him, showing his dry humor. "Well, yes sir, I'm pretty sure I did."[18] Blalock knew the elegance of Thomas's surgical skills, but now he was awed. He stood there, silent and stunned. Giving him the highest praise he could, Blalock turned to squarely face Thomas. "Well, this looks like something the Lord made," he said.[19]

Augmenting the miraculous atmosphere, he walked over to Thomas's handwritten protocol notes, found an empty space on the first page, and wrote, "This is an operation devised by Vivien."[20] It was the first and only time that Blalock gave full credit to his lab assistant for an entire surgical procedure.

Then Blalock turned and asked Thomas to repeat the surgery for him because he wasn't sure how Thomas had brought it off.[21] The only thing to which he objected was the rubber band that Thomas had ingeniously placed on the improvised instrument, so after his demonstration, he ran the instrument over to the machine shop and had a pressure spring added.

Thomas, without the benefit of assistance from Blalock, knew he was truly responsible for the whole creation of this surgery that would let TGA babies live. Later, he wrote of his entire career saying, "My biggest single contribution was the development of a bloodless method for producing an interatrial septal defect in a search for palliative surgical treatment of the transposition of the aorta and pulmonary artery."[22] Notably, he did not cite his TOF blue baby operation as his most important surgery, although it certainly has been the one that most people identify as his, just as Blalock had wanted to be remembered for the treatment of traumatic shock, which continues to save an uncountable number of people, but instead is known for the TOF blue baby surgery.[23]

It was extremely innovative work; Thomas had created an opening that redirected the course of oxygenated blood and he'd found a way that didn't interrupt the infant's circulation. He did it by himself, alone,

Theft and Deception

without any particularly helpful ideas or magical solution from Blalock when they'd gotten stumped. Perhaps that's why Thomas was taking an unusually proprietary interest in this surgery. He could call it entirely his own.

Thomas's heady sense of triumph was not to last. Soon, Blalock brought one of his surgical fellows, C. Rollins Hanlon, to the lab and asked Thomas to demonstrate the surgery for Hanlon. Thomas remembered, "I had not known of Hanlon or seen him up to this time," but he operated with Hanlon watching.[24]

Afterword, Rollo Hanlon suggested that Thomas should remove more of the septum. Thomas said that it would cause too much bleeding, but he attempted it on his next dog. The blood loss was terrible.[25] Next, Hanlon tinkered around and came up with another modification that was helpful because it resulted in a smoother, easier surface on which to sew the sutures and his idea improved the success rate of the surgery Thomas had invented.[26]

Of course, Blalock, with his eye always on publication, asked Hanlon to borrow Thomas's research notes to rewrite the experiments and outcomes in a medical journal format. In August 1948, the article "Interatrial Septal Defects," which described Thomas's innovative surgery, was published.[27] Thomas was a realist and he assumed that its sole author would be Alfred Blalock; certainly he knew not to anticipate any reference to him in the publication. Yet when he read it, he was smacked sideways when he saw that his work was attributed not just to Blalock, but also to C. Rollins Hanlon, who received credit as the second author. The article even included an image of Thomas's special curved clamp, but there was no mention whatsoever of Thomas, not even in a note.[28]

Thomas had created the surgery, known then and now as the Blalock-Hanlon surgery, before he'd even met Hanlon. Now he knew why Blalock had not asked him to review the article for accuracy, as he'd done so consistently before; Blalock might have anticipated that Thomas might protest the attribution to Hanlon. As angry as he could ever be, Thomas objected to Hanlon's authorship through a cold but precise memo for the record, which he wrote carefully and thoughtfully, beginning: "For the sake of the medical archives, I am giving my account of the production of the atrial septum defect" for the TGA newborns.[29]

No doubt, Blalock preferred that one of his students who had a future—rather than an uncredentialed Black lab tech, who had no prospects, apparently—obtain the benefit of Thomas's achievement. The young surgical men dependent on Blalock delighted in how he called them "his boys," as if they were his sons,[30] but Thomas, once again, remained a caged bird, one longing for freedom but unable to fly.

In January 1950, Blalock and Hanlon again published an article discussing Thomas's atrial defect operation: this time, the publication discussed both Thomas's surgery on dogs and Blalock's use of this surgical approach on TGA children, on whom he'd been operating since 1948. (It also covered Blalock's use of anastomosis techniques to produce a shunt that increased oxygen-rich blood flow, which, in some children, improved chances for survival.) In this publication, "The Surgical Treatment of Complete Transposition of the Aorta and the Pulmonary Artery," Blalock and Hanlon complimented the skills of Miss Olive Berger, who had skillfully anesthetized the fragile children who underwent surgery: once more, the article made no mention of how Thomas had created the dog surgeries and originated the initial atrial septum defect surgery.[31]

Over the years, others have confirmed that the first palliative surgery to treat transposition of the great arteries, called the Blalock-Hanlon surgery, was Thomas's work. In 1987, Clarence Weldon, MD wrote, "Throughout my training years at Hopkins, there had been frequent and persistent rumor that it was Thomas himself who had invented the technique." Added Weldon, "The role played by Vivien Thomas should surprise no one, for in 1946 and 1947, he was possibly the most skilled and experienced cardiac surgeon in the world."[32] Denton Cooley also has weighed in, saying, "The Blalock-Hanlon surgery is entirely the work of Vivien."[33] Dan Nokawama went even further and charged that naming the surgery for Blalock and Hanlon was "an act of academic larceny."[34]

Its significance was described by Marathe and Talwar, who said that Thomas's bloodless surgery was "so totally innovative and so audaciously

Theft and Deception

creative as to constitute an act of surgical genius."[35] Its outcome reinforced that surgery on babies, as well as heart surgery, was feasible and beneficial, verifying to the medical community what they'd learned from the TOF blue baby surgery in 1945. Thereafter, Thomas's work helped lay the foundation for future medical breakthroughs in cardiology and thoracic surgery. Although Thomas's TOF blue baby surgery is still performed in a modified manner, his TGA palliative surgery was a stopgap measure to allow these children to survive. By 1958, a different procedure for TGA children would be introduced and, later, varied surgical techniques were selected, based on individual cardiac defects.[36]

As time passed, Hanlon flew skyward up the professional ladder, eventually leaving Hopkins in 1950 to head surgery at Saint Louis University and later to serve as the president of the American College of Surgeons. Before leaving for the Midwest, Hanlon placed Vivien Thomas's name as the third coauthor of a June 1950 article describing the apparatus that Thomas had created and built for administering positive-pressure anesthesia during his experimental procedures on dogs.[37] This was the first time that Thomas was listed as a coauthor in a scholarly publication. While far from being as an important article as the original Blalock-Hanlon 1948 publication, at least it gave Thomas a little bit of recognition, although certainly not the acknowledgment that he sought and deserved.

Apparently, when Hanlon left for St. Louis, he grabbed the surgery's department's TGA files and took them with him.[38] The purloined material must have included all of Thomas's handwritten notes as well as the page where Blalock had written that the operation was devised by Vivien Thomas. No matter how many times Thomas searched the files, nothing remained that could have established the surgery as his.

To Thomas's lifelong anguish, the credit that rightfully belonged to him was given by Blalock to his one of his protégés. It is known as the Blalock-Hanlon TGA surgery to this day. What should have brought Vivien Thomas great joy would instead bring him only frustration, anger, and misery over the years.

CHAPTER TWENTY-SIX

A Lulu of a Meeting

The plethora of pediatric heart surgery news at Hopkins caught the attention of animal rights activists and they were outraged. What right did surgeons have to experiment on dogs? The animal rights groups pressured the Baltimore city council in 1949 to pass a bill that would prohibit dogs from being used in medical research. The council held a public meeting on using animals for medical research and it was the most turbulent hearing Baltimore had ever held.[1] The usually staid *Washington Post* reported that the meeting "was really a lulu."[2] The reporter's assessment may have been understated.

In modern times, a fresh wave of protest had begun right after World War I, led by people who wanted to mitigate, minimize, or just plain stop the use of animals for research. The most influential of them was William Randolph Hearst, who used his power to "promote an antivivisection agenda" through his newspaper chain.[3] In Baltimore, Hearst's *News-Post* stood against using animals for research while the *Baltimore Sun* took a stance for it, as did the country's burgeoning pharmaceutical corporations.[4]

In the mid-thirties and the decades following, Blalock made a considerable splash when he jumped into the movement for animal research and against anti-vivisectionists, who believe that any surgery on animals, even while using pain-numbing anesthesia, causes distress. He had first taken up this cudgel in 1935 while he and Thomas were at Vanderbilt; it was the year that a bill was introduced in Tennessee's state assembly that would have made it illegal to use animals for research. Vanderbilt's dean of medicine had asked Blalock "to serve as the organizer and chief directing influence in opposition to the anti-vivisection movement in Tennessee."[5] He also wanted him to investigate "the importance of vivisection to scientific experimentation."[6] Blalock was in wholehearted agreement, even though the dean's request distracted him from battling Cannon over the cause of traumatic shock.

Because Thomas had not received any credit for his experimental animal surgeries, he happily remained unidentified by the antivivisectionists who had dogged Blalock for a decade. One complaint voiced loudly was about shock research, particularly the crushing of dogs, which they described as "torture and slow death" without pain relief anesthesia.[7] Here, Vivien Thomas's anonymity protected him for he had firsthand knowledge and could have contradicted the anti-vivisectionists' charge that his canine experiments were conducted without anesthesia.[8] Of course, Hopkins would never have agreed to a Black man as its spokesman, nor would the antivivisectionists have shown him any respect. His presence would have been incendiary.

Those outside the medical community were surprised to learn that publicly owned animal pounds supplied "almost one-third of the nation's medical schools" with lab dogs.[9] The private pounds run by such anti-vivisection organizations as the Society for the Prevention of Cruelty to Animals (SPCA—the US organization is the ASPCA) would not sell stray dogs to medical schools. Instead, they killed them outright. When the pound became crowded with too many stray dogs and cats, the pound master would conduct a mass asphyxiation. Staff would put the animals in large, closed containers and gas them with a straight infusion of carbon monoxide until they suffocated. Most pounds were cramming a dozen or so animals into the same box, which panicked the dogs even before carbon monoxide was pumped in. In Maryland alone, the SPCA in the 1940s had been suffocating about 14,000 stray dogs and cats each year.[10]

Baltimore and Washington, DC, were among the first cities to feel the wrath of the anti-vivisectionists when they learned that the medical schools were outwitting the restrictions imposed on them by protestors. In Baltimore, the city had awarded the contract to collect strays to the local SPCA, which then refused to sell its dogs to such local medical schools as Hopkins or the University of Maryland medical school, also located in Baltimore. Out of necessity, the two schools began to purchase their animals from locations outside the state.[11] This was not a problem only in Maryland: throughout the nation, thirty-four of the country's fifty-four medical schools reported experiencing an experimental lab animal shortfall.[12] The end run by Baltimore's medical schools against the anti-vivisectionists worked for a short time, until the furious opponents realized that these schools were obtaining dogs from a private Pennsylvania pound.

The leader of Hopkins's pushback was Alan Chesney, the dean of its medical school, who was tireless in his efforts to keep animal research viable. His letters to faculty strongly encouraged them to write in protest to council members and to ask ten of their closest friends to do the same. Chesney leapt into action and wrote city council members and members of the city's Board of Estimates, who were tasked with awarding the next city pound contract.[13] No one was against the SPCA managing Baltimore's pounds but Blalock and the physicians wanted the city to amend the wording of the upcoming contract so it would be mandatory for the SPCA to give or sell about 3,000 of its stray animals to medical schools.[14]

On November 16, 1949, Baltimore's legislative committee held its public meeting to hear people's thoughts on animal research before the contract for the city's animal pound was awarded for 1950. There also would be a public referendum on the issue. To accommodate a crowd at the hearing, for animal rights was known to be a controversial subject, it was scheduled for the city's capacious War Memorial Auditorium. Between 3,000 and 4,000 people jammed into the auditorium, most of them already screaming at each other while they were still lined up outside the building.[15] (Earlier animal rights hearings in London had been more violent because each side attacked the other with their umbrellas.[16])

The US military was particularly active in animal research because its goal was improving survival rates for those wounded in war. As a result, many men in uniform were in attendance. The Baltimore protestors recognized the uniformed Gen. James Devereux, who was renowned as battalion leader of the Marines at Wake Island. The Japanese had captured him and made him suffer through four years in a barbaric prison camp. Apparently, that wasn't enough punishment; the animal rights supporters screamed at him, "You should have died!"[17]

The topic was controversial, but no one had expected the hearing to be so rowdy or so acrimonious. Some animal rights supporters held up photos of a medical surgeon holding a hatchet over a dog's head. A cute and friendly looking dog was shown on a poster that read, "Should dogs and cats be cut up for experiment?"[18] A sympathetic former surgeon from Bellevue Hospital in New York claimed that he had witnessed dogs being literally "baked to death" in experiments involving X-rays. One anti-vivisectionist tried to hit a sensitive spot by positing that operating on dogs was "unmanly." Another intoned with *gravitas*, "The eyes of the American people rest on you today for a decision that will decree either death or life for helpless dogs."[19]

Hopkins medical students had been bused in for the hearing but the city council, after taking a good look at them, confined them to the auditorium gallery. Sure enough, the students howled and stamped their feet in derision when anti-vivisectionists held the floor. Several times, the meeting's chairman threatened to muzzle the chaos by clearing the hall.[20]

The protestors heard the physicians identify a litany of diseases and illnesses that had been fought through animal research: shock, diabetes, malaria, meningitis, syphilis, diphtheria, typhoid fever, infections, and smallpox were just some. It was true, they admitted, that research to fight a tropical parasite that caused malaria involved dog deaths. But, the doctors asked, would the protesters have preferred that Marines die, instead? The uniformed men in attendance, who also had been bused to the hearing in strong numbers, out-shouted the decibel level of everyone with their "Ooh-Rahs!" The animal rights supporters remained unmoved by the patriotic assertion that "almost 48,000 American boys" in World War II "owe their lives to medical progress," and, in turn, jeered at the Marines.

Unfortunately, the Pennsylvania supplier of pound animals attended the meeting and had been identified by the protestors. Now it was time for them to show their strength. The SPCA had sworn out a complaint against the supplier and arranged for him to be arrested halfway through the meeting, which only inflamed the ill will on both sides. Chesney put up bail for the man and used his own house for collateral.[21]

Through meticulous scene-setting, Hopkins medical school confronted the animal-rights activists as dramatically as they could without appearing unprofessional.[22] Doctors arrived with children whose lives had been saved by the blue baby surgery and paraded the little ones before the unsympathetic antivivisectionists who cried out to the little ones, "Shame, shame," and "Thou shalt not kill."[23] The blue baby mothers tried to speak—some tearfully and others outright weeping—but it was nearly impossible to hear them through all the pandemonium.

As the TOF children were brought in front to face the antivivisectionists, their doctor asked the audience, "A child's life or a dog's?" He was shouted down by the activists' resounding, "A dog's life!" Even Sister Jessica, a nursing nun and caregiver to institutionalized children at St. Gabriel's Home, was booed as she spoke.[24]

The only Hopkins physician who made a hit with the activists was Helen Taussig. She brought her beloved fluffy black-haired poodle to the front of the hall and told the demonstrators that without the blue baby surgery, her curly-haired dog would have died from congenital heart problems. The activists heartily cheered her and her poodle.

The legislative committee listened intently to testimony from administrators of Baltimore's medical schools, who warned that banning medical research on dogs would result in the city's universities and hospitals being shunned by medical students and physician-researchers. To the relief of the medical community, the city council recommended that the bill to end the use of dogs for medical research should not be adopted.

The *Baltimore Sun* trumpeted the news in its front-page headline: COUNCIL PASSES DOCTORS' DOG BILL. The price boost that Baltimore's US Steel had just announced was relegated to a secondary head, below the dog news.²⁵ In the wake of the council vote, a public referendum was held in Baltimore a few months later, in 1950. The administrators at Hopkins understood the value of good publicity and it paid Stark-Films to produce a short film about Anna, Thomas's favorite dog, that was the first to survive both phases of the crucial blue baby experiments. Anna was Thomas's responsibility, and he was so fond of her that he undoubtedly was her handler during production. *Anna, Her Story*, was produced "on short notice to be aired on local television prior to the Baltimore Dog Referendum."²⁶ Leaving nothing to chance on election day, Hopkins sent its medical students to hand out pamphlets at the polls.²⁷ To the pleasure of Blalock and Thomas, the referendum resulted in 80 percent of Baltimoreans voting in support of using animals for medical research.²⁸

The medical schools had won this round but the public's sensitivity to the treatment of lab animals had been heightened. The debate persisted.

CHAPTER TWENTY-SEVEN

Too Much Southern Comfort

As Thomas and Blalock eased into the 1950s, neither man had a hint that within the decade, a burgeoning civil rights movement would begin to change American lives. Despite Thomas's brother's legal victory for equal pay that invoked change, things remained pretty much the same more than a decade later at Hopkins. The city of Baltimore, though, was creeping forward, centimeter by centimeter, as a coalition of religious and community leaders pushed for improvement in the treatment of African American customers by white owners of local restaurants, hotels, and department stores.[1] Still, in 1952, when Thomas built his family a new pink stucco house on 1113 Springfield Avenue, where he and Clara planted lush flower gardens, vegetable gardens, and fruit trees,[2] he was amazed to learn that no Black men in the city were permitted to be certified as electricians or plumbers.

To commemorate its 1,000th blue baby surgery, Hopkins honored Blalock—but not Taussig—in 1950 by commissioning the Canadian photographer Yousuf Karsh to capture his likeness. Renowned for his creativity in black-and-white photography, Karsh had portrayed such inimitable subjects as Winston Churchill, Pandit Nehru, and Frank Lloyd Wright. The photographer trailed his subject for several days around the medical campus while he pondered the best locations to photograph the physician.³

Finally, in 1975, only twenty-five years after Karsh shot Blalock, Hopkins realized that perhaps it should have a Karsh photo of Taussig, too, and it rehired Karsh. Hopkins will display the two Karsh photos together and one assumes the photos were taken concurrently, which would explain why Taussig, who was one year younger than Blalock, looks so much older than he.

Karsh complained to Thomas that Blalock wanted to take off his glasses for the picture.⁴ The portraitist refused; Karsh's trademark portraits were famous for their realism. The photo that was selected captured Blalock with his glasses in place, gazing forward with a slight smile on his face, his right hand prominently placed holding his cigarette holder and burning cigarette.⁵

On the night before Karsh's departure, the Blalocks threw him a large party and invited everyone associated with the blue baby breakthrough, including Thomas. This time, the lab tech could sit down and slurp Chincoteague oysters on the half shell rather than tending bar, which the Blalocks had declared would be BYOB and self-service. To the best of anyone's knowledge, this was the first time and only time Thomas was invited to a social occasion in a surgeon's home and he finally was able to enjoy the experience of just being another guest. Karsh's photo proofs were passed around and it was Mary Blalock who settled on the ultimate photo of her husband.

Later, Blalock presented a copy of the Karsh photo to Thomas and signed it, "All good wishes to Vivien Thomas, to whom I owe so much."⁶

The *leitmotif* of the 1950s was heavy social drinking. The first to be hit hard was Mary Blalock, who had suffered her husband's years of neglect. Her escape through alcohol had accelerated as a result. She could barely face the day without a drink before breakfast. One surgeon pointed to her main issue: "Blalock must have been a horrible husband, working night and day, never home."⁷ The Blalock marriage, now in its second decade, was noticeably unhappy and sometimes embarrassingly so. Perhaps the liquor loosened her tongue: when she was asked how her husband spent his summers, she replied, "Why, he spends them the way he does his winters—working."[8] This was a slight exaggeration, as she and Blalock took off the entire month of August to spend at Maryland's Eastern Shore on Gibson Island.[9] Still, Denton Cooley, who'd struggled growing up with an alcoholic father, noted, "We used to say Mrs. B. could drink Dr. B. under the table."[10]

Mary was drinking herself sick. Blalock would refer to Mary's health woes to his colleagues at work or in his letters home, but he never mentioned their root cause, alcoholism.[11] It became the elephant in the room, just sitting there in clear view every time he would tell someone that she had been admitted, once again, to the Hopkins hospital. She'd lost so much weight that Bill Longmire wrote of bumping into her, "My, what a shock! She was nothing but a bag of bones."[12] Blalock himself was also drinking heavily, despite his own tottering health.

Thomas, too, was coping with dark moods, still frustrated by his absence of recognition, by his inability to get another research job, by his low pay, by his lack of authentic friendship with the surgeons with whom he worked and by his rejection by his own community due to his Hopkins job.[13] It seemed inevitable that in this soused atmosphere, Thomas would develop a drinking problem. He turned to alcohol for consolation and, given a family history that included a few heavy drinkers, he got hooked but good.[14]

Clara was holding the Thomas household together to compensate for her husband's drinking and did her best to keep arguments out of the girls' hearing. At Clara's firm suggestion, Thomas began to see a psychiatrist. He recognized that Alcoholics Anonymous meetings would also have been helpful but said he was too self-conscious to attend. Still, he was able to stop drinking for a few years, saying, "I got a hold of myself rather than the booze having a hold on me."[15]

Thomas might have been aided in his victory by the gratifying surprise of seeing his name listed as coauthor in the journal *Circulation* in 1951. A young Canadian surgeon, Raymond Heimbecker, MD, submitted an article on reversing capillary circulation and listed Thomas as second author and Blalock as third.[16] This was Thomas's second authorship but it was the first time that Thomas's name was included with the name of Alfred

Blalock—a significant event that chipped away at the barricades in which Blalock had enclosed Thomas. In fact, Thomas confided to Mark Ravitch that one of the things that made him most proud was "After twenty years, I became a co-author with the Professor."[17] Finally, some solid recognition he could use to prove his capabilities and contributions.

Thomas knew, however, that the attribution was Heimbecker's idea and not Blalock's, a difference he attributed "to a Canadian versus American way of thinking."[18] Heimbecker had not been trying to make any social statements; he had naturally assumed Thomas would always have credit on papers where he had created the experiments and instruments.

Thomas kept his authorship credit, in what he called a "highbrow" scholarly journal, to himself. He showed the article only to Clara, believing that mentioning it to friends and neighbors would automatically generate more criticism about his role at Hopkins. He remained unrecognized: at work, no one attributed his breathtaking surgeries to him, and, in the neighborhood, people faulted him for letting Hopkins take advantage of him. His grit and endurance allowed him to move forward, and, in 1957, he was astonished when Morgan State University, which had denied him college credit in the mid-1940s, now asked him to give guest lectures to students in the Department of Biology. He, of course, gracefully accepted their request despite their history. He saw no reason to turn them down and demonstrated his willingness to move on from the past.

Now, with his more visible status, the surgeons who had observed Thomas's talent with animals brought their four-pawed companions to Thomas if their pets needed complicated surgery. They nicknamed him "master of the hounds" and, acknowledging his expertise, joked that Thomas was the "first full time veterinarian at Hopkins."[19] When he could, Thomas worked with such Maryland animal doctors as Harold Burton, DVM who called him "unquestionably the best canine surgeon of the time. His physical dexterity was phenomenal. His fingers were long and elegant, and his hands just followed. He made everything look so simple."[20]

Burton described arriving at the Hopkins lab with a dying St. Bernard, recently struck by a truck, asking that Thomas operate. The dog made it. When it came time to take the dog home, the owner happily forked over $300, which Burton gave to Vivien, who nearly fell on the floor with surprise. Burton explained, "They paid him next to nothing at Hopkins, and there were weeks and months when he had made more from me than he had made from Hopkins."[21]

As these things happen, Thomas's work was gaining unwanted attention from local vets, who griped at a meeting about Thomas operating without a veterinarian's license. Harold Burton came to his defense. "I could see where this was going, so I stood up and said, 'This man is a better surgeon than all of us in the room put together.' That was the end of that!"[22]

Rather than shine credit on Thomas for his exceptional canine surgical skills, in December 1957, Hopkins Hospital literally colluded with several Baltimore newspapers to set up a story that falsely described Blalock operating on a seriously ill dog. The feel-good piece told the readers all about the "world renowned surgeon" who worked for ninety minutes to save the life of Squeaky, a Rottweiler with intestinal injuries or, as another paper said, "mixed-up insides."[23]

In truth, it was Thomas who performed the surgery with Gardner Smith, MD, a surgical fellow, assisting at his side. Thomas recalled, "Dr. Blalock stood by looking over our shoulders until we were near completion of the operation" and then Blalock stepped in so that Hopkins could promote their heart-of-gold surgeon and the benevolent hospital.[24] The news photograph accompanying the story showed Smith, the "laboratory aide" as it identified him, examining poor little Squeaky.[25] Thomas was slighted, never mentioned in the article and certainly not or shown in the photo.

Adding a veneer of credibility to Hopkins's duplicity was the venerable newsmagazine *TIME*, which picked up the carefully crafted story later that month and ran the item as its weekly Medicine column update. Headed "Squeaky in Surgery," the piece gave full credit to "Famed surgeon Alfred Blalock for operating on the dog for 90 minutes at Baltimore's Johns Hopkins Hospital." *TIME* concluded, "The patient did fine."[26]

CHAPTER TWENTY-EIGHT

Power Moves

Even as Vivien Thomas was watching his responsibilities grow, Al Blalock was feeling redundant. He was a man in his fifties and his health, never robust, was failing him. He was losing his edge; he would never again achieve anything as great as his shock research.[1] He lamented to his son Dan Blalock that most people would associate him only with the blue baby operation.[2] With a long face, Blalock suggested to Bill Longmire that he should stop operating, that being a surgeon was better suited to younger men. "His greatest fear," said Longmire, "was that he would get old and start to slip."[3] Blalock echoed the same sentiment to Thomas, who, on the other hand, had just turned forty and was in good health. Nothing was bothering him, and his productivity level reflected this.

Blalock, despite his personal fears, was dead set on keeping cardiac surgery as a highly ranked Hopkins specialty. New developments in heart surgery were racing along and he was nervous that his department was falling behind such other excellent academic research hospitals as Case Western University School of Medicine. As unlikely as it had seemed just a decade earlier, heart surgery was moving fast, applications to enter surgery were snowballing, and people were already thinking beyond palliative closed-heart surgeries to the possibility of corrective open-heart surgery. (In fact, his former student Denton Cooley would be the first surgeon to implant a totally artificial heart in 1969.)

One new quest for Hopkins was to stem a flood of cardiac deaths due to rapid irregular heart contractions. Everyone has certain cells in their hearts that will start an electrical signal moving at rapid speed through the heart. These electrical pathways allow the heart to pump blood to the lungs and through the body's circulation. If these signals are interrupted, and the heart fails to beat, a person will die without intervention.

Blalock had already brought Jerome Kay, MD on board as a surgery fellow to work on cardiac surgery experiments with Thomas. He challenged Kay to find his own specific project within cardiac surgery and Kay, after perusing the research, decided to work on preventing cardiac death during surgery. Most surgeons thought that if a patient went into cardiac arrest while on the operating table, either drugs or other stimuli should be administered.[4] At this time, there was no best solution for keeping a person alive during a heart attack. Although there was a potential role for electrical intervention or for heart massage if a patient seized, the research was slim, and few doctors were aware of interventions that could save a life.

Kay had an idea. Why not, he asked Blalock, enlist the critical expertise of William B. Kouwenhoven, PhD, an electrical engineer teaching in the graduate school at Hopkins? After electricity was captured by Thomas Edison and electric lighting made popular, a neophyte electric lineman would accidentally receive a volt of electricity that made his heart stop. Death followed immediately. New York's Consolidated Edison Electric Company sponsored research to minimize the risk of these catastrophic shocks to electric lineman and the man they sought was Kouwenhoven. Before meeting Blalock, he had already made seminal contributions to the field.

Kouwenhoven knew that an additional jolt of electricity, even a low voltage, could get the heart going again. Kouwenhoven's experience pushed the cardiac medical group's work forward in what would be techniques of electric countershock and heart-lung resuscitation. Although he was already sixty-four years old, he was soon receiving research funds from the manufacturers of the latest invention, television, who feared electrocution of their novice TV repairmen. Also, as the number of surgical operations soared in the fifties, so did heart attacks during surgery, and Hopkins and other hospitals also would benefit from some type of mechanism that would reverse a heart that stopped during surgery by administering an electric jolt.

The first research team working on cardiac arrest in 1950 and 1951 at Hopkins included Kay, Kouwenhoven, Thomas, and G. Guy Knickerbocker, who was an engineering student at Hopkins working toward his PhD. With the help of Kouwenhoven, Kay and Thomas put together a mighty odd-looking, patched-together electrical defibrillation unit (a closed chest defibrillator) that could restore a heartbeat with an additional electrical shock (countershock). Even Thomas would describe it as "essentially a collection of [four metal] parts" built on a sheet of wood, with two electrodes attached.[5]

One day, Thomas and Kay were operating on a dog that went into cardiac arrest. The experimental defibrillator was nowhere around, so Kay began massaging the dog's heart to keep it alive while Thomas ran downstairs to grab the defibrillator and climbed the stairs to bring it up to the lab. After three or four minutes of Kay's massaging the dog's heart, Thomas had set up the unsophisticated but effective defibrillator. It shocked the dog and the animal survived. Neither man had the opportunity to build on their work because Blalock reassigned them to other functions, Kay to the hospital staff as assistant resident and Thomas to different research.

Kouwenhoven and Knickerbocker continued working on a remedy for cardiac arrest with the assistance of James R. Jude, MD, an assistant resident. These three men persisted with the experiments on the heart message technique and showed that massage could raise a dog's blood pressure just enough to keep its blood circulation flowing, which was vital to surviving cardiac arrest. This technique became known as CPR.

Later, however, Knickerbocker would unknowingly assume that he was the first to massage a dog's heart and apply defibrillation, rather than Kay and Thomas, and he received credit.[6] Because Thomas and Kay were pulled off this research, the three who continued are the ones known as the "Fathers of CPR," Kouwenhoven, Knickerbocker, and James R. Jude. As Kay later wrote Thomas, "Others received the credit, but it was Dr.

Kouwenhoven, you and I who accomplished this. This was the beginning of closed heart massage and external defibrillation."[7]

When surgeon Mark Ravitch, who was then working at Mount Sinai Hospital in Manhattan, learned of Thomas's role, he noted, "You and Kay, in fact, had been doing closed cardiac massage in the laboratory several years before Guy Knickerbocker came upon it independently. That's a real eye-opener."[8] An eye-opener for sure, but one of those for which Thomas and Kay received minimal recognition although Kouwenhoven gave credit to Thomas for making those "closed chest defibrillators."[9]

Thomas, with Kay, had also been doing some other cardiac assignments relating to babies and others with congenital heart defects. They worked on new discoveries concerning septal defects (openings in the heart), pulmonary stenosis (obstruction of blood flow to the lungs), and hypotrophy (thickening of the heart muscle). In quick succession, Thomas was made coauthor on three more scientific papers for this work with Kay: one in *Surgery, Gynecology and Obstetrics* in 1953,[10] and two articles in 1954 in *Archives of Surgery*.[11] However, Blalock himself never included Thomas's name with his own.

Thomas had been so touched by Kay putting his name as coauthor on these articles that he wrote him, "I don't know what it took, integrity, audacity, or just plain guts to submit manuscripts to the Professor with his name as coauthor. You will have noted that of all the other fellows who came through the lab, none of the others did [except Heimbecker].

"Even if no recognition had ever come, I would feel forever grateful to you that you did have whatever it took, that is something that I really can't describe."[12]

That same year, Vivien Thomas's name, if only his first name, became known to the public for the first time when the AMA awarded its Gold Medal Distinguished Service Award to Blalock. The AMA was spurred to write a fictionalized radio script that had aired about the first blue baby surgery. It included a mention of "Vivien," without a last name.[13] This was the very first time the public learned that someone named "Vivien" had played a role in that seminal surgery. His name was mentioned so quickly, though, that no one followed up on who "Vivien" was or what he had accomplished.

At Hopkins, Thomas was becoming revered by medical students for both his surgical skills and his graciousness, which insulated him against overt racism by these mostly Southern surgical students. Despite his rising status in the lab, however, a few of the established surgeons and physicians on campus felt free to use their racist sense of humor to humiliate him.

His younger daughter, Theodosia, was visiting her father at work one time and as they walked outside the buildings, one of the physicians called out, loudly. "If you want a woman who is a little older, I can show you where to go," he said to the father in front of his teen daughter. Then the doctor laughed at his own humor and at the father and daughter's discomfort. Theodosia, like any sensitive teenage girl, was deeply embarrassed and looked down at the ground. Her father, however, was used to putting on an emotional mask at work. "How he kept his temper," Theodosia said, "I'll never know.

"But he just kept walking and pretended that he hadn't heard anything. I wondered, 'How can he keep himself under such tight control?'"[14] Undoubtedly, he knew that complaining would accomplish little.

As head of lab personnel by now, Thomas's greatest hurdle in hiring and retaining lab assistants, he said, was Hopkins's "ridiculously low pay scale" for lab workers.[15] Neither Blalock "nor the institution seemed to realize that you get the quality personnel you are willing to pay for."[16] Thomas was concerned with more than their work quality; he also cared about the staff's personal goals and often recommended them for higher-paying positions at other hospitals. He kept hoping that their departure would spur Blalock to raise salaries.[17]

Thomas made himself adept at finding talent among the African American staff whom Hopkins had placed in low-ranking jobs. He trained, for example, one of the hospital's elevator operators in lab techniques and then promoted him to the lab. Blalock gave Thomas a high level of independence to make these lab personnel decisions. As Blalock put it, do it "any way you want to. I have enough problems of my own."[18]

Julius Mayo, for instance, was a Black operating room orderly who had been, according to Thomas, "forced to leave" the hospital after he voiced his displeasure at being barred from the orderly locker room and washroom because Hopkins had designated it for whites only. (There was no washroom designated for Black orderlies.) Hopkins fired Mayo when he refused to descend to the basement's "colored" facilities meant for Black people of all ranks.

Thomas hired him for a lab spot and told him he could use the lab bathroom just as Thomas did, even though it was designated for white workers. Mayo became so proficient that when he took a position at another hospital, even Blalock noticed his absence. Thomas felt some pleasure in telling the professor that he had left for a better salary.[19]

On his own initiative and without formal permission, Thomas began a summer program for Black Baltimore high school students who were interested in science careers, and he worked with the high schools to identify those who would benefit. Blalock, when he learned this, did not cancel Thomas's new and very different program. Thomas was delighted and proud when two of his former high school student-employees graduated from college and ultimately became physicians. He himself didn't make it but he did his best to make sure that a younger generation could. That was his way.

CHAPTER TWENTY-NINE

THE HEADACHE MAN

For most of the country, the 1950s were fantastic boom years: the economy was bustling like never before and the future looked golden. For Vivien Thomas, the times were not so good. With Blalock's grudging support, he had gained a better salary a few years earlier, but it still wasn't enough to put his family solidly in the middle class. It wasn't that Blalock begrudged him earning more, but rather that the surgery chief didn't want any more of his wages come out of his departmental budget. To this end, Blalock was helpful giving Thomas ideas for outside income, but he also made it clear "that he didn't necessarily want to know about other employment" once Thomas started his extra jobs.[1]

Seeking part-time employment as a salesman, Thomas approached a local medical supply company that had never been successful capturing Hopkins Medicine as a client. He was quickly rebuffed because he was Black. "This attitude was a sad state of affairs," Thomas remembered, "but unfortunately it was common at the time."[2] He decided to fight back a few years later, when one of the company's white salesmen visited him in his lab. He patiently allowed the salesman to pitch his products and even encouraged him by asking questions. Finally, he told him that he wouldn't be ordering anything from the company because of its refusal to hire Black salespeople. In his understated way, told the salesman to tell "his boss to be careful of what they say to people."[3]

When Thomas was new to Baltimore and wanted a physician, he naturally asked Blalock. The surgeon's response was immediate: Ralph J. Young, he said, who he declared to be "the best doctor in town, colored or white."[4] Thomas and Young soon developed a warm friendship and, through Young, Thomas learned that he could become a "detail man" for a local small pharmaceutical company. He could work part-time as his Hopkins schedule allowed, making cold calls to Black physicians in Baltimore to introduce new products. As he went about his visits, the physicians he met were surprised by his knowledge of medicine: his successful presentations brought the company greater profits. Thomas was pleased that after seeing his sales records, the company decided to hire more Black detail men.[5] Again, he was utilizing his philosophy of setting a good example rather than one of confrontation. Thomas ran into doctors who queried him, as he said, "Couldn't Hopkins pay me for what I did?"[6] When they realized the paucity of his salary, they soon offered him a full time job at a higher pay rate than Hopkins. He felt he had to turn them down: he had promised Blalock that he'd stay at Hopkins if he received a raise, and he was a man of his word.

Thomas also reproduced his new surgical devices for other hospitals, with Blalock's permission. A self-starter, Thomas sold, without advertising and solely through word-of-mouth, 125 positive pressure anesthesia machines for $139 each that he'd manufactured. A few years later, he'd would be billing hospitals $250 for each external defibrillator unit he'd built. He made the devices in his home basement and he set his younger daughter, Theodosia, to work with him in a two-person assembly line.[7] The reasonable prices of his equipment were a bargain to the hospitals: one industrial sales rep told him that he should be charging five times as much. Thomas kept a third of the profits for himself and the rest went back to Hopkins. In 1954, he was earning $400 from his machines. The extra money he made from his inventions was a significant boost and he duly reported his extra income to the IRS.[8]

Even after he made a sale, Thomas helped surgeons with their questions; he responded to one physician who'd written him about an unexpected outcome with one of his defibrillators, "The case you mentioned was quite interesting," Thomas answered. "With padded and saline-soaked electrodes, you would have not gotten the searing of the myocardium as there would have been better contact."[9] This from a man who was earning the current equivalent salary of a worker whose most frequent question is, "Do you want fries with that?"[10]

In an interview, Thomas was asked why he never patented any of his inventions. He emphatically responded, "I never, never even thought about it."[11] His daughter Theodosia had asked him the same question and "He said that he would never make money on an instrument that saved lives."[12]

There were many other occasions when Thomas exercised amazing self-restraint and generosity of spirit. By this time, Blalock had given Thomas free hand in purchasing all lab supplies. As a result, Thomas often came upon medical supplies salesmen wandering around the lab, hoping to pitch their products to "Mr. Thomas," all the while looking past him as they sought a white man. Sometimes, if a salesman brusquely barked at Thomas, "Where's your boss?" Thomas would give them a good-natured runaround. He'd send them to Blalock's office, where Mrs. Grebel would tell them promptly to return to the lab. In the end, Thomas decided to stop his teasing.[13] Thomas excused them with his usual graciousness, "Certainly, an African American man at Hopkins could not have purchasing authority."[14]

Thomas, by now, had his own private office in the lab complete with a coat closet and he supervised the other lab workers. "He was in his own world on the lab floor," said one surgeon. "He had created his own world."[15] A world that he kept safely apart from the hostile stares and condescending demeanor of many Hopkins surgeons and physicians.

Despite the increasing acknowledgment of his work, Thomas was still chained to Blalock, and he did not foresee any other medical research job options for himself outside of Hopkins. He had good reason to be gloomy about his lack of prospects. In 1953, he visited A. Glenn Morrow, MD, a former Blalock and Thomas student who was now chief of surgery at the National Heart Institute at the National Institutes of Health (NIH), which is located in Bethesda, Maryland, about an hour away from Baltimore.[16] Having heard that Morrow was looking for a surgical lab tech, Thomas hoped that he might be able to finally leave Hopkins. A job at

NIH would allow him to escape his oppressive Hopkins surroundings in addition to getting a great leap in pay as a federal government employee.

Morrow, though, to Thomas's dismay, refused to hire Thomas. The NIH heart surgeon unabashedly admitted that he would not offer him the job because, as Thomas related, "even though his relations with the professor were extremely good, he knew all that would change if I went with him, that his career would end before it had even a chance to begin. He preferred this not happen to him."[17]

How far Vivien Thomas could rise and even control his own professional life apparently relied on his strange ancillary relationship with Alfred Blalock, whose power was so great that, even unknowingly, it locked Thomas out from any future independent of him. Still, it wasn't within Thomas to hold a grudge; when Morrow called to say he'd hired a new lab worker and could he send this man, Alfred Casper, to Hopkins for a few days so that Thomas could train him, Thomas agreed.[18] Later, he noticed that on research articles that came from NIH's Heart Institute, Casper's name appeared as second author, with Morrow's name given first. Thomas surely realized that working at NIH would have given him the recognition than Hopkins never did.

A story traveled through Hopkins about how Caspar was later working on a project with a young Alex Haller when Caspar congratulated him on his surgical skills. Haller boasted, "I trained with Dr. Blalock." Then Haller returned the compliment, commenting on Caspar's surgical skills. With a twinkle in his eye, Caspar explained, "Well, I trained with Vivien."[19]

Thomas's creativity helped him excel at solving problems in the lab or in his other jobs. "I am the headache man," he later described himself. "Anyone who has a headache brings it to me."[20]

One headache for sure was that 1915 Hunterian doghouse, which was embarrassingly outdated. When Hopkins approved a new surgery building, Thomas, on Blalock's orders, stopped his research for three months to work with a Hopkins architect and engineer on a state-of-the-art dog lab, which included flying to the Mayo Clinic and the University of

Chicago to look at their labs.[21] In 1955, the dog lab moved into the new surgical building later named for Alfred Blalock.

As the more typical workdays resumed, more than 95 percent of the second- or third-year medical students took a hands-on class in operative animal surgery. The lab surgery lessons were taught by two medical school instructors and Thomas, although he was not recognized by Hopkins as an instructor: he received neither the title of instructor nor instructor pay. The new lab that he'd planned had the capacity to run as many as eight surgeries at a time and sometimes supervision ran thin. When Thomas was overseeing a team of students, he put his gloves on only when they had gotten themselves into real trouble.

A good proportion of medical students, said Alex Haller—and here he included himself—"were surprised to be taught by a Black man, particularly those from the South who had never seen a Black man in that type of position."[22] Haller defined Thomas's special talent as a teacher when he revealed Thomas's secret: he could break complicated surgical operations into little steps for the students. "In that way, you could teach it to anybody—even me," he joked,[23] additionally ranking Thomas as a vitally important part of the teaching of cardiac surgery at Johns Hopkins. The super-surgeon Denton Cooley remarked, "Even if you'd never seen surgery before, you could do it because Vivien made it look so simple."[24] Lazar Greenfield, MD emphasized that he asked Thomas to call him by his first name (one of very few surgeons who did) and spoke of his character, "He was very special, revered in the lab, so gracious and such a good surgeon."[25] Rowena Spencer, the only female surgeon that Blalock trained, went even further: "Many times in my career, I was complimented about my surgical technique, and I will admit that a good many people were shocked when I told them that I learned surgical technique from a Black man who had a high school education only."[26]

CHAPTER THIRTY

BLALOCK'S NADIR

Alfred Blalock was ill, and no one knew why. He had fever and pain so persistent that he was repeatedly admitted to the hospital, but even the Hopkins physicians couldn't understand their causes. Anything that hit him seemed to be enhanced: a respiratory infection hung on for four weeks, leaving him first burning with a fever and then shaking with cold.[1] There were also little problems here and there—a red swollen polyp that had to be removed from his sinus cavity and an ulcer on his cornea—but nothing that explained the constant sickness.[2] He suffered from frequent recurring urinary tract infections.[3] He was also bothered by a large hernia but waited until 1956 to have it removed because he hated to stop working, even when it was for his own good. Yet he was beginning to miss medical meetings or appear at them weaving drunkenly in the mornings.[4] Longmire, his admirer, realized, "He thrives on crises and often has periods of deep but not pathological despair."[5]

Some of the crises seemed to be of his own making. He always seemed to be in the midst of constant arguments and disruptive feuds, with one surgeon commenting, "His lust for power in the affairs of the medical school became excessive and he could not tolerate an opinion contrary to his own."[6] He faced off with the hospital's anesthesiologists, arguing that during an operation the surgeon should have complete decision-making power. He managed to completely alienate the anesthesiology staff to the point that some left Hopkins rather than work with him.[7]

Depending on how much he'd had to drink, he would make abusive late-night calls to his residents, staff, and even to Hopkins administrators. The next day, he'd remember his behavior and make it a habit to call or visit his latest victim, acting as if nothing had happened and turning on his Southern charm. It upset the young residents terribly because they were never sure whether they were talking to Dr. Jekyll or Mr. Hyde. Vivien Thomas was used to his mercurial moods and noted of the professor, "The battle of the booze, it really took its toll."[8] In short, Alfred Blalock was no longer Hopkins's golden boy, and he knew this, and became more embittered.[9]

Thomas had known Alfred Blalock longer than nearly anyone else at Hopkins and could read him well. He described him as polite, soft-spoken, and congenial, even charming, "in most normal circumstances."[10] Insisting always they were never friends, Thomas said they'd chiseled out a generally functional professional relationship. "Neither of us went too far out of our way to do favors for each other, it was almost strictly business."[11] Yet they'd have disagreements at work, with Blalock screaming at Thomas, "Why can't you try it my way for once?" Another time when they were arguing, Blalock told him, "What's was wrong with you is that you drink too damn much."

Thomas responded sharply, "Look who's talking."[12]

Nor was Blalock helped by the extent of his wife's insobriety. Mary was in and out of the hospital even more than her husband. In 1958, Al detailed her continuing ill health in his letters to his mother. In February, he said, Mary was back in Hopkins hospital for surgery on an intestinal obstruction.[13] In April, she returned because of "a bout of bleeding" from esophageal varices.[14] In November, Blalock wrote, "Mary is in the hospital again and is rather ill."[15] In December, he thanked his mother for sending Mary flowers and said, "I am afraid it will be quite a while before she is able to leave this hospital."[16] No one would address her alcoholism, the root cause of her health woes.

Mary, in perhaps a last-ditch effort to get hold of herself, told her husband that she was unhappy being alone much of the time in the Blalocks' large house, now that their older two children were adults and Dan was away at school. According to a letter Blalock wrote to his mother in 1957, Mary wanted to sell the Guilford place and buy a cottage on peaceful Gibson Island.[17] He understandingly balked and procrastinated for a year because the move would mean a good extra hour's commute to Baltimore.

Blalock was in Los Angeles the following year with Bill Longmire when Mary phoned him. After the call ended, he turned to Longmire and, obviously soliciting his sympathy, said that Mary, without telling him and without his knowledge, had sold the house in Guilford. Of course, this went beyond exaggeration as he not only had full knowledge of the upcoming sale but the house couldn't have been sold without his signature. He received the empathy he'd sought: Longmire appeared shocked and appalled. In his diary Longmire wrote, "My heart went out to him."[18]

The couple did move, but it was too late to do any good. Mary died of cirrhosis of the liver on December 13, 1958. She was only forty-nine years old, with her youngest child still in high school. Blalock, already struggling with his own addiction to alcohol, was distraught. A few days later, returning to work, he was so unsteady on his feet that he had to firmly grasp the stair railing, hand over hand, to pull himself up each step to get into the hospital, observed Jack Zimmerman, MD.[19]

With his wife's death, Blalock found himself on the rocks. Longmire reported, "He spoke of being lonesome and of how much he missed Mary; he was drinking heavily."[20] His alcoholism was widely known. The booze had control of him. Blalock even admitted to Longmire, "I have just got to get ahold of myself. I am afraid of what's in the bottle."[21]

Within six months, Blalock—a man who was incapable of dealing with matters both practical and emotional—remarried. His new wife was Alice Waters, a widow who had been a good friend of Mary's. The marriage reduced his loneliness, but not, sadly, his need for liquor. Thomas was worried about Blalock's alcoholism and felt compelled to help him out. Deciding that he needed to speak to Blalock outside the Hopkins campus, Thomas traveled uninvited and unannounced to the Gibson Island house to deal out some straight talk. This is how far Vivien had come: by now, he was unafraid of speaking his mind.

That weekend, Thomas arrived on Saturday morning around eleven. Blalock's wife told him Al was still in bed. Around noon, Blalock shuffled downstairs in his robe, unkempt and unshaven. Vivien laid it out straight. People were talking about his drinking, not just at Hopkins but also other surgery departments throughout the country. He had to change. Then he generously shared his experiences visiting a psychiatrist and begged him to get help.[22]

Blalock didn't want to hear it, possibly from Vivien Thomas, of all people.

CHAPTER THIRTY-ONE

BETRAYAL AT THE SOUTHERN HOTEL

It was early 1960 and in most communities in Baltimore, people were talking about the cataclysmic events taking place in the South, as they watched evening news clips on national television narrated by broadcasters David Brinkley or Walter Cronkite. Just a few years before, the Little Rock Nine had defied Governor Orval Faubus of Arkansas and entered Central High School under the protection of federal troops and the National Guard.

In February, four college students in Greensboro, North Carolina, had held the first civil rights lunch counter sit-in as a protest against segregation. Sit-ins flashed throughout the South with mercurial speed in Nashville, Richmond, Houston, and Atlanta. Other civil disobedience protests followed and, just as fast, the targeted restaurants and stores hastily desegregated. In Nashville, Pearl High School students were permitted to go to the local demonstration at Woolworth's and Fifth Avenue, escorted by a sympathetic teacher for the teenagers' own safety. That teacher happened to be Vivien's sister-in-law, Ootsie (Lillian) Dunn Thomas, his brother Harold's second wife.[1]

Race discrimination was an easy topic to ignore in Baltimore, where institutional racism prevailed through the fifties as if encased in amber. The same conditions created both: tremendous pressure and high heat.

The exhausted surgeons were focused on their work and professional standing. Nearly all the surgeons working at Hopkins hospital and medical school were basically unconcerned and uninterested in the nation's civil rights struggles. Lazar Greenfield, who was at Hopkins during the crucial years of 1961–1966, said that he "had never heard civil rights discussed at Hopkins."[2] That Blalock was their chief pretty much guaranteed that they remained untouched by any social movement, especially this one. Levi Watkins, who would study medicine there, remembered, "Some of the good ol' boys at Hopkins were flat-out racists."[3]

What the surgeons, though, were anticipating was the upcoming April 2 celebration of Alfred Blalock's sixtieth birthday. Hospital staff chattered about the hundreds of prominent physicians from around the world who were expected to attend. The party was to have been held the year before, in 1959, when Blalock had turned sixty, but it was postponed when Mary died.

The tribute dinner was said to be a surprise, but its planners consulted Blalock on every important decision. The organizers were all Blalock's former students, two of whom were local: David Sabiston, the only member who was currently working at Hopkins, and A. Glenn Morrow, the NIH cardiac director who'd refused to hire Thomas for fear of Blalock's retaliation. The remaining members, Henry Bahnson and Mark Ravitch, were coming in from out of town. In reality, Blalock was an unofficial fifth member of the committee, who had the last say on who would be included in the guest list and who would not be invited.[4]

Vivien Thomas was aware of who was attending: "The guest list included all of [Blalock's] former residents, his professional friends and associates from throughout the US and foreign countries, doctors who had spent fellowships on his clinical service and in the laboratory, old school ties, personal friends, the Johns Hopkins professional and operating room staffs down in rank to scrub nurse staff, and, of course, his family."[5] There were nearly 400 people in all.[6]

As the preparations intensified and the date grew nearer, Thomas wondered if he would receive an invitation. Although it seemed impossible for the organizers not to include Vivien Thomas among the invited, he tried to put the entire situation out of his mind and not dwell on it.

With the dinner date growing closer, Thomas realized that he and Mrs. Thomas were not going to be asked to join. He initially thought, "It would not be the first time that I had been left out and surely would not be the last."[7] If things had been left as they were, Thomas would have given the incident little thought; it would be just one more slight to endure as a Black staff member at Hopkins.

The dinner was to be held at the aptly named Southern Hotel, Baltimore's most exclusive hotel. The site it stood on had been at the intersection of Light and East Redwood streets (the latter known as German Street until World War I) and had been continuously used for lodging since colonial days. During the War for Independence, George Washington and his staff stayed at its Fountain Inn and, during the War of 1812, Francis Scott Key repaired there to finish the poem that became the lyrics of the national anthem, "The Star-Spangled Banner."

When the Southern hotel opened in 1918 in the financial center, it boasted of its fourteen floors and 400 rooms, and its "girl" elevator operators. The building was buff brick on the outside and displayed gilt filigreed walls within. Tradition was paramount here. The dining rooms offered such local fare as Maryland fried chicken, blue crabs, oysters, baked ham stuffed with greens, Smith Island cake (ten thin-sliced layers of yellow cake frosted with chocolate icing between the layers and on the top and side), Lady Baltimore Cake (a white cake with boiled white meringue frosting, liberally sprinkled with nuts and dried fruit), and Lord Baltimore cake, the same as the Lady but with egg yolks added to the batter for a yellow color. These cholesterol-high meals were served on china printed with the hotel's name and its fabricated coat of arms.

White Baltimore quickly nicknamed the swank Southern, "The Queen of Light Street." Black Baltimore, however, called it less endearing terms. Its record of race discrimination was infamous; Black residents would prefer to cross the street in heavy rain rather than walk directly past the Southern because both its white and its Black doormen would harass and insult anyone passing by who was not white.[8] Despite the Southern Hotel's hateful reputation among the Black community and civil rights advocates, the committee and the sponsoring Hopkins medical school did not hesitate to choose its grand ballroom for the Blalock dinner.

By the late fifties, all Baltimore hotels had opened their dining facilities to African Americans. Some hotels and dining rooms were completely integrated while other hotels initially allowed Black guests to dine only with greater numbers of white people. The Southern Hotel allowed this mixed, if unequal, seating to appease the conventions that came to Baltimore for conferences or sporting events; otherwise, these organizations would have chosen a different city. However, by 1960, all hotel dining rooms in Baltimore except for the Southern had already progressed to accepting a guest of any race regardless of the dining room's racial balance. The Southern hotel was the only one that still required Black guests to dine only in a group constituted of a majority of white people.[9] Still, nothing about the Southern Hotel self-imposed segregation policies would have prohibited the Thomases from attending the large Blalock celebration dinner as no other Black guests had been invited.

The four committee members—Sabiston, Morrow, Bahnson, and Ravitch—scanned the names of final invited guests and noticed the obvious absence of Mr. and Mrs. Vivien Thomas. They wondered if this was a purposeful omission or whether Blalock would want Thomas to be at the party. Hoping against hope that the Thomases had been accidentally excluded, they were still nervous about raising the topic to Blalock. They were aware of Blalock's background, his feelings about race and his support of segregation, and they accepted these attitudes without question. The men chose Sabiston to take on the unenviable job of approaching Blalock because he was one of his closest colleagues.

Sabiston went off to speak to Blalock, optimistic that Thomas's exclusion was an oversight. No such luck. Blalock, despite the flourishing and ever-widening civil rights movement, was still a son of the Old South. (A few years later, Blalock suggested that his niece's newborn daughter be named "Tara," after the name of Scarlett O'Hara's plantation.) He immediately responded to Sabiston's query by refusing to invite the Thomases; his words, as repeated by Sabiston to Ravitch, were that inviting Blacks to dine with whites was "simply something that isn't done."[10]

When Sabiston reported back, the committee was left with a conundrum. "In point of fact," said Ravitch, "we wanted Vivien there."[11] Ravitch even wrote a note about this for the record and appended it to a copy of the dinner's printed program.[12] In any case, they sent Sabiston back a second time in quest of a reversal. Of course, if they had been more open or sincere about their desire to have Thomas present, they would have shared their thoughts with Blalock. None of the men would speak out on the racial injustice toward the one man who had been essential to Blalock's successful career and, also, to their own. Particularly not Sabiston, who was taking great care not to offend Blalock in any way, as he hoped that the professor, so close to retirement, would endorse him as his successor.

There could be no doubt that this was an occasion sponsored by Hopkins. Its plans were typed on Johns Hopkins Hospital letterhead by Blalock's faithful secretary while she was at work. All the dinner guests were invited to a day-long symposium held at Hopkins's medical campus and, at the dinner, the Johns Hopkins Hospital Board of Trustees was to award Blalock with the Johns Hopkins University Distinguished Service medal.[13] Still, it would be another four years before Hopkins's exclusion of Thomas would become illegal under federal employment law and so it was free to continue its long history of discrimination.

Once the four surgeons were convinced that Blalock was immovable in his refusal to seat Mr. and Mrs. Thomas for reasons of race, they tried to circumvent this sorry state of affairs. The men decided that the thing to do was for Thomas to sneak into the hotel and hide where he could watch the dinner proceedings without Blalock's knowledge. This, for the four men, would be the best of both worlds; he could be present but hidden. They thought Vivien should duck behind the potted palms and the curtains in the rear of the ballroom. As for Blalock, their plan was that he would never know that Thomas was present if he could not see him.

This time, the committee sent Hank Bahnson to deliver its last-minute proposal to Thomas.[14] As Thomas sarcastically said, he received "a special invitation" to the dinner.[15] Bahnson waited to visit Thomas in the lab until the day before the festivities, on Friday, April 1—certainly it became April Fool's Day for Thomas—and told him that the reason he had not been invited was because the Southern Hotel *would not let him* sit at a dining room table. Bahnson, who throughout his life touted his strong morals and his Moravian Christian upbringing in Winston-Salem, North Carolina, blatantly lied to Thomas.

Bahnson wrongly assumed that Thomas would not know any better and would therefore just accept his fabrication. What Bahnson and most white Baltimoreans did not grasp, or care to concern themselves with, was that Black residents in Baltimore were far more attuned to the nuances of racism in their city then its white residents, who had no need to learn Baltimore's twisted byways.

As Bahnson talked, Thomas began to steam. The oblivious Bahnson chattered away, claiming that the Southern hotel had generously *allowed* Hopkins to offer Thomas a separate arrangement. Thomas was appalled but initially suppressed his anger at "this most gracious back door invitation" as he sarcastically called it. Thomas tried to keep his cool.[16]

The surgeon began detailing how the committee were going to sneak Thomas into the Southern without anyone knowing by pretending that he was a valet of one of the guests. Then he'd be taken through the kitchen to the back ballroom and hidden so that he could peek out from among its decorative palms. From there, he could watch the guests dining on fresh prawns with cream sauce, consommé bouillon, and broiled filet mignon of beef served with new potatoes, mushrooms, and green beans. Then he could view them as they finished their salad with creamy Roquefort dressing and, finally, their steaming coffee with meringue pecan pralines and petit fours.[17] Hearing this, Thomas's stronger emotions took control. He shouted, "No, thanks." Then, "I informed him that the days they had in mind were past and gone." He said that he could pay the price of two tickets ($9 per guest) "for my wife and myself and that we had been invited through the front door often enough to have my own tuxedo."[18]

Vivien realized that for the first time, his last vestige of his respect for Bahnson and "for almost everyone" in the department was gone. "This did it," he said.[19]

Bahnson was shocked and completely unprepared for Thomas's fury. After all, Thomas had always put up with whatever Blalock as well as Hopkins and its surgeons had thrown at him. Bahnson never dreamed that Thomas would call his bluff and he was clueless about how to respond. The only thing Bahnson could think of to do was to beat a hasty retreat from the lab while he gratuitously lied once more.

As Thomas reported, Bahnson stopped at the door and turned to say, "'I want you to know that Dr. Blalock didn't have anything to do with this.'"[20]

Bahnson never told the other committee members about Thomas's emotional pushback nor of Thomas's stated refusal to attend as a "special" guest. So far as Ravitch, Sabiston, and Morrow assumed, Thomas *had* agreed to their plan and did hide in the back of the ballroom. The photographs of the occasion, though, show that this scheme would have been impossible: each one of the scanty three-foot-high potted palms was placed singly in the four corners of the room. Black and white photographs of the dinner show that there never was a lush tropical display of tall palm trees with their wide fronds offering full coverage for hiding out.[21] For a man who was six feet two inches, crouching unseen would be a feat worthy of Houdini.

Mark Ravitch, who considered himself a good friend of Vivien's, excused the committee's actions later. "We all felt regret and thought it was a pity, but I don't remember that I felt, or any of us expressed, moral outrage."[22] Then he added, "Vivien might possibly have attributed his exclusion to us rather than to the Professor, or simply to the custom of the times, which it surely was."[23]

CHAPTER THIRTY-TWO

Shattered Illusions

At first light on April 2, the temperature was in the low forties with fog: not a favorable omen for what was hoped to be a delightful spring day. Blalock woke up, feverish, and could stomach only toast and tea. In the early evening, as he was leaving his house for the big party, he vomited outside his car. His family and the committee were beside themselves because guests from the Americas, Europe, and Scandinavia were already in Baltimore. Those in the know feared that he would not be at his best, but at least he was on his way.

Arriving at the Southern, he looked weak but behaved normally during drinks and cocktail period and at the dinner ceremony, where they were seated at 7:00 p.m. Several people paid him homage, including his old friend Tinsley Harrison, and finally the president of the hospital bestowed Hopkins's Distinguished Service Award on him. The celebration was a splendid affair for his guests and for Blalock, despite his lethargy.

Around 9:00 p.m. Blalock stood and approached the microphone to address and acknowledge, one by one, nearly all the attendees. Speaking from his typed notes, Blalock first thanked the guests by name, adding personal details of their relationships. This took twenty minutes. Toward the end, he skipped an entire paragraph of his prepared speech, probably because he was feeling wan and listless. Some of the omitted names included Helen Taussig, his secretary Frances Grebel, and "my technician, Vivian." No last name and a misspelled first name.¹

That night, Thomas sat at home, mulling things over.

At the lab on Monday, William Kouwenhoven, who had worked with Thomas on the cardiac defibrillator and massage, walked into the lab to query Thomas. "Where were you?" he asked. "You weren't at the big party."²

Thomas honestly and candidly responded that he hadn't been invited. The electrical engineer appeared confused and didn't seem to understand the full gist of what Thomas had said. Instead, he volunteered that the Thomases could have sat at his table. Thomas did not respond.

Kouwenhoven was not the only guest who came by the lab, puzzled by Thomas's absence. Within the hour, a senior member of the surgical staff Richard Shackelford made the same inquiry and received the same reply. Shackelford, on the other hand, caught it immediately. "The smile disappeared from his face, his expression becoming very grave," Thomas said. "He stood and looked at me for a long moment, turned and walked away, speechless."³

"Maybe," Thomas reflected bitterly, "Hopkins wasn't ready. It was only 1960 and I had only been there a little over 20 years."⁴

As time went on, Thomas pondered that special invitation to sneak in and hide in back of the ballroom and he contemplated Bahnson's gratuitous statement that Blalock had nothing to do with his exclusion. "If I had been ignored," he said, "I would not have given it a second thought but their action, to me, was as if I were a thorn in their side, not to be completely ignored."⁵ Even though it pained him, he visited and revisited the slight. He also heard from others that he had not been included in Blalock's acknowledgments. That was painful. He said, bitterly, to his Clara, "I would have thought he would have mentioned me."⁶

Everything he had been told about Blalock not having been the person to exclude him sounded false. Thomas thought about the thirty years of work he had given Blalock, times that were often unpleasant for him at both Vanderbilt and Hopkins universities, and the many ways in which his shockingly low income had resulted in his family going without even the basics of life, so well enjoyed by his white colleagues. "During the next several months," he noted, "I gave quite a bit of thought to the matter. These were the people with whom I had worked and been associated for years. Was I proud of this association? Dr. Blalock had pointed out to me that one of the advantages of the job I had was that I would be associated with intelligent people. Were they?" he wondered.[7]

Then he decided to talk to someone who'd been in the surgical resident group. He chose Alan C. Woods, saying, "I felt that we were close enough friends that we could talk in a no-holds-barred manner." The two men met in his small office off the laboratory; Thomas pushed the door until it snicked shut. "I started out by telling him how great I thought doctors were," said Thomas.

"They were among the best educated, they had studied long years, had had psychology, psychiatry, and anatomy, and were supposed to be up to date on the workings of man's mind and body. I told him they were the intelligentsia, the leaders of society, that they expected to be and were the most respected profession.

"I then related to him how I had received the back-door invitation to the Blalock party. I let him know that I did not know at what point he [Woods] may have actually been a part but asked how he could justify the action of the group.

"Normally, Dr. Woods is never at a loss for words, but this time it took him a little while to come up with any kind of explanation. We had quite a long discussion about race relations, segregation, not just at Hopkins but on a national level."[8]

Thomas then pinned Woods down: why wasn't he invited? Woods began to hem and haw. Then, to shift the responsibility from Hopkins and the committee members, he claimed, "Oh, yes, I know what it was, they [the hotel] wouldn't serve you."[9]

Immediately, Thomas rejoined: "Oh, come on, Dr. Woods, I won't buy that, the hotel is in business. I don't believe any hotel in these days is going to turn down a banquet for 500 people because two people are not white. They don't serve that size banquet every night."[10]

Woods had no response, for there was nothing he could say.

Thomas then spoke heartbreaking words to Woods. "[I] let him know that my attitude and feeling toward the entire group had been altered as a result, that it makes one ashamed rather than proud to be associated so closely with such a rotten bunch.

"As far as respect, were they due it?" he asked.[11] Woods remained silent.

On April 26, 1960, only twenty-four days after Blalock's party, the Southern Hotel announced that it would join every other Baltimore hotel and desegregate completely by stopping its racial percentage limit of their diners. "We've removed all restrictions," proudly heralded the hotel's owner to the *Afro American* newspaper, the most popular source for news about Black Baltimoreans.[12] It was too little, too late. Only four years later, the outmoded Southern Hotel went out of business. The building was sold to be a nursing home[13] and, a few years later, resold to the Maritime Engineers Beneficial Association, which used Baltimore's former *grande dame salons* as its training rooms.[14] In 1984, one of its seamen shut off the lights and left the formerly proud edifice empty.

On a cold day in December 1999, after fifteen years of standing vacant, the building that had housed the Southern Hotel for most of the century was torn down to make way for a parking garage. The wrecking crew had an unexpected audience: dozens of Baltimore's Black residents decided that the demolition of the former Southern Hotel, and all the racial hatred it had stood for, was something they wanted—even needed—to watch.[15]

Despite the weather, the crowd stood patiently until an iron ball struck the building. Then the group's first cheer went up. The demolition crew worked hard, hitting the highest yellow bricks over and over until the decorative interior plaster peeked out. The audience stared for hours, mesmerized, as the building was split open, battered, smashed, wrenched apart, gutted, and pulverized. The dust and smoke raised by the demolition coated everyone who stood watching with gray ash, and they coughed and covered their mouths with handkerchiefs or winter scarves. Still, they stayed.

Finally, at the end of a long day and when darkness descended, most of the building had been torn to rubble. The demolition machines that had ravaged it were shut off. Before going home, the spectators gave out one last hurrah. A few men walked forward and spat on the crumbled devastation of an era.[16]

Ultimately, the Southern Hotel and all that it stood for was gone, no longer a visible reminder of the ugly history of racism. Still, the dust of its demise would continue to cloud the tale of Vivien Thomas and his betrayal by those who owed him the most.

CHAPTER THIRTY-THREE

The End of an Era

Blalock was shocked and distraught to realize that he had become the lion in winter. He had hand-picked David Sabiston to succeed him as surgery chief, but the Hopkins search committee and department heads had grown tired of Blalock and his imperious ways, and they resolutely ignored his recommendation.[1] Hopkins was no longer considered tops in surgery and the committee sought a surgery chair with a fresh approach. It plucked thirty-six year-old George Zuidema, MD, a Hopkins medical school graduate from the University of Michigan, where he was serving as associate professor.

No one would describe Al Blalock as a graceful loser and, in the years before his retirement, he wasted eighteen months politicking against Zuidema, which included his circulating a seventeen-page rebuttal and pejorative critique of the man. Then he formed cabals of surgeons to join him, including, of course, many of the nation's surgery chiefs who'd trained at Hopkins under Blalock and who owed their careers to him. Zuidema was sure that Blalock opposed him because he'd left Hopkins after receiving his MD degree and chose to train in surgery elsewhere: "I jumped ship," Zuidema remembered.[2] The furor was becoming known at other hospitals, too, and soon no one wanted to return a call from a Hopkins surgeon department member for fear of being pulled into its whirlpool of dissent.[3]

THE END OF AN ERA

Having lost a battle to put his favored successor in place, Blalock declared that he would retire from Hopkins in 1964. As a result, Thomas said, "By fall 1963, we were in a state of winding down and closing out all of Dr. Blalock's research."[4] Thomas juggled his administrative tasks, but the slower pace of research studies suited him just fine as he tried to imagine life without Blalock. However, despite Blalock's drinking and his fragile health, which had been worsening for reasons that no one could pinpoint, he talked about leaving Hopkins to become a professor of surgery at another university. Thomas was startled when he told him of his plans. Was Blalock implying that he thought Thomas would want to continue their working relationship? Thomas set him straight: "I preferred that he not include me in any plans he might consider."[5] Thomas still hoped to continue working at Hopkins for another decade so he could collect his retirement pay and he had no desire to stay with Blalock or to move to a different city.[6] At this point, Baltimore was home, where his adult daughters and their families lived.

Changes started at Hopkins as soon as Zuidema arrived in the spring of 1964. On his first day of rounds, he desegregated the hospital's surgery patients for reasons of efficiency and made it clear that he didn't want his action to be construed as advocacy for the civil rights movement.[7] It wasn't that he was against it, but neither was he a proponent. Still, this was a welcome change from his predecessor, "who never once thought of this," said R. Robinson Baker, MD, a former Hopkins student and professor.[8]

Thomas was unsure whether Zuidema would want to keep him in the lab, not knowing that the new department head was cognizant that Blalock had "left the major contributions of protocols, procedures and operations to Vivien" or that Thomas's contributions to surgery "were enormous."[9] Thomas, though, flashed back to his shock years earlier when Barney Brooks at Vanderbilt told him that he'd be out of a job when Blalock left for Hopkins. Thomas preferred to stay at Hopkins and keep his pension safe, but he feared that he was too closely associated with Blalock. He decided to find a backup position, just in case.

The situation was that Thomas had relatively few paper credentials to his name and his greatest accomplishments were largely unknown outside of Hopkins. Perhaps he underestimated the power of his influence over the doctors he had taught. From his point of view, he worried that the many men he'd trained who were now surgeons working throughout the country would still fear Blalock's waning power and would refuse to hire him, as had Glenn Morrow at the Heart Institute at NIH ten years earlier. They all knew that Blalock's reach was long and could be unforgiving. Thomas, feeling limited in his job search, reached out to only two men, one at Vanderbilt and the other at Indiana University.[10] Each jumped at the chance to hire him. Still nervous about Blalock's reaction, he decided to wait until two weeks before the professor's retirement to tell him of the job offers. He was correct in doing so. Blalock bristled at the news and appeared querulous that Thomas could find two staff positions without his help.

Thomas also had a problem of his own making: soon after the 1960 Southern Hotel party, he broke his vow to his wife and went back to drinking. Charles Manlove's daughter, Gwen Clarke, summarized it as, "Thomas was spiraling downward after Blalock took all the fame, fortune, and success. It was a combination of his entire life's disappointments coming into him all at the same time."[11]

Vivien wasn't the only person who had been affected by the racial prejudice of the Southern Hotel extravaganza. His loss of faith following the Southern Hotel incident upset Clara, also. Her physician, James P. Isaacs, MD, wrote Mark Ravitch, "This [the Blalock dinner] affected Mr. Thomas and his family in *deep personal ways* that I knew well, because I attended his wife for a stress goiter and *observed the psychological problems that appeared in the wake of this and related disappointments.*"[12] (Emphasis added.)

Naturally, Thomas would try to hide his drinking but, just as inevitably, he wasn't fooling anyone. John Cameron, MD remembers nearly being knocked down by the smell of alcohol on Thomas's breath in surgery class.[13] One morning, Jean Queen, Thomas's talented lab colleague, accidentally picked up Thomas's coffee cup and took a big gulp. She was jolted when she swallowed the hot coffee mixed with cheap grain alcohol.

The End of an Era

She acknowledged, "He was walking a very fine line."[14] Regardless, Zuidema wanted Thomas to stay at Hopkins, as he told him in a friendly chat. Afterward, he sent Thomas to meet with the surgery department administrator, Louise Cavagnaro, who spoke to him about getting help for his drinking problem.[15] In a no-nonsense voice, she told Thomas that everyone knew he was abusing alcohol and that his drinking had to stop, then and there. One well-placed Hopkins surgeon remembered her telling him, "If you come to work one more time with any drink on your lips, you are fired."[16]

Cav, as she was nicknamed, had arranged for Thomas to enter a Pennsylvania addiction center that Hopkins used for staff. He was not to return to the Hopkins medical campus until he'd completed the program and was willing to stay clean and sober.[17] Clara drove him to the treatment center, Chit Chat Farms, now part of Caron Addiction Centers, and dropped him off for a several-month stay.[18] Vivien pulled himself together, stayed the course and stopped drinking.

Hopkins hospital celebrated its seventy-fifth anniversary in 1964 and used the occasion to honor Alfred Blalock by renaming the new clinical science building for him. By now, he was sixty-five years old and his various illnesses had caught up to him. He'd recently had surgery to remove a vertebra in his spine, but it didn't ease his back and flank pain and he began using a wheelchair for transport. He wrote his brother, "I have a great deal of pain which makes it difficult to sleep at night."[19] He could barely stand or walk due to severe back pain and his back brace didn't seem to lessen his misery.

After the event concluded, Thomas pushed Blalock's wheelchair to the lobby where Alice Blalock was bringing the car around. When Blalock stood, he was bent at a 45-degree angle and was obviously in great discomfort. Thomas, now newly sober, rejoiced that Blalock hadn't fortified himself with liquor before this last Hopkins ceremony in his honor. As he said of the professor, "Except during hospitalizations, I'm not sure he ever completely sobered [up] except on special occasions."[20]

Soon, Blalock was back in the hospital, and it appeared unlikely that he would ever be well enough to be discharged. Blalock's fading star still shed enough light to attract a pilgrimage of his disciples. As word of his deterioration spread, his favorite former students—"Longmire, Hanlon, Bahnson, Sabiston," according to Ravitch[21]—flew to Baltimore to express their thanks and say goodbye and pay homage to the man who'd mentored and coached them, and who'd accelerated their careers. Bill Longmire was heading the surgery department at UCLA; Rollo Hanlon, at St. Louis University; Hank Bahnson, at the University of Pittsburgh; Dave Sabiston, at Duke University; and Mark Ravitch was a professor at Hopkins as well as being surgeon in chief of Baltimore city hospitals. Even this demonstration of loyal affection did not have the power to cheer Blalock, who was in deep pain. His profound unhappiness and even his bitterness was obvious to them all. During that long summer, he never received any visits from Vivien Thomas.

Among the topics Blalock raised to his star students when he felt well enough to speak was his regret at not having facilitated Thomas's return to college and medical school.[22] His remorse did not rise to the level of sharing it with Thomas, however, only those who were already Blalock's partisans. They, to a man, granted him absolution and never, ever let Thomas know that Blalock had finally repented, which might have given Thomas some satisfaction. It was an open secret in Hopkins surgery's Old Hands Club, but one not ever divulged to Vivien himself, even though Thomas would live a quarter-century beyond Blalock's death.[23]

In September 1964, Vivien braced himself and walked over to the hospital, stopping outside Blalock's room. He left when the nurse told him that Blalock was asleep. Though he worked only a short distance away, Thomas never returned. "I made no further attempt to see him," he said.[24]

Alfred Blalock died on September 15, 1964, "in utter agony,"[25] said Longmire. He was sixty-five years old. His old fear that he would die of TB before he was thirty was unfounded; his autopsy showed that he'd died of cancer. When they opened him up, the surgeons saw widespread metastatic cancer of the stump of the ureter, which might have been not excised properly at his nephrectomy (kidney removal) in the early 1920s at Hopkins. Blalock had spent his life dying as the cancer that had developed

The End of an Era

in the ureter stump metastasized throughout his body, accounting for his years of pain and illness.[26]

Ravitch dashed off a telegram to each of the Old Hands Club members and, in response, they sent hundreds of condolence notes to his widow, Alice. In this collection, for reasons only Thomas knew, there is no note from Vivien Thomas.[27] Perhaps if Mary Blalock had been alive, a woman he respected and had great compassion for, he would have written Blalock's widow.

Coincidentally, on the day of Blalock's death, Helen Taussig was at the White House to receive the country's highest civilian honor given for a body of work, the Presidential Medal of Freedom. President Lyndon B. Johnson praised her for both the blue baby surgery and her actions to tighten the oversight of such potentially harmful drugs as thalidomide. As a result of her timely award, Alfred Blalock's obituaries included references to Taussig and her just-won Medal of Freedom, an honor never bestowed on him.[28] That her award was mentioned in Blalock's obituaries would have tortured him no end. He had been frequently heard saying that he had earned his crown in heaven for putting up with Taussig.

No one knows if his assertion proved accurate.

CHAPTER THIRTY-FOUR

Token Recognition

In 1969, Vivien Thomas was astounded to learn that the Old Hands Club, a group of current and past Hopkins surgery residents, wanted a portrait painted of him to display on the Hopkins medical campus. Alex Haller, who headed the project, had asked the members for contributions and, in response, had received twice as much money as needed to pay the painter they'd hired. After all, as Haller put it, "All of the other important surgeons at Hopkins had portraits."[1]

One of the physicians knew the work of a local man, Bob Gee, who was white but "had successfully painted Negroes before."[2] When George Zuidema called Vivien into his office to give him the good news, Vivien's first reaction was surprise and amazement. He thought, "It just could not happen to me. This must be a dream."[3]

Then he mulled it over. The previous April had been a month of tragedy. On April 4, Rev. Dr. Martin Luther King, Jr. had been assassinated in Memphis, Tennessee. People were furious at the murder of the civil rights leader and, in Baltimore, the reaction jolted Hopkins out of its tranquility and comfort about segregation. The rest of white America was astounded to see the actions of some very frustrated people as they broke storefront windows to protest or looted and set fires in area neighborhoods. Despite traditional claims that "it couldn't happen" in Baltimore, it did.[4] The Maryland National Guard protected the Hopkins medical campus, but some overly fearful physicians sent their wives and children out of town.⁵ It was an eye-opener for Hopkins as it attempted to gauge the anger of those who felt they had been treated as second-class citizens since the university had opened.

Was there, Thomas wondered, a causal relationship between the 1968 protests and his portrait recognition? He jotted down a few questions to himself. "Would this have been done if I were white? Would it have been done except for the civil unrest? Was it done as a front to try to improve the image of the institution in its Black setting?"⁶ And, although he was sincerely touched by the gesture, he did wonder, "How much did the civil unrest lead to the effort to upgrade the image of the institution? Was the portrait a part of this effort?"⁷ He concluded, "Without the racial situation being what it was, the chance was slim that I would have been singled out for recognition. There are strong doubts."⁸

The sad thing was that the Old Hands Club had never considered Thomas for membership or even for honorary membership, although he, too, had been trained by Blalock. And, following that, Thomas had helped train the members of the club! The men apparently never thought to include him in their club, which hurt Thomas terribly although he said nothing to them; only his wife and his friend Gwenn Manlove Clarke knew his true feelings.⁹

Now, at least, they were commissioning his portrait. Posing for his picture, he fidgeted a little as he sat there, under the eyes of artist Bob Gee, who called Thomas "very humble and genuine."¹⁰ Since the money collected was several times Gee's fee, a check for the extra $470 was given to Thomas afterward. It's unfortunate that the sum collected wasn't used to pay a better painter, because the image is awkward looking and doesn't capture the intelligent look that others saw in Vivien's eyes. It was a good enough likeness, though, and it would have to do.

However, since Hopkins as an institution hadn't been involved in this activity, the administration was not convinced that the portrait of Vivien Thomas should hang in public view. The issue turned contentious between members of the Old Hands Club and Hopkins administrators. While these struggles were ongoing, the painting was completed and shrouded in brown wrapping paper while Haller and the rest awaited word from the administration. In the meantime, the club members didn't know what to do with the painting, so it was brought upstairs to Thomas's lab office and pushed to the back of his closet, where it remained for two years while Hopkins wrestled with the decision to hang it or not. Its presence served as a daily reminder to Thomas of his shaky status.

As time passed, Haller became truly peeved and decided to write to the dean of the medical faculty to emphasize Thomas's importance. He cited a number of his contributions to surgery and also dubbed him "the first full time veterinarian of Hopkins"[11] and ended, "He has remained truly loyal to Johns Hopkins for almost thirty years, and I think his recognition, by the hanging of his portrait alongside the other major surgeons in the Johns Hopkins medical institutions, is in keeping with his important contributions."[12] Zuidema stood behind Haller's effort and pushed his proposal until the university agreed.

"It was the right thing to do," Zuidema said, downplaying any role that the civil rights movement had on the decision by the department and its surgeons to honor Thomas for the first time in a public way.[13]

The presentation took place, at last, on February 27, 1971.[14] The original thought was to hold the ceremony at the Maryland Club as part of an Old Hands Club meeting but, as Zuidema pointed out, Thomas and his family could not be admitted because of their skin color. Instead, the painting was presented to Thomas in the Turner auditorium, which was filled to capacity with more than 1,000 people during a biennial Hopkins physician reunion.[15] Cooley was there from Dallas, along with Longmire from Los Angeles, Ravitch from Pittsburgh, Hanlon from Chicago, and even Sabiston from Duke University, where he had become head of surgery after failing to succeed Blalock. When he left Hopkins, he took Blalock's secretary with him, and she brought to Duke all the Blalock files that she had kept so meticulously. To Thomas's great regret, his fellow lab workers were not released from their duties to attend their supervisor's ceremony.[16]

The portrait presentation remarks, ironically, were made by Thomas's old nemesis, C. Rollins Hanlon, who had accepted credit for the TGA surgery.[17] Hanlon appeared very gracious in his remarks, saying, "In a certain sense, Dr. Blalock stood there because of Vivien Thomas and in the same restricted sense, Vivien Thomas stands here because of Alfred Blalock. Each was greater because of his dependence on the other."[18] He disingenuously added, "It was my good fortune, some years ago, to work closely with Vivien Thomas."[19] He neglected to mention his having made off with the papers documenting Thomas's seminal work.

When it came time for Thomas to speak, he started off with a whammy. "First of all, I do want to thank Dr. Hanlon and the others for the most kind and complimentary remarks. Dr. Hanlon and I did work at some length in the laboratory, as he said, and we understand each other pretty well. Dr. Hanlon was even kind enough to include me as co-author in *one* of his papers."[20]

Thinking back to Hanlon's taking credit for his work, Thomas paused, then let it rip, "I always thought he should've included me on *two*."[21]

Hundreds of surgeons howled with, as Thomas put it, "knowing" laughter and applauded his comment.[22] It was the most enjoyable part of the ceremony for everyone save Hanlon.

When Vivien wound down his comments, the surgeon, Richard Shackelford, said that he'd received "the greatest ovation I have ever heard given to anyone at Johns Hopkins. The applause on three different occasions was tremendous and lengthy. Furthermore, never have I seen an entire audience rise to its feet while applauding on three different occasions during the ceremony. I thought it was wonderful."[23] Yet among all of this acclaim for Vivien Thomas, Hopkins didn't bother to send a photographer to memorialize the occasion, although two Baltimore newspaper reporters and photographers were there.

Despite this, Thomas said, "Of course, I was elated; it had been the most emotionally gratifying experience of my life."[24]

At the coffee hour that followed, Clara and a grown-up Olga and Theodosia, with children of their own, chatted with the physicians. Local news reporters and photographers were in attendance because Hopkins had sent out a press release, dated February 22, 1971, which was the first time that the institution had ever attributed any of the blue baby work to Thomas or had mentioned his name.[25]

One young Southern surgeon tried to put Thomas down a bit, saying, "I didn't believe you would be able to talk with all those 'wheels' around."²⁶ Thomas's measured response was, "I knew all of those 'wheels' when they were small boys, like you."²⁷

Thomas, unassuming as always, had told no one outside his immediate family about the portrait. Still, everyone saw the press coverage in the newspapers the next day. One friend called to tell him, "Well, if someone was going to put my portrait up somewhere, everybody would have known about it."²⁸

Originally, the portrait was hung in the lobby of the Blalock building and could be seen all the way to the area where patients and visitors waited for the elevators. Thomas became uncomfortable in the morning as he waited for the lift to arrive; people would notice his portrait, and then stare at him and then study the portrait again. They kept doing double-takes. Were their eyes deceiving them? Some days, Thomas just decided to take a different elevator in the Halsted building instead and walk through the buildings' connecting tunnel.

Though flattered and a bit overwhelmed, Thomas was clear-eyed. He later divulged to his lab staff that he thought Hopkins should have paid for the portrait rather than relying on donations from the Old Hands Club.²⁹ He wasn't a man to hold his hand out and he also saw the institution's delay in hanging the picture as a sign of their ambivalence about honoring him.

A few weeks after the ceremony, Thomas wrote his sister-in-law Ootsie, the Nashville teacher, opening with, "I know this whole package will be quite a surprise to you. The event as such was a surprise to me, too, except that I've known about it for two years."³⁰ He'd never even told his Nashville kin about the portrait until after the ceremony. Although Thomas had consistently said throughout his life that he did not seek recognition, in this case he did ask Ootsie to see if she could get an article written in the Nashville papers about his Hopkins portrait. If so, he asked if he could receive two copies "for my file since I'm starting a file on me (smiles)."³¹ Vivien Thomas, finally, was aware that his work should be recognized and he yearned for approbation, no longer willing for Hopkins to keep his role in medicine hidden.

TOKEN RECOGNITION

One interesting consequence of Thomas's portrait was that it was immediately noticed by a young Black man who had arrived on campus in 1971 to begin his medical residency. His name was Levi Watkins and he had an upper-echelon pedigree. His father was president of Alabama State College and the family worshipped at the Dexter Avenue Baptist Church in Montgomery, Alabama, where Rev. Ralph Abernathy had baptized Watkins. As a teenager, Watkins had participated in the Montgomery Bus Boycott that was closely associated with Mrs. Rosa Parks's civil disobedience and he served as a volunteer driver for the Rev. Dr. Martin Luther King.

Although Watkins was Hopkins's first surgical resident who was Black, he was used to being a "first." After college, the University of Alabama, his home state's flagship university, preferred to pay his full private-school tuition at Vanderbilt University rather than admit him to the state medical school. Watkins, though, was the first Black medical student at Vanderbilt University and he endured a rough time. His classmates, seeing him walking outside the dormitory, played such pranks as throwing their feces down from their windows at him and, worse, celebrated boisterously when they learned that King had been assassinated.

On arrival at Hopkins, Watkins was both weary and wary. Delighted to see a portrait of an African American man on the wall of the Blalock building, he introduced himself the second he spotted Vivien Thomas in the cafeteria. The men had several things in common, including time spent in Nashville, where Watkins had graduated from Tennessee State University, which was where Thomas had once hoped to study. The men became fast friends, despite their different perspectives on how to approach life at Hopkins.

Thomas had a personal interest in seeing a young Black resident emerge unscathed from a thorny Hopkins. Watkins became a frequent guest at Clara's wonderful meals at the Thomas house. At Thomas's firm suggestion, Watkins moderated his controversial comments and protestations. The older man had little desire to change the student's point-of-view, he merely wanted him to be given a chance to succeed. "One thing I learned from Thomas," said Watkins, "was to watch the mouth."[32] After finishing his program and doing advanced work at Harvard, Watkins returned to Hopkins and stayed his entire career. He repaid any debt he had to his mentor, explaining, "After Blalock died, it was a tough time for Thomas. He was lacking purpose and was a bit lost. I connected him to a new project, and it gave him a real mission and meaning."[33]

The new project was an important one. For more than a decade, work had been ongoing at Mt. Sinai Hospital in Manhattan to develop an implantable cardiac defibrillator (ICD), which was designed for use in patients with such problems as irregular heart contractions (ventricular fibrillation) or a pathologically rapid heartbeat (ventricular tachycardia). A defibrillator, the size of a cigarette pack, could potentially detect an irregular heart rhythm and reset it by automatically delivering electric shocks to prevent cardiac arrest.

The defibrillator team working on this at Hopkins needed to conduct more animal research before it could try to implant such a device in a person. "So, I went upstairs," said Watkins, "and who was the person to help? It was Vivien, still in the lab, still around, still giving advice."[34] Together, the men tested the device on dogs by putting a defibrillator on one side of the dog's chest to cause irregular heartbeats and, on the other side, implanting a defibrillator to readjust the heartbeat back to normal. After years of work, Watkins became the world's first surgeon to implant the automatic battery-operated defibrillator in a human being. It began saving as many as 300,000 lives in the US alone. Or, as one news reporter dramatically put it, the device would bring people to life back from the dead.

Still, Hopkins demonstrated how deeply it wanted to keep Vivien Thomas in the shadows. In 1974, the university had produced a film, *A Crisis in Medical Education SOS,* complete with a jazz soundtrack and a voice-over that encouraged young African Americans to choose careers in health care.[35] Its emphasis, though, was to show Black nurses, doctors, and lab techs happily working in environments that were completely segregated. Yes, it seemed to advocate for African Americans to serve in health care but only if they did not treat white people. Some of it was shot at the historically Black Provident Hospital in Baltimore.

The twenty-seven-minute documentary included a scene of Vivien Thomas in his lab, talking about his work in medical research. The credits at the end of the film included Vivien Thomas's name but, unfortunately, Hopkins was apparently reluctant to be identified with this Black man. In a gesture that seems nearly unbelievable, the 1974 film's credit lines state that Thomas was an employee of Baltimore's historically Black Provident Hospital—and not Johns Hopkins Medicine. And his first name was misspelled as Vivian. No one looking at the credits in this Hopkins film could ever have realized that, by then, Thomas had been an employee of Hopkins for thirty-four years.

CHAPTER THIRTY-FIVE

VIVIEN THOMAS, LLD

I f anyone deserved to make the leap between a high school diploma and an honorary doctorate degree, it would be Vivien Thomas. This event was kicked off by Alex Haller, who was one of the surgeons who heard Blalock's confession and deathbed regrets about stymieing Thomas's hope to return to college. The subject had resonated with Haller, who had genuine affection for Thomas as shown by his leadership in getting Thomas's portrait painted and hung. He thought it would be a great idea if Hopkins awarded an honorary bachelor's degree in science (BS) to Thomas. He went to Zuidema to talk it over since there was no groundswell of support for Thomas displayed by any of the other surgeons.[1]

Unknown to them, a much greater honor was in the works, but not from Johns Hopkins University. As Thomas tells it, "In late March 1976, a gentleman came unannounced to my office."[2] The mystery man introduced himself as George H. Callcott, PhD, the vice chancellor of academic affairs at the University of Maryland. He told Thomas that the university's administrative and faculty-student committee had nominated him to the university regents to receive an honorary DSc (doctor of science) degree.

Thomas was staggered and amazed, and he would never know that this award had been kicked off two years earlier by a Maryland professor whose child had successfully undergone heart surgery at Hopkins.[3] A few days later, a letter from Callcott arrived at Thomas's Hopkins surgery department workplace confirming the endorsement, saying that the official vote was to be held on April 9.[4]

Then, in an astounding reversal, Thomas received another letter from Callcott dated April 12 that said, "It is a matter of great personal embarrassment and sadness to have to report to you that the Board of Regents of the University of Maryland did not approve the recommendation that you be awarded an honorary Doctor of Science degree."[5]

Callcott, more than fifty years later, remembered the incident as an "embarrassing episode, a shameful episode" for the University of Maryland.[6] Apparently, when Thomas's name was submitted and the regents learned that he was Black, they objected because the university was already awarding an honorary degree that year to a Black man. (He was Andrew F. Brimmer, the first African American man to serve as governor of the Federal Reserve System.) "It wasn't necessarily that they were against awarding degrees to two Black men," said Callcott, "but rather that they wanted to stay apart from the whole [racial] issue."[7]

Thomas was disappointed but he claimed that he shrugged it off: after all, he had told no one about the honorary degree but Clara. He graciously wrote Callcott, explaining that his skeptical "Let's wait and see" attitude made "my disappointment not nearly as great as it might have been."[8] He also noted, in his typically kind way, that his consolation came from the nomination itself. "To me this consideration and recommendation is in itself an honor."[9] In the meantime, Thomas took both letters from the other university to Zuidema because, he claimed, the degree rejection issue had perplexed him. He said that he hoped his surgery chief could make sense of what had happened. It's also possible that Thomas, who'd grown more attuned to the political ramifications of university behavior, had wanted the department to realize that he'd at least been considered for an honorary doctorate.

Surprisingly, Zuidema reviewed the letters and responded, "That's too bad, but if it will keep you from feeling too badly about it, you had better keep May 21 open."[10]

"For what?" Thomas asked.[11]

Zuidema told him that Hopkins University planned to award an LLD degree (in the US, an honorary doctor of law) to Thomas at spring commencement. Now Thomas was confounded. He asked Zuidema if there'd been some type of collusion between the two universities, which the surgery head denied.[12] Although Zuidema gruffly would note later that "the civil rights era played zero role in Vivien Thomas's recognition and I was dealing with an individual who deserved recognition," he also admitted that the degree "was the right thing to do at the time."[13]

However, as Thomas privately continued his investigation into why Hopkins was suddenly giving him a degree, he noted that his name had not been submitted with other nominees but rather came up later from "a special faculty committee."[14] He learned from several Hopkins secretaries that the University of Maryland had been making inquiries of the Hopkins personnel office in the months before Callcott had visited him. He was sure that once Hopkins had learned of the University of Maryland's intentions, it realized that it would lose its chance to be the first university to honor Thomas with an honorary degree if it didn't act quickly.[15]

Thomas naturally was delighted with the forthcoming honor but remained skeptical of Hopkins's motivation. His son-in-law Harold Norris said he "always believed it was the letter from Maryland that started everything at Hopkins."[16] He thought that "Hopkins felt embarrassed" by the possibility of being shown up by another university.[17]

As the commencement ceremony grew closer, Vivien was no doubt amused by the form letter he received from the university asking what type of academic regalia would he be wearing? He realized how uncommon it was for the university to award honorary doctorate degrees to mere high school graduates. To one Hopkins physician who knew about the upcoming honor he joked, "Hopkins is really a tough place—it has taken me thirty-five years to get a degree out of them."[18] Still, there was some regret in losing out on the chance for a doctorate in science, which the University of Maryland had held out to him, and instead receiving a doctorate in law, which is a sort of catch-all degree intended to reflect on a person's character or contributions to a general area, rather than any accomplishments in science.

Helen Taussig was belatedly receiving an award at the same ceremony for her distinguished service to Hopkins. The university had treated her very poorly over the years, as shown in part by its failure to promote her to a full professorship until 1969, a few years before her retirement. Her pension was so small that she could not afford to keep her summer house in Cotuit, Massachusetts. Johns Hopkins, apparently embarrassed by her financial problems, bought her house and property, and allowed her to stay there as a "grace and favor" dwelling, meaning that she could remain until her death.[19]

Unlike with the portrait ceremony that Vivien had kept hidden from his Nashville family, this time Thomas invited his some of his family to his commencement. Vivien was extremely reluctant to invite his outspoken brother Maceo, a successful Nashville businessman who invested in properties, owned a small hotel and a record label, and also owned a roller-skating rink that, on weekend nights, starred such headliners as Chuck Berry, Little Richard, and Ike and Tina Turner. When his sister-in-law Ootsie Thomas said, "I want Maceo to come," Thomas replied, "I'm not going to invite Maceo."

Ootsie was a strong-minded woman, said her daughter-in-law Truly Jackson, and Ootsie replied, "Please. That's your brother."[20]

Thomas was heated. "No, he'd get up before the president" and say something about how his brother should have been treated fairly and equally.[21] So Maceo stayed behind in Nashville.

On May 21, 1976, a beautiful sunny commencement day, in her gold and sable regalia, Taussig received the Milton S. Eisenhower Medal for Distinguished Service (named for the Hopkins University president who was also former US President Dwight Eisenhower's brother). President Richard S. Ross intoned about Taussig's long career, particularly emphasizing her responsibility for the blue baby surgery. Of course, he also talked about Dr. Blalock's courage in conducting the surgery. For whatever reason, even though Vivien Thomas was sitting on the dais behind him, a few seats away from Taussig, Ross never mentioned Thomas nor gave him any recognition for his integral part in the blue baby operation in Taussig's citation.[22] It must have seemed surrealistic to Thomas, sitting there listening to a rendition of the blue baby surgery that excluded any reference to him. Still, he overlooked this slight. A few minutes later, the university president read Thomas's citation, which was appropriately salted with mentions of the contributions of both Blalock and Taussig.[23]

Thomas, wearing the gold and sable robes of Hopkins, was nearly overwhelmed when he received his LLD. The ovation "was so great that I felt very small."[24] Afterwards, he wrote Zuidema a sweet yet rueful note, saying, "It was truly a great day in my life. I feel now that I am really a part of Hopkins."[25]

One accomplishment mentioned in Thomas's citation was the part he had played over the decades teaching surgery and animal experimentation to young Hopkins medical students. Now he realized that he could play Hopkins against itself and made an appointment to speak with Zuidema a few weeks later.[26] He approached him, saying, "I had expressed my opinion that in as much as I had been recognized as a teacher of surgeons, that I should be put in that category and serve in that official capacity as a faculty member."[27] He added, "I pointed out that it would be to my financial advantage and be greatly appreciated to be put in a position to receive the higher salary."

Zuidema hadn't anticipated his request, especially as Thomas was close to retirement. He realized, though, that it was important "to see that Thomas get proper recognition before he stepped down."[28] The well-paid chief surgeon said loftily that "it was not a pay issue."[29] But to Thomas and his family, after so many years of miserly pay, it certainly was about the money. Thomas had already warned Jean Queen, his trusted lab colleague, that "no Hopkins pay increase would ever come easily."[30]

He was correct about needing patience while he waited for a decision. It took a full six months in 1977 before the dean of the medical faculty signed off on the arrangement that retroactively appointed Thomas an instructor in Surgery. Zuidema backdated the promotion by six months, albeit without the pay. As Thomas commented of Hopkins, "official wheels turn oh-so-slowly."[31] Thomas, although he was eligible for retirement, planned to work a few more years, most likely because he needed to take advantage of his higher annual salary.[32] Beginning in 1977, Thomas was paid a new salary of $16,000.

Thomas retired on July 1, 1979, and was given the title of instructor emeritus a little later. His farewell party was thrown by the surgery department and was held in the doctors' dining room. Laboratory workers could not dine in this room, obviously, and no surgeon thought to make an exception and invite Vivien's laboratory technicians to attend.[33]

CHAPTER THIRTY-SIX

PIONEERING RESEARCH IN SURGICAL SHOCK AND CARDIOVASCULAR SURGERY

Well before his retirement, Thomas was pitched a flattering idea by Hopkins surgeon Richard Shackelford: he insisted to Thomas that he write a book about his pioneering years in cardiovascular and shock research.[1] Why not, asked the surgeon? Thomas had been a critical part—and sometimes the sole creator—of a half-century's worth of research and surgery on shock, the closed heart surgeries on the TOF blue babies (the Blalock-Taussig procedure) and on the TGA babies (the Blalock-Hanlon procedure), as well as cardiac resuscitation and other studies. Thomas was stunned: it was something that he'd never imagined writing, yet he never doubted his ability to finish this project. Still, until he left his job at Hopkins, the book idea remained just a tickle in the back of his mind.

Now retired, he talked the notion over with Mark Ravitch, who was head of surgery at University of Pittsburgh and its Montefiore hospital. Over the years, the men had become friends of a sort. As with all the surgeons Thomas had trained, theirs remained a cordial but oddly hierarchical relationship. During the summers at the Ravitch's place in Martha's Vineyard, they would entertain Clara and Vivien as houseguests. Despite

Pioneering Research

their weeklong stays, Thomas always addressed his host as "Dr. Ravitch," whereas the surgeon called him "Vivien."

Jumping on the idea of a book about Thomas's work, Ravitch told him that he'd help him get it published. Thomas worried that people would be surprised by what he had to say, especially about Blalock: "I know this will make you wonder how many other places I have 'covered up' for him [Blalock]."[2] He also feared for the chances of getting the book accepted by what he called "99 percent white-owned and operated" publishing houses.[3] If he were going to write about his research, he said, he wanted it to be factually accurate. He told Ravitch that he certainly was proud of his work, but he was anxious because it had never been properly documented. He worried, "My concern is that by the time the decision is made [whether to publish], some 'reader' [of the manuscript] decides he can't let a Negro take credit for something a white man already has credit for."[4]

Fortunately, his interest in telling his story was piqued by two invitations he received in 1981. Baltimore's Provident Hospital honored him by giving him its "Unsung Hero" award. At the awards ceremony, Thomas talked about his work at Hopkins, opening it by telling his audience, "After working behind the scenes for so long at another institution, it is quite gratifying to be brought on stage by *this* institution."[5] Everyone laughed, knowing that his words about "working behind the scenes" referred to his anonymity at Hopkins. Acknowledging his independence in the lab, he spoke gratefully of how he set the protocol (rules) for each experiment and, for the most part, worked alone, saying that in time he'd been able "to sing [my] own song,"[6] coincidentally using the words of Walt Whitman. Then, a month after this award, he received a letter from Thomas Turner, the head of the Hopkins's Alan Mason Chesney Medical Archives. Turner asked him to donate his papers to the archives, which would "enrich" the collections because Thomas had played "a long and distinguished role on the faculty and staff."[7] Vivien Thomas felt greatly complimented.

However, without constant noodging from Ravitch, Thomas would never have kept at his book, which was eventually titled *Pioneering Research in Surgical Shock and Cardiovascular Surgery: Vivien Thomas and*

His Work with Alfred Blalock.[8] During the five years Thomas took to complete his manuscript, he sent his writing, section by section, to Ravitch for comment. Many surgeons believe Ravitch's greatest accomplishment was bringing the USSR's surgical stapler innovation to the US in 1958, where he introduced it, with minor adjustments, to American surgeons.[9] But perhaps Mark Ravitch's most important act was to introduce Vivien Thomas to the world by insisting he write *Pioneering Research*.

As for Thomas, he ached to leave a record of his work and so he plugged away. He would often talk about how history could "get so fouled up" and how important it was to be accurate in narrating the process of heart surgery and shock research.[10] It was a challenge, not because he had to struggle with his writing skills—he was a good writer, especially for a scientist—but he remained a bit trepidatious about where his book would find a home.

His natural modesty and his low-key personality made him hesitant to highlight his work. Also, his history of being overlooked by Vanderbilt and Hopkins universities had done nothing to boost his ego. For a man who liked being active and on his feet, the new project required long hours of sitting. Clara had hoped that after his years of working at Hopkins into the night, they'd finally have some time together; she was not particularly pleased to see her newly retired husband disappear into the depth of their basement each morning to write.

At least she had other company in the house. Their daughter, Theodosia Dullea, was in the process of a divorce and had moved back to her parents' house with her two young daughters, Ursula and Marcia.[11] She had graduated from business school and was working full time, grateful for her parents' assistance. Their older daughter, Olga Thomas Norris, was a graduate of Morgan State University and was also living in Baltimore with her husband and daughter Nena. The girls' grandparents made sure that the young ones weren't indulged and encouraged them to show discipline in their behavior. Their grandfather was their role model: whatever had happened to Thomas at work that day, he never came home looking discouraged. "Don't let hurt define you," Clara and Vivien emphasized.[12] Their granddaughters were encouraged to focus on their schoolwork and to look ahead for success in their careers, rather than to be distracted by the world outside them, including the civil rights issues of the day. The message they heard was to take care of yourself first and then improve the world.

Taking a pause from writing, he brought his much-younger cousin, Koco Eaton, to an informal meeting with the Hopkins's medical school admissions chief. Eaton, who always addressed Thomas as "Uncle Vivien" due to their age difference, would be graduating college in 1983 and hoped to go to medical school.[13] Levi Watkins remembered that the Hopkins surgeons had hoped to admit Thomas's nephew but were unsure of his credentials, showing the same attitude as when they'd had underrated Thomas's high school education. As Levi Watkins said, "Whoo, were we relieved when we learned he was graduating from Columbia University! That was the big time."[14]

Ever diligent, Thomas continued writing his book and joked to Ravitch that he'd "thought that retirement was going to be a time of leisure but I haven't seen any of it loitering around here during this past year."[15] Ravitch responded, encouraging him to "work like hell" because "(1) You owe it to yourself and your family; (2) You owe it to history; (3) Ravitch predicts it will bring you an impressive sum of money."[16]

At this point, Thomas was completely free to be as candid as he liked and felt no restraints. Also, the civil rights movement had opened up greater opportunities to speak out about discrimination. Perhaps, too, his emerging health problems—he had trouble digesting food due to his irritable stomach and he'd started losing weight—gave him a more acerbic point-of-view. As he started to write his first handwritten draft, he began to unleash his suppressed fury at his racially prejudicial treatment. He had stored up thirty-nine years of anger, frustration, and resentment and now all the past injustices poured from him onto the page. Purging himself of his most bitter thoughts provided emotional catharsis. His most stinging comments centered on three issues: his red-hot fury about being excluded from Blalock's Southern Hotel party, his lack of credit in Blalock's journal articles for his traumatic shock surgical experiments and others, and how Blalock handed over credit to Hanlon for the transposition of the great arteries surgery that he himself had created.

He wrote and wrote about his unfair treatment, sometimes sounding bitter and sometimes sarcastic. On deep reflection, he censored his most angry thoughts and did not send them to Ravitch. In the end, *Pioneering Research* included a dialed-down version of his criticism of Blalock for not giving him credit for all his work, particularly for the transposition surgery. However, his searing write-ups of the Southern Hotel incident and his traumatic reaction to his exclusion due to his race were never sent to Ravitch. His book didn't mention Blalock's party, not once. It was if it had never happened, although in his notes for the manuscript he drafted page after page of his bitter thoughts. Before he sent his book manuscript to Ravitch, he removed the lines where he sadly summarized the reason for his absence at the party, even distancing himself from his pain by writing in the third person:

"He could not attend.

He was not white.

That person was me."[17]

Why would Vivien Thomas keep back certain aspects of his history? Perhaps he was reluctant to be completely candid with Ravitch, the man whose assistance he needed to get his book published. After all, Ravitch was a member of the Old Hands Southern Hotel party committee and he'd once served as director of Hopkins's segregated blood bank, all the while admitting that there was no valid reason to separate blood based on race but that doing so was "deemed best."[18] If Ravitch became offended, Thomas would have no support for his book: he was completely unknown with no credentials, no contacts, and no clout.

He did embrace a discussion about his lack of credit from Blalock, but censored most of his angry comments. Particularly bitter about his anonymity, he had earlier said that the one and only time Blalock acknowledged him in one of his articles was not sufficient. He had even complained in an interview conducted for the Johns Hopkins Chesney Archives about it, "That little fine print at the bottom. Fine print I was talking about."[19] Thomas's first handwritten book draft had detailed

Pioneering Research

Blalock's refusal to give him fair credit, or any credit at all, for his own surgical experiments. He described how only two of Blalock's many hundreds of journal publications from 1930 onward listed him as a coauthor. "I have been what you call hidden in the medical world," he said, adding, "I personally performed *all* the experimental surgical operations and research procedures for Dr. Alfred Blalock from 1930 to 1964. In most laboratories, this work is done by post-graduate fellows."[20]

He insisted, "Dr. B. worked from my protocols. We had the discussions and *he* published as sole author."[21] Thomas noted that it would have been "physically impossible for him to spend the amount of time in the laboratory that would be required for the amount of work published under his name as single author."[22] In an understatement, he presaged, "I feel that I will be a controversial figure among the medical historians."[23]

Thomas had good reason to be dissatisfied by not having received proper credit for his work. Under current guidelines of the International Committee of Medical Journal Editors, which defines how participants in published research projects should be acknowledged, Thomas warranted being listed as a contributor or a coauthor on a great many of Blalock's articles.[24] Other medical journals have also clarified that all contributors should be named as authors.[25] Thomas remembered how, as early as the 1930s at Vanderbilt, Tinsley Harrison had made his own lab assistant a coauthor of his articles she had researched.

In the handwritten pages that Thomas never sent Ravitch, he raged at Rollins Hanlon for taking credit for his experimental surgical work on the transposition of the great vessels. Thomas explained that as early as 1974 and for the next decade, he had repeatedly tried to get Hanlon to return Thomas's surgery notes and had written the surgeon many letters over the years, to no avail. A typical message from Thomas to Hanlon was, "Several months ago, I wrote to you and... I told you that I would like to have the protocols on the production of the ASD which, as you said, were in my own handwriting."[26] Then Ravitch contacted Hanlon in a futile attempt to have him return the papers.[27]

Hanlon always rebuffed both men, claiming that he couldn't locate any of the original notebooks, including the one where Blalock wrote that Thomas had devised the surgery.[28] When Hanlon moved to Chicago to work at the American College of Surgeons, he used his relocation as a defense for "losing" Thomas's material. Then Ravitch, who'd never seen these notebooks, was nervous that Hanlon might interpret Thomas's book as libelous or slanderous.

Perhaps Ravitch was uncomfortable including Thomas's accusations about a man with such high status that he was president of the American College of Surgeons. As Thomas wrote, "This is serious business" and insisted that Hanlon was a "liar."[29] He maintained that Hanlon had probably destroyed Thomas's original research records. Referring to the audio tapes at the center of the Watergate scandal, he said, "I'm sure Rollo is not as stupid as Nixon and they won't be found."[30]

Ravitch decided to ask other surgeons who were there at the time for their memories of Thomas's work, and it was their unanimous support that convinced Ravitch that Thomas was being truthful. Over the years and on multiple occasions, Denton Cooley always insisted, "the Blalock-Hanlon procedure was all the work of Vivien."[31] Jerome Kay wrote, "I remember very well your production of atrial septal defects; in fact, I must have mentioned the story of your creating atrial septum defect without Dr. Blalock's ever knowing."[32] Both Alex Haller and Rowena Spencer agreed, too.[33] Since that time, a number of articles have declared that the surgery was Thomas's alone and it credited him with laying "the foundation of the surgical treatment of transposition of the great arteries."[34]

Finally, when Thomas realized that Hanlon would never send him back his original surgery protocols, he drafted but never mailed several heartbreaking letters, not mentioned in *Pioneering Surgery*. Had Thomas known that Hanlon would publish an article on ethical principles in health care, he would have noted the irony.[35] He also reacted to how Hanlon had always assumed the façade of a virtuous Catholic by piously making it known to his colleagues that he attended Mass every day.

Thomas decided to pen Hanlon a letter which he never mailed: "I am not a Catholic but maybe you should talk to Mother Mary—maybe she'll only want for you to say a few 'Hail Marys' and a Rosary to intercede for you and everything will be alright. You've lived so long with this system of penalties that I guess that by now you can *live with yourself*.

"Fortunately or maybe unfortunately, I still have a conscience to live with."[36]

By now, Ravitch knew that Thomas had withheld writing that criticized Hopkins and some of its surgeons, but it didn't seem to bother him: in fact, he seemed to encourage Thomas to hold information back, questioning him closely about any incidents at work that readers might interpret as racist actions. Thomas teased Ravitch with some tantalizing hints. "Oh, yes," he wrote, "About my censoring, after all of this is over and gone to press, I'll tell you much more of the story possibly in writing. Sorry about my reticence. But I have to maintain my diplomacy."[37]

Then he explained his thoughts about avoiding the issue of racism at Hopkins. "One of the things that slowed down my writing was how to keep it 'race free.'"[38] In perhaps his most devastatingly candid comment, he said, "Hopkins is presented as a progressive liberal institution, which it is not."[39] He further alerted Ravitch to his lifelong dilemma in academe: "I've really been walking a tightrope."[40]

Ravitch did not ask to read or ask about any of this race-related material, although he did go back and forth with Thomas with questions and comments about many other topics. In fact, he commended him, writing, "At all events, while you bring the racial issue in from time to time, you do it quite obliquely and your comments are all the stronger for that."[41] At least Thomas ensured that his more candid history eventually would be discovered by keeping his unpublished handwritten drafts among his personal papers that would be given to Johns Hopkins Chesney Medical Archives.

The preparation and editing of the *Pioneering Research* manuscript would become a family affair. He had asked Theodosia to type the manuscript pages he gave her, after holding back some of his more personal writing. She made suggestions for his consideration as did her cousin, Valeria Thomas Spann, Harold's daughter.[42]

Now it was time for Ravitch to find a publisher for *Pioneering Research*. The dilemma in selling the book to publishers was twofold: Thomas was an unknown entity outside of Hopkins and the book he wrote was technical. It was an intricate description of his research and was not at all a memoir. One clear indicator of its scientific value was the inclusion of more than fifty surgical drawings illustrated by Hopkins's famed medical illustrator, Leon Schlossberg. No memoir or autobiography could ever accommodate such technical drawings.

Ravitch, recognizing that hardly anyone outside of Hopkins University understood what Thomas had created in his lifetime, first submitted Thomas's manuscript to Johns Hopkins Press at the beginning of 1985. One might have assumed that the Johns Hopkins University Press would leap at any opportunity to publish Vivien Thomas's book, which reflected all his work there, as well as Blalock's. However, Thomas was terribly disappointed to receive a *pro forma* rejection letter from the Hopkins Press on the dubious grounds that although the press published biographies, it did not publish "personal memoirs."[43] Of course, *Pioneering Research in Surgical Shock and Cardiovascular Surgery* was not a memoir, which was made clear by its title. As Thomas's son-in law Harold Norris remarked, "Interesting that the book was not published by Hopkins. Enough said."[44]

Pioneering Research was sent to other publishers and initially received the usual handful of rejections. It was a hard book to classify, which does not appeal to editors. Most of the manuscript was technical, but there were some elements of autobiography (Thomas's) and some of biography (Blalock's). Then, through a colleague, Ravitch approached the publisher of the University of Pennsylvania Press, Thomas Rotell. This Ivy League publisher was eager to accept the book that Hopkins had turned down. Thomas was ecstatic that his research book would be published by a prestigious publisher. However, UPenn Press remained concerned that sales might not break even with publishing costs. Printing any type of visual scientific information is very costly and here were those fifty-plus Schlossberg drawings. At the time, it was not uncommon for academic publishers to request an initial subsidy to tide them over until they are out of the red. Ravitch told the Press that he was willing to pay the $5,000 the press had requested to offset publication costs because he so strongly believed in the book's importance.[45]

Pioneering Research

Then Ravitch had another idea and wrote Richard S. Ross, MD who was the vice president for medicine at Hopkins, to remind him of his earlier remark that Hopkins might put up some money to support the book.[46] Ross then asked Nancy McCall, who was then an assistant archivist and, later, the head archivist of Chesney, to independently review the submitted manuscript and she wrote a stunningly enthusiastic review. She said that it "clearly merits publication on the basis of both style and content" and describes its "richly significant detail and good writing."[47] With her recommendation, Ross decided that Hopkins would pay half; Ravitch then had his own surgery department in Pittsburgh pay the other half.[48] Of course, Ross knew that the Hopkins University press had rejected the book; perhaps his gesture was an attempt to make amends. In any case, Penn Press's Rotell explained in a letter to Ravitch, "We propose to repay the subvention by $5 per book to Pittsburgh and Hopkins on all copies sold from the point of break-even until the $5000 subvention is repaid."[49] After that, Thomas would begin receiving the royalty payments. Unfortunately, Ravitch never disclosed this financial situation to Thomas, once again leaving him in the dark.

After the reimbursements were paid back in full, the book is still earning royalties for the Thomas family. Most books, unfortunately, retain a shelf life shorter than a carton of Mochi ice cream, but *Pioneering Research* has remained in print since its publication and is still selling nearly four decades later.

Thomas had anticipated that *Pioneering Research* would be the most significant endeavor of his life. For once, he would achieve full and sole authorship. He had dedicated the book to Clara and had told others that he couldn't wait to see her expression when she saw her name. All through the fall of 1985, Thomas awaited early December, when his book would land in bookstores and on library shelves throughout the country.

Alas, only a handful of days before *Pioneering Research* was published, Vivien Thomas was dead.

CHAPTER THIRTY-SEVEN

STONY SILENCE

Six months earlier, in the spring of 1985, Mark Ravitch, worried about Thomas's plummeting weight, pushed him into making an appointment with his internist, Philip Tumulty, MD. As Ravitch, Thomas, and, certainly, Clara had secretly feared, the news wasn't good. Tumulty suspected pancreatic cancer and sent Thomas to see John L. Cameron, who had just become Hopkins's surgery chief in 1984 when Zuidema left to become vice-provost at the University of Michigan after spending twenty years at Hopkins. Cameron diagnosed a malignant tumor in Thomas's pancreas, which is the six-inch-long organ behind the lower stomach. Pancreatic cancer is very difficult to recognize in its early stages because its symptoms are the common problems of indigestion and back pain. Even though pancreatic cancer is common in alcoholics, Thomas's disease had nothing to do with his former drinking episodes, according to Cameron.[1] Regrettably, this form of cancer quickly spreads to nearby organs and, indeed, Vivien Thomas's cancer had already metastasized throughout his body.

Cameron removed the pancreatic tumor in late summer 1985. At some point during the surgery, Thomas threw a blood clot, resulting in a stroke. He was unconscious, lying in his hospital bed, when Cameron received a call from Mark Ravitch, who was extremely excited: he had just received the final page proofs of *Pioneering Research*.[2] "Tell Vivien," Ravitch commanded Cameron. "Tell him the book looks terrific." Cameron explained that Thomas was in a coma; he could not understand anything that was said to him. Still, Ravitch persisted, urging the doctor, "Tell him!"[3]

As a favor to Ravitch, Cameron went to Thomas's bedside. As the surgeon remembers, he put his mouth close to Thomas's ear and said, "Dr. Ravitch just called to say that he's got the proofs of your book and everything looks great."

The experienced surgeon said in amazement, "Thomas opened his eyes and smiled."[4] Cameron was flabbergasted that the news brought Thomas back to consciousness, even for a few brief seconds. "I've seen this happen only twice in my life," he said. "In a fleeting moment, he was conscious, with his synapses fired." Thomas's quick awakening and then his immediate return to unconsciousness was so unusual that Cameron said, "People thought I was making this up."[5]

After a long number of days, Thomas recovered full consciousness and returned home to recover as best he could. At the beginning of November 1985, Ravitch flew in to see him and reported that he seemed unfocused, but he went ahead and told him that *Pioneering Surgery* would be in bookstores at the end of the month and he shared UPenn Press's plans to publicize it. Thomas tried to respond to Ravitch but settled for smiling contendedly.[6] It would be the last time the men saw each other. Soon Clara, heavily burdened by Thomas's need for twenty-four-hour care, arranged for him to move into a nursing home.

On November 25, 1985, Vivien Thomas passed on, while in his wife's arms. He was seventy-five years old. He and Clara had been married for fifty-two years.

Thomas's pastor from the Madison Avenue Presbyterian Church came out of retirement to preside over his memorial service.[7] Jean Queen, who became Thomas's successor at the Hopkins lab, said, "Dr. Cameron asked me to go to represent the Department of Surgery and I went with two surgeons."[8] Clara and her daughters asked Levi Watkins, for whom Thomas had acted as a mentor, to give the eulogy.

At the service, Watkins homilyzed, "Even in this moment of pain, God is still good through His power and love and magnificence. He took a little Black boy from Louisiana and transformed him into a giant among men."⁹ After his funeral, his family had his tombstone engraved "Dr. Vivien T. Thomas" because he'd been so proud of his honorary doctorate.

Clara received many condolence notes, but the two most engaging were from Denton Cooley and Helen Taussig. The Texas heart surgeon was the only physician unpretentious enough to handwrite his condolence note and sign it with his first name. Helen Taussig's message made clear the reason for her respect: "Vivien was a very real and important man on the [blue baby] surgical team and perhaps the only man who stood up to Dr. Blalock." She spoke of him as being known as "the best vascular surgeon in Baltimore." At the end of her letter, she summed up his character, "I admire the way he stood up to Dr. Blalock and would not tolerate his temper—of course, he was in the right, and he would not have been able to work with him all those years if he had repeatedly had to endure his temper. As his father had before him, Vivien had a keen sense of right and wrong and stood for what was right and just."¹⁰

Thomas's obituary ran in newspapers in the mid-Atlantic states and an AP story was printed in a few papers around the country. The coverage focused on how Thomas had made the famous blue baby operation possible. Then, Johns Hopkins issued its news: "Vivien Thomas, Hopkins Pioneer Surgical Technician, Dies."¹¹ Remarkably, the Johns Hopkins's announcement referenced Thomas's work that Blalock had attributed to Hanlon: "During his years at Hopkins, Thomas was instrumental in developing procedures in animals that would later be applied to several heart defects in children and adults. Among them were the blue baby procedure and the [TGA] Blalock-Hanlon procedure that corrected defects of the great arteries."¹² This was the first time—and perhaps the only time—that Hopkins acknowledged Thomas's creation of the Blalock-Hanlon procedure.

Reviewers praised the *Pioneering Surgery* book in more than a half-dozen important medical journals in the US and the UK. The *New England Journal of Medicine*'s write-up designated it "as a classic account of laboratory investigation"¹³ and the American Medical Writers Association awarded an Honorable Mention to *Pioneering Surgery* in its category of—get this— "best book written by a physician."¹⁴ In contrast, the reaction on the

Hopkins medical campus to the Thomas book was stony silence, despite the book's many accolades. Both George Zuidema and Cameron said that Hopkins surgeons were unfamiliar with it. Zuidema stated, "There was no reaction to Thomas's book one way or the other,"[15] while Cameron said that he "was not sure there was anyone who read it or cared to read it."[16]

Why didn't the Hopkins surgeons bother to take even a quick glance at *Pioneering Research*? Perhaps the reason is that they couldn't get hold of it: unbelievably, the Hopkins medical campus bookstore refused to stock *Pioneering Research*. Ravitch contacted its manager, who told him that "he'd never heard of Vivien or his book." Ravitch was outraged. "I told him it merited a *display*."[17] UPenn Press hit the same roadblock: when its sales rep paid a visit to the campus bookstore, he got nowhere with the manager. Then, its marketing manager took up the cause and called the manager himself. Alas, to no avail. The edict stood, even though one of Hopkins's own publications had given it a favorable review.[18]

It seems unimaginable, given Hopkins's current touting of Vivien Thomas, but for nearly twenty years after his death, Hopkins remained hesitant to identify Thomas's achievements and even his presence at Hopkins. Six years after Thomas's 1985 death, in 1991, Hopkins held a daylong "Symposium in Honor of Alfred Blalock," which went the entire day, but the printed program never mentioned Thomas, despite its fifteen-minute discussion of the work at the Hunterian Lab. Ironically, the speaker discussing the lab work was Rollins Hanlon.[19] Then, in 1995, the anniversary year of the surgery's public announcement, Hopkins observed another symposium called "A Celebration: 50th Anniversary of the Blalock-Taussig Shunt."[20] The program got underway with a "Tribute to Helen Taussig," followed by a "Tribute to Alfred Blalock," and then a presentation about the "First Patient," Eileen Saxon, to undergo the surgery. There was no tribute nor presentation about Vivien Thomas for his vital contributions to the blue baby surgery.

The obscurity of Vivien Thomas by Hopkins in the late 1990s is difficult to believe now that Hopkins, in the 2000s, continually promotes Thomas's name whenever it is even marginally relevant. Yet as recently as 2019, Hopkins issued a press release announcing the seventy-fifth anniversary of the blue baby surgery that included a photo of the blue baby participants in the operating room. Unfortunately, it cropped this photo so that Vivien Thomas's head cannot be seen. He is still invisible.[21]

It had been a perfect storm: first, Hopkins paid Thomas a poverty-level salary and refused to acknowledge any of his work until 1971. Next, his book manuscript about his years at Hopkins and Vanderbilt was rejected by the Johns Hopkins University Press. After *Pioneering Research* was published by UPenn Press and had received wonderful reviews, the JHMI campus bookstore adamantly refused put his book on its shelves. Then, Hopkins virtually ignored him in its two pivotal blue baby anniversary celebrations. At least Thomas was not alive to see these last institutional rebuffs of him and his work.

Finally, something happened that even Hopkins could not overlook. A talented and determined writer named Katie McCabe introduced Thomas to the world in a fascinating magazine article skillfully edited by Jack Limpert that ran in 1989 in two regional publications, the *Baltimore* and *Washingtonian* magazines.[22] Although the feature was only published regionally, the story of Vivien Thomas was so extraordinary that it caught the public's attention and, with it, McCabe won the prestigious National Magazine Award for Feature Writing.[23]

By 2003, PBS had picked up on people's interest in Vivien Thomas's story and devoted an episode of its documentary series, *The American Experience,* to him.[24] Narrated by Morgan Freeman, it was called "Partners of the Heart," referring to the allegedly warm Blalock-Thomas relationship. The show was heavily influenced by information gained from the Hopkins surgeons who minimized the effect of the discrimination Thomas faced. In fact, the Hopkins's *Gazette* story about the show's opening proudly emphasized that Hopkins had "defied racial barriers" in its treatment of Thomas.[25] The PBS documentary wrongly attributed, among other things, that Thomas's exclusion from Blalock's extravaganza was due to the Southern Hotel's alleged barring of Black guests. In fact, the voice-over by Freeman intoned that no hotel restaurant in all of Baltimore City allowed an African American person to dine, which was utterly untrue. However, it was a prestigious series, watched by many millions of people. UPenn Press promptly changed the name of *Pioneering Research* to *Partners of the Heart* to take advantage of the interest in the widely publicized PBS show.

In the meantime, McCabe had sold her magazine rights to HBO, which released *Something the Lord Made* in 2004.[26] It was a wonderfully entertaining made-for-television movie, if inauthentic, advertised as based on true events, but it did not follow the storyline of McCabes's article. It was shot at the Hopkins medical campus and, again, its surgeons provided considerable input. The feel-good movie had a top rate cast starring Mos Def as Thomas, Gabrielle Union as Clara Thomas, and Alan Rickman as Blalock. The story it portrays is both intriguing and inspirational but is similarly fictitious; among its errors was its stress on a friendship between Thomas and Blalock that never existed.

In a completely fantasized scene at the Southern Hotel ceremony, Thomas is seen hiding in the back of the room, weeping among a forest of palm trees. The movie also shows him receiving an honorary "doctorate in medicine," rather than the generic degree that was bestowed upon him.[27] Again, toward the end of the movie, an older Blalock is portrayed stumbling over a few words of regret to Thomas about his not encouraging him to attend college, another incident that never happened.

When Levi Watkins and the Thomas family members read the script, they had pleaded with HBO to cut all its concocted feel-good drama about how Blalock defied racial barriers and befriended Thomas.[28] Their comments were mostly ignored because the truth would have marred HBO's need to present a sudsy sentimental movie. Certainly if Thomas were alive, he would have been enraged by the use of Blalock's words, "This is like something the Lord made" to describe the blue baby surgery rather than to Thomas's transposition of the great arteries surgery, from which it derived.

As an indicator of the movie's positive spin, Johns Hopkins University sponsored the show's premiere. It was an eye-opener to his grandchildren, who knew very little about their grandfather's contributions to medicine. Marcia Rasberry Smith, Theodosia's daughter, said, "My sister [Ursula Rasberry-Dijkhoffz], and I were just floored" as they watched the premiere. It was the first time they truly "recognized the significance of our grandfather's work."[29]

Although many family members attended the Baltimore opening, the person who was most knowledgeable about Thomas's life refused to be there. Clara Thomas had read the script and *would not be part* of this biopic fabrication. She made her feelings about it perfectly clear to its producers. Still, HBO sent a car and driver for her, and the driver sat outside her house for several hours, waiting and waiting, before he was told to give it up and drive away.[30]

In 2005, Clara Thomas died. She had been two decades a widow and at least was able to enjoy her last years, despite missing her husband's companionship. Right after her husband's death, she was understandably depressed, she wrote to Nancy McCall, and wasn't up to pulling Vivien's papers together for the Chesney archives for several years.[31] She eventually rallied round and donated box after box of materials.

She continued to cherish her three granddaughters. Fortunately, Vivien's pension was higher than expected due to his last-minute promotion to the rank of instructor. Clara Thomas savored her first cruise and traveled internationally. Back home, she would treat herself to a tall cup of hot black coffee, the strong highly caffeinated type that she and Vivien had craved, at the Towson Starbucks counter in Barnes & Noble.[32] Clara and Vivien Thomas were survived by their two daughters, three granddaughters, and, later, three great-granddaughters.

CHAPTER THIRTY-EIGHT

Unsung Hero

This is what Vivien Thomas accomplished during his professional life: in the 1930s, he carried out the great majority of surgical experiments on the physiology of traumatic shock that supported Blalock's groundbreaking medical journal articles. During World War II, the work he conducted for Blalock helped save countless lives and contributed to the defeat of the Third Reich and the Empire of Japan.

In the 1940s, he created the medical instrument that is known as the Blalock clamp and other important tools and machines, as well. He devised, without any medical literature available on the topic relevant to an operation, the surgical procedures that made the blue baby surgery (the Blalock-Taussig operation) possible, snatching tiny babies from the jaws of death while perched on a step stool behind Al Blalock. Afterward, he coached that head of surgery through the first hundred-plus operations. In doing so, he virtually created the first techniques necessary for closed cardiac surgery, opening the way to the era of successful open-heart operations that followed his work. Afterward, he stayed on call for another decade in case any other Hopkins surgeons ran into blue baby problems in the operating room.

So many tens of thousands of lives have been saved by his blue baby operation and have gone on to lead full lives. Most grew up to be everyday people, but occasionally you see them in the news. Shaun White, the red-haired snowboarder and skateboarder who brought home three Olympic gold medals, had been a TOF baby. More recently, Jimmy Kimmel's son, Billy, was born with a TOF heart and was saved by the current blue baby surgery, based on Thomas's innovative operation.

Also in the 1940s, Vivien Thomas created another operation for TGA babies, who had even a higher chance of death (the Blalock-Hanlon operation). Then he had to watch as his long-time surgery chief gave away the credit he deserved. In the fifties, Thomas worked on cardiac massage and designed, as an integral member of a three-person team, a closed-chest defibrillator that made heart-lung surgery possible and sold his creation to hospitals throughout the US and Canada. Toward the end of his career, in the late seventies, he assisted in the development of procedures for the world's first automatic defibrillator implanted in a human being.

Oh, and he also taught the techniques of surgery to hundreds of physicians, many of whom became leaders in the field. One expert said that his greatest contribution was that he "helped train the next generation of American surgeons."[1] Although it was Blalock's influence that placed his best surgeons in top jobs around the country, it was Thomas's instruction that assisted them in becoming the directors of surgery departments and surgery divisions of more than twenty-five university medical schools and hospitals. He, with Blalock, produced an amazing number of surgeons—nine in all—who became presidents of surgical associations.[2]

During his long career, he coauthored eight papers published in medical journals.[3] These represented only a fraction of the work that should have borne his name. Nearly all of his experimental research was credited to Blalock alone or to Blalock along with other physicians.

Reviewing Blalock's publications and comparing them to Thomas's experimental work shows that hundreds of the surgeon's research papers should have named him as second or third author. There have been a few attempts to give Thomas his overdue credit by referring to the Blalock-Taussig-Thomas surgery (and also the Blalock-Thomas-Hanlon surgery)—for example, the children's hospital at the University of Toronto renamed the blue baby surgery "the Blalock-Thomas-Taussig procedure"[4]—but these have been individual voices.[5] Only the institutional support of Johns Hopkins could permanently rename these two operations and, to date, it has not shown the leadership that would bring about this change.

No one with a high school diploma will ever be able to surpass the medical feats of Vivien Thomas, explained John Cameron: "Vivien Thomas came along during an era when new ideas needed to be worked out in the laboratory."[6] Medical research has become so complex, so complicated, and so refined that a person must be highly educated to do groundbreaking work. Nor would any hospital today allow someone without specialized training the freedom that Thomas had to carry out solo surgical experiments and to interact with patients and their families. He was unique. We will never see his like again.

The distinguished orthopedic surgeon Koco Eaton proudly boasted of his cousin, "He did the absolute most with the opportunities he had."[7] Was it his character that allowed him to be so incredibly productive in the hostile environments that were impossible for him to escape? His resilience was extraordinary. He coped throughout the stresses and adversities that might have caused others to surrender. His younger daughter, Theodosia Thomas Dullea, said that she could not understand how he was able to take the demeaning way he was treated at work and accept a poverty-wage salary.[8] Throughout it all, however, he remained optimistic. He accepted his second-class treatment so that he could continue the work that gave his life meaning and satisfaction.

His tenacity derived in large part from his background as a youngster in Nashville. Certainly, his own parents were an example of how to successfully cope in segregated communities. They looked ahead and kept working for future goals and never acted as if they were helpless victims of their circumstances. The Black community in Nashville, particularly the Pearl High School teachers, was also highly supportive of its children. Their friends and neighbors promoted the young people's resiliency by giving meaning to their sacrifices and by showing an example of self-confidence to their children. Eaton put it, "Your generation had it better than the generation before you and your kids can have a better life than you did. You endure the hardships for the next group."[9]

Vivien Thomas had a strong moral compass that he used to guide his personal behavior. Some of it derived from his religious belief and the rest from his basic sense of decency toward others. In his book on his experimental work, he never called anyone at Vanderbilt or Hopkins a racist, even though it's clear that they acted as if they were. Instead, in his own positive way, he refrained from insulting anyone and managed to always keep his cool. He could find the humor in even the most trying circumstances. He could rise above it all and cope with nearly any situation without losing his temper or becoming bitter by keeping his eye on what he saw as his purpose. Thomas uncomplainingly and graciously took second and third jobs to continue his experimental surgery work at Hopkins. As he explained, "It was the challenges that kept me in the lab almost 50 years."[10] He was creative and could improvise with whatever materials he had on hand. He was so disciplined and had such a robust healthy ego that he didn't need to brag about his incredible medical work. "He was a scientist. He let his work speak for itself," observed Eaton.[11]

His close relationship with Clara, his only confidante, allowed his wounds to heal. A different, less-traditional spouse might have complained or criticized her husband's decisions but that wasn't Clara's way. Fortunately, she could rely on her own deep vein of grit. And, together, they raised their daughters and grandchildren not to ruminate on their problems, "Never come home from work sad," according to granddaughter Marcia Smith.[12]

Perhaps these suppressed emotions ultimately led to Thomas's periodic episodes of depression, which he then attempted to self-heal with alcohol, as his niece, Valeria Thomas Spann, noted.[13] Clara, however, put a check on his drinking as had George Zuidema, and Thomas had the courage to seek out the help he needed to straighten himself out. In addition to all this, his son-in-law added, with tears in his eyes, "I want people to understand that he was the most kind and the most steady person I have ever met."[14]

Some might criticize him for not being more assertive, for not trying to openly lead any visible civil rights movement. That just wasn't his way. Instead, he ignored the "colored" men's washrooms typically found in the basements of Hopkins's buildings and quietly used the "white" men's room on the floor near his lab and didn't make an issue of it. As soon as he had the opportunity, he hired other Black lab workers and set up a program that he ran each summer in his laboratory for Baltimore high school students interested in a medical or scientific career. He would continue to mentor them, justifiably proud of the ones who became physicians or went into science. He hired a worker whom Hopkins had fired for his insolence in refusing to use the "colored" bathrooms and trained him as a lab tech. And he taught all his male workers to never acknowledge a surgeon who addressed them as "boy."

Given the magnitude of Vivien Thomas's creativity, surgical talent, and self-discipline, if he could have financed his medical school education, he very well might have made even greater contributions to medicine than he did. Of course, Thomas might have been content to be a family doctor, which was his original intention. Yet he so closely resembled the blood-type originator Thomas Drew in his aptitude and capacity that he could have made Drew's level of contributions to the world and would have been an honored and recognized medical pioneer. With a degree, Vivien Thomas would not have needed Alfred Blalock to become an outstanding physician-scientist and a trailblazer in whatever specialty he chose.

Thomas's history of missing the higher education that he sought is recognized by today's medical community as it starts to use his name to motivate and assist thousands of students with medical training. Each year on a warm day over the summer months, students—both male and female, minority and not—begin their medical education at schools and medical colleges throughout the country. They have one thing in common: they are taking part in a program named for Vivien Thomas.

In Atlanta, dozens of students begin the Vivien Thomas High School Research Program at the Morehouse School of Medicine, even though the school has never had a connection to him. In Baltimore, hundreds of high school students enter the Vivien T. Thomas Medical Arts Academy on North Calhoun Street.

At Johns Hopkins University, one of four medical students enters the Vivien T. Thomas College Advisory Program. Hopkins also had administered a Vivien T. Thomas Fund to increase diversity at the school of medicine. When Bloomberg Philanthropies donated $150 million to Hopkins in 2021 for this purpose, it was renamed the Vivien Thomas Scholars Initiative. The fund provides scholarships to students who earned their undergraduate degrees from historically Black colleges and universities.

Similarly, each year at Vanderbilt University, a selection of the incoming medical students is placed in the Vivien Thomas Medical Training Program. Vanderbilt also gives a Vivien Thomas Award for Clinical Research to an employee whose work demonstrates excellence. Vanderbilt finally hung a copy of the Hopkins portrait of Vivien Thomas in 2017 and was instrumental in having the state of Tennessee issue a proclamation honoring him as a pioneer who devoted himself to bettering humanity. It also changed the name of a campus street from "Dixie Place" to "Vivien Thomas Way." Meharry Medical College, also in Nashville, began the Vivien Thomas Endowed Scholarship. Even the United Kingdom's Institute for Technical Skills and Strategy launched a Vivien Thomas Technical Leadership program.

Professional medical organizations have started recognizing him, too. The American Heart Association confers on exemplary postdoctoral students a Vivien Thomas Young Investigator award. Thomas is included, with Watkins, in the Association of Black Cardiologists "Roll Call" of African American contributors to the advancement of cardiovascular medicine.

The Congressional Black Caucus foundation, with financial backing from the mega-pharmaceutical company GlaxoSmithKline, gives a Vivien Thomas Scholarship for Medical Science and Research. The National Medical Association, formed for the Black physicians who were barred from the American Medical Association, bestowed a Posthumous Scroll of Merit on Vivien Thomas in 2003. Also, the Society of Thoracic Surgeons sponsors an annual lecture in his name.

Wouldn't Thomas be deeply pleased—and perhaps surprised—that Hopkins named a Black man, Robert S. D. Higgins, MD as surgery chair and surgeon-in-chief in 2015? Higgins has noted that as a department head, he had achieved the highest rank at Hopkins that a Black person has ever held.[15] He remained at Hopkins for only eight years before being taking a more prestigious position and he is now president and chief academic officer at Rush University in Chicago.

Higgins reflected on his experiences at Hopkins, saying that the Thomas story "resonates with me"[16] and he purposely kept a copy of *Pioneering Research* in his office on campus. Higgins is affected by more than Thomas's inspirational story; he stressed that, after graduation from Dartmouth College and Yale University medicine, he was a resident in surgery at the University of Pittsburgh under Henry Bahnson. To Higgins, this meant, "I am touched by the legacy of Vivien Thomas since he taught surgical techniques to Bahnson, who helped teach me at Pittsburgh."[17]

Vivien Thomas was able to come to a sense of peace about the opportunities in life that he had lost due to his race. "At this point in my life, I feel that I have helped more people than I would have if I had realized my hopes."[18] And he gave this statement his own special emphasis: "Health or lack of good health is no respecter of race. All research benefited thousands of us in the *Human Race*."[19]

His life is a timeless story of struggle and triumph. Modest to the end, he summed up his medical miracles, saying, "As for me, I just work here. I've thoroughly enjoyed the role I have played and only tried to be me."[20] He explained, "I had lived with the personal inner satisfaction that I was helping to solve some of the numerous health problems that beset all mankind."[21]

Thomas would never have anticipated that anyone would write his biography or make a television documentary or television movie about his life. Nor would he have dreamed that numerous medical schools and associations would keep his name alive through their programs and awards. "Vivien saw himself just trying to make a life for himself and his family," said Watkins, the Hopkins surgeon who worked with him and delivered his eulogy.[22]

Despite this—or perhaps because of it—Watkins concluded, "He was an unsung hero."[23]

ENDNOTES

INTRODUCTION: THE MAN BEHIND THE MEDICAL WONDERS
1. Alfred Blalock and Helen Taussig, "Surgical Treatments of Malformations of the Heart Which There Is Pulmonary Stenosis or Pulmonary Atresia," *J. of the American Medical Association*, May 19, 1945.
2. Alex Haller, Interview by author, Glencoe, Maryland, July 30, 2014.
3. Gwendolyn Clarke, Interview by author, White's Creek, Tennessee, July 17, 2017.
4. William Longmire, *Alfred Blalock: His Life and Times*, self-published, 1991, p. 104.
5. C. Forenzc, "Reflections on Her 88 Years in Historical Milestones, Helen Brooke Taussig, 1898–1986," *J. of American College of Cardiology*, 1987, 10: 262–271.
6. William Longmire, *Alfred Blalock: His Life and Times*, p. 98.
7. Denton Cooley, "First Blalock-Taussig Shunt," *J. of Thoracic and Cardiovascular Surgery*, 2010.
8. Lisa Yount, *Alfred Blalock, Helen Taussig and Vivien Thomas*, Chelsea House, 2012, pp. 54–57.
9. Vivien Thomas, *Pioneering Research in Surgical Shock and Cardiovascular Surgery: Vivien Thomas and His Work with Alfred Blalock*, University of Pennsylvania Press, p. 92.
10. *Ibid.*
11. Levi Watkins, Interviews by author, Baltimore, Maryland, August 22 and Sept. 14, 2014.
12. "New Operation Helps Doomed 'Blue' Babies," *Des Moines Tribune*, Dec. 20, 1945.
13. Photo of Blue Baby Operation, Johns Hopkins U. Chesney Archives.
14. Vivien Thomas, *Pioneering Research*, p. 115.

15. Ibid., 114–129.
16. Victor Baum, "Pediatric Cardiology: An Historical Appreciation," *Pediatric Anesthesia*, 2006; 16: 1213–1225; Frank Gerbode and G. Sharma, "Recent Advances in Surgery of Congenital Heart Disease," *The Western Journal of Medicine*, 1970 May; 112(5): 25–31.
17. Don Nakayama, "Vivien Thomas: Surgical Researcher and Innovator." *Black Surgeons and Surgery in America*, American College of Surgeons, Chicago, Illinois, 2021.
18. Levi Watkins, Interview by author, Baltimore, Maryland, Aug. 22 and Sept. 14, 2014.

CHAPTER ONE: COMING UP IN NASHVILLE

1. Jack White, "Poorest Place," *TIME*, Aug. 15, 1994, 144:7, pp. 34–36; John Sutter, "Lake Providence Income Inequality," http://www.cnn.com/2013/10/29/opinions/sutter-lake-providence-income-inequality.
2. M. Booth and G. Gordon, "Interview with Vivien Thomas," Oct. 2, 1976, Johns Hopkins U. Chesney Archives.
3. Loren Schweninger, "A Vanishing Breed: Black Farm Owners in the South, 1651–1982," *Agricultural History*, 63(3), Summer 1989, 41–54; "Sharecropping, Black Land Acquisition and White Supremacy." *World Food Policy Center, Duke U.* http://wfpc.sanford.duke.edu/north-carolina/durham-food-history/sharecropping-black-land-acquisition-and-white-supremacy-1868-1900/.
4. Theodosia Thomas Dullea, Conversations with author, telephone.
5. Gwendolyn Manlove Clarke, Interview with author, Whites Creek, Tennessee, July 17, 2017.
6. Roy Garis, "The Negro in Nashville," *Social Science*, 23(1), Jan. 1948, p. 38.
7. Reavis Mitchell, Interview with author, Nashville, Tennessee, July 20, 2017.
8. Booker T. Washington, "The Atlanta Compromise," *The Future of the American Negro*, Dreamscaped Media, 2022.
9. J.R. Lind, "The Rich History of Black Landowners and Farmers Here in the South," *Nashville Scene*, Nov. 5, 2020, p. 2.
10. Richard Pride and J. David Woodard. *The Burden of Bussing, The Politics of Desegregation in Nashville, Tennessee*, University of Tennessee Press, 1985, p. 49.
11. Vivien Thomas, *Pioneering Research*, p. 4.
12. Bobby Lovett, *The Civil Rights Movement*, University of Tennessee Press, 2015, pp. 12–13.
13. Vivien Thomas, Unpublished MS material, Johns Hopkins U. Chesney Archives.

Endnotes

14. Southern Advertising Agency, *Nashville Negro City Business Directory,* 1925.
15. Reavis Mitchell, Interview with author, Nashville, Tennessee, July 20, 2017. Reavis Mitchell, "Meharry Medical College," *Tennessee Encyclopedia of History and Culture.* http://tennesseeencyclopedia.net/entries/meharry-medical-college. "Julius Rosenwald Fund." Tennessee Encyclopedia of History and Culture, http://tennesseeencyclopedia.net/entry.php?rec=728. http://tennesseeencyclopedia.net/entries/julius-rosenberg-fund.
16. Bobby Lovett, *The Civil Rights Movement,* 2015, p. 90.
17. Reavis Mitchell, Interview with author, Nashville, Tennessee, July 20, 2017.
18. Vivien Thomas, Unpublished MS, material, Johns Hopkins U. Chesney Archives.
19. Vivien Thomas, *Pioneering Research,* p. 4.
20. Gwendolyn Clarke, Interview with author, White's Ford, Tennessee, July 17, 2017.
21. Vivien Thomas, *Pioneering Research,* p. 4.
22. Thomas J. Ward, *Black Physicians in the Jim Crow South,* University of Arkansas Press, 2003, p. 28; "Black History Month," Duke. U. http://guides:mclibrary.duke.edu/blackhistorymonth/education.
23. Kenneth M. Ludmerer, *Time to Heal: American Medical Education from the Turn of the Century to the Era of Managed Care,* Oxford U. Press, 1999, p. 63.
24. Andrew Maraniss, "The Legacy of Pearl High School and Its Success During Desegregation." http://theundefeated.com/features/the-legacy-of-pearl-high-school; see Andrew Maraniss, *Strong Inside: Perry Wallace and the Collision of Race and Sports in the South,* Vanderbilt University Press, 2014; Connolly, Patrick. "Pearls of Wisdom." *Tennessean* (Nashville, Tennessee), July 26, 1998.
25. "Graduation Program, Pearl High School 1929," Tennessee State Archives, Nashville, Tennessee.
26. Afi-Odelia E. Scruggs, *Claiming Kin: Confronting the History of an African American Family,* St. Martin's Press, 2002, p. 26.
27. "Drake Inspires Students." http://www.nashvillescene.com/music/photo-of-the-week-drake-speaks-at-martin-luther-king-jr-magnet-school/article_e76b263c-56e0-a720-bd1829f443f0.html.
28. See Frederick Patterson, "Foundation Policies," *J. of Educational Sociology,* pp. 290–291. And Ulin Leavell, "Trends of Philanthropy," *J. of Negro Education,* pp. 41–43.
29. Joy Wallace, "Places That Matter," Orlando (Florida) *Sentinel.*
30. Pride and Woodward, *Burden of Busing,* p. 49.
31. "Tennessee's School System," *Tennessean,* Feb 13, 1932.

32. Valerie Spann, Interview with author, telephone, Aug. 29, 2017; Gwendolyn Clarke, Interview with author, White's Ford, Tennessee, July 17, 2017; Melvin Black, Interview with author, Nashville, Tennessee, July 18, 2017.
33. Vivien Thomas, *Pioneering Research*, p. 5.
34. "Pearl Graduation Program," Tennessee State Archives, 1929.
35. Melvin Black, Interview with author, Nashville, Tennessee, July 18, 2017.
36. "A Visit with Vivien Thomas," Oct. 28, 1974, Johns Hopkins U. Chesney Archives.
37. Vivien Thomas, *Pioneering Research*, p. 6.
38. "Exercises," *Tennessean,* June 15, 1929.
39. "A Visit with Vivien Thomas," Hopkins U. Chesney Archives.
40. Ibid.
41. Tennessee A&I State Teachers College, "The Bulletin," November 1929/1930.
42. "The Meharry Medical College Catalogue," Meharry Medical School, Nashville, Tennessee, 1931, p. 35.
43. "Tennessee A&I," *Tennessean,* June 15, 1930.

CHAPTER TWO: THE TURNING POINT

1. Reavis Mitchell, Interview with author, Nashville, Tennessee, July 20, 2017.
2. Vivien Thomas, *Pioneering Research*, p. 11.
3. Gwendolyn Clarke, Interview with author, Whites Creek, Tennessee, July 17, 2017.
4. Ibid.
5. Ibid.
6. Ibid. And "A Visit with Vivien Thomas," Oct. 28, 1974, Johns Hopkins U. Chesney Archives.
7. Ibid.
8. Ibid.
9. Vivien Thomas, *Pioneering Research*, p. 9.
10. Ibid.
11. Ibid., p. 11.
12. Ibid., pp. 10–11.
13. Alfred Blalock, "Mechanism and Treatment of Experimental Shock: Shock Following Hemorrhage," *Archives of Surgery,* 15(5), Nov. 1927, p. 762.
14. Alfred Blalock. "Experimental Shock: The Cause of the Low Blood Pressure Produced by Muscle Injury," *Archives of Surgery,* June 1930.
15. Dan (Dandy) Blalock, Email to author, June 9, 2017.

16. Vivien Thomas, *Pioneering Research,* p. 11. The current equivalency of the any dollar amount given was calculated using "What Is a Dollar Worth?" as defined by the Federal Reserve Bank of Minneapolis, Minnesota http://www.minneapolisfed.org.
17. Ibid.
18. Reavis Mitchell, Interview with author, Nashville, Tennessee, July 20, 2017.
19. Vivien Thomas, *Pioneering Research,* p. 6.
20. Ibid., p. 11.

CHAPTER THREE: STARTING OFF: EXPERIMENTS IN TRAUMATIC SHOCK

1. Christo Kleisiaris, Chisanthros Sfakianakis and Ionna Papathanasiou, "Health Care Practices in Ancient Greece: The Hippocratic Ideal," *J. of Medical Ethics and History of Medicine,* 2014(7): p. 6.
2. Henri Francois Le Dran, *Treaties on Reflection Drawn from Practice on Gun-Shot Wounds,* (translation), 1743.
3. Samuel Gross, *A System of Surgery,* 1862; Sidartha Mukherjee, "Bodies," The *New Yorker,* 2018, p. 30.
4. Ibid.
5. S. Riva-Rocci, A. Zanchetti, G. Mancia, "A New Sphygmomanometer Technique," *J. of Hypertension,* 14(1), pp. 1–12.
6. Karina Soto-Ruiz, "George Washington Crile, A Visionary Mind in Resuscitation," *Resuscitation,* 2009.
7. Walter Bradford Cannon, "Studies in Experimental Toxic Shock IV, Theory, Evidence of a Toxic Factor in Wound Shock," *Archives of Surgery,* 1922, pp. 15–18.
8. Theodore Brown and Elizabeth Fee, "Walter Bradford Cannon," *Am J Public Health,* Oct. 2002, 92(10): pp. 1594–1595. http://www.ncbi.nlm.nih.gov/pmc/articles/PMC1447286.
9. Walter Cannon, *Traumatic Shock,* Appleton, 1923.
10. Vivien Thomas, Unpublished MS deletions MMR, Mark M. Ravitch Collection, National Library of Medicine, NIH.
11. Mark Ravitch, *Papers of Alfred Blalock,* JHU Press, 1966, pp. xxii–xxiii.
12. Vivien Thomas, *Pioneering Research,* p. 14.
13. Christo Kleisiaris, et al., "Health Care Practices in Ancient Greece," *J of Med Ethics and Hist of Med,* 7:6, March 15, 2014.
14. Nuno Henrique Franco, "Animal Experiments in Biomedical Research: A Historical Perspective," *Animals,* 3, no. 1, p. 18.
15. Ibid.
16. Vivien Thomas, *Pioneering Research,* pp. 12–13.
17. Ibid., p. 13.

18. *Ibid.*

CHAPTER FOUR: AT LAST, ON HIS WAY
1. Vivien Thomas, *Pioneering Research,* p. 13.
2. Peter Olch, Oral History Collections, "Interview with Vivien Thomas," April 20, 1967, National Library of Medicine, NIH, p. 8.
3. Vivien Thomas, *Pioneering Research,* p. 13.
4. Gwendolyn Clarke, Interview with author, White's Ford, Tennessee, July 17, 2017.
5. Vivien Thomas, *Pioneering Research,* p. 18–19.
6. *Ibid.,* p. 19.
7. *Ibid.*
8. *Ibid.,* pp. 18–19.
9. *Ibid.,* p. 19.
10. *Ibid.,* p. 19.
11. *Ibid.,* p. 41.
12. *Ibid.*
13. Vivien Thomas, Unpublished MS material, Johns Hopkins U. Chesney Archives.
14. Vanderbilt U. Dept. of Surgery, "Surgery Budgets, 1930–1939," History of Medicine Collections, Vanderbilt U.
15. James Pittman, *Tinsley Harrison, MD: Teacher of Medicine,* NewSouth Books, 1991, pp. 112, 136.
16. Alfred Blalock, "Letter to Barney Brooks," Nov. 28, 1933. And __, "Letter to Barney Brooks," Dec. 1, 1934. Both History of Medicine Collections, Vanderbilt U.
17. *Ibid.,* History of Medicine Collections, Vanderbilt U.
18. Vanderbilt U., Department of Surgery, "Surgery Budget," 1928–1929, 1929–1930, 1930–1931, 1931–1932, 1932–1933, 1933–1934, 1934–1935, 1936–1937, 1937–1938, 1938–1939, 1939–1940, History of Medicine Collections, Vanderbilt U.
19. Thomas, *Pioneering Research,* pp. 44–45.
20. *Ibid.*
21. Alfred Blalock, "Letter to Brooks," Dec. 3, 1937, History of Medicine Collections, Vanderbilt U.

CHAPTER FIVE: COMING UP EASY
1. A. McGehee Harvey, "Alfred Blalock 1899–1964, Biographical Memoir," *National Academy of Sciences,* 1982, p. 1.
2. "Surry, Smith's Fort: Warren House," National Park Service, 2023. http://www.nps.gov/articles/smiths.htm.
3. *Ibid.*

Endnotes

4. Carole Scott, "The Troubled World of Antebellum Banking in Georgia," *B>Quest,* 2016. http://www.westga.edu/~bquest/2000/antebellumGAbanks.pdf.
5. Bobby Lovett, *Of Promises Kept,* R.H. Boyd Publishing; Reavis Mitchell, Interview with author, Nashville, Tennessee, July 20, 2017.
6. Joe Moore, *Partners of the Heart,* American Experience, Public Broadcasting Station. http://www.pbs.org/wgbh/americanexperience/films/partners/.
7. William Longmire, *Alfred Blalock: His Life and Times,* p. 24.
8. *Ibid.,* p. 26.
9. Mark Ravitch, "Biography of Alfred Blalock," History of Medicine Collections, Vanderbilt U., pp 23, 25.
10. *Ibid.,* p. 29.
11. Mark Ravitch, Papers of Alfred Blalock, JHU Press, 1966.
12. Anne Edwards, *Road to Tara: The Life of Margaret Mitchell,* Ticknor & Fields, 1983.
13. Kathyrn Kemp, *Historic Clayton County: The Sesquicentennial History,* Historic Publishing Network, 2009, pp. 66–68.
14. State of Georgia, "Property Tax Digest Digests, 1793–1892," for Zadock B. Blalock.
15. State of Georgia, "Returns of Qualified Voters Under the Reconstruction Act of 1867–1869," for Zadock Blalock.
16. James Geisen, "Sharecropping," *New Georgia Encyclopedia,* 2018.

CHAPTER SIX: STAYING ALIVE

1. Kenneth Lundmerer, *Time to Heal: American Medication from the Turn of the Century to the Era of Managed Care,* Oxford University Press, 1999, pp. 30–31; Robert Bruce, *The Launching of Modern American Science,* Knopf, 1987, pp. 281 and 335.
2. *Ibid,* p. 13.
3. *Ibid,* p. 19.
4. *Ibid,* p. 19–20. And see Keith Wailoo, *Dying in the City of the Blues: Sickle Cell Anemia and the Politics of Race and Health,* University of North Carolina Press, 2001. Alondra Nelson, *Body and Soul: The Black Panther Party and the Fight Against Medical Discrimination,* University of Minnesota Press, 2013.
5. Lundmerer, *Time to Heal,* pp. 30–32.
6. Percentage of Southern classmates include those from Maryland, "Johns Hopkins University Medical Circular, 1921–1924," Johns Hopkins U. Chesney Archives.

7. James Pittman, *Tinsley Harrison, MD: Teacher of Medicine*, NewSouth Books, 1991, p. 78. Warfield Firor, Oral History Collections, "Vivien Thomas," National Library of Medicine, NIH p. 33.
8. William Longmire, *Alfred Blalock: His Life and Times*, p. 33.
9. Mark Ravitch, *Papers of Alfred Blalock*, JHU Press, 1966, p. xix. For a different outlook, see Walter Merrill, "What's Past is Prologue," *Annals of Thoracic Surgery*, Dec. 1999, pp. 2366-2375.
10. Ibid.
11. Ibid., p. xxi.
12. Blalock, Alfred, "A Clinical Study of the Biliary Tract Disease," *J. of the American Medical Association*, 83: 2057, Dec. 27, 1924; "A Statistical Study of 881 Cases of Biliary Tract Disease," *Johns Hopkins Hospital Bulletin*, 35: 391, 1924; with S. J. Crowe, "The Treatment of Chronic Middle Ear Suppuration," *Archives of Otolaryngology*, 1: 267, March, 1925; "The Effect of Changes in Hydrogen Ion Concentration on the Blood Flow of Morphinized Dogs," *J. of Clinical Investigation*, 1: 547, Aug. 1925; "The Incidence of Mastoid Disease in the US," *Southern Medical J.*, 18:621, Aug. 1925.
13. William Longmire, *Alfred Blalock*, p. 41.
14. Alfred Blalock, "Letter to Barney Brooks." Feb. 6, 1925, History of Medicine Collections, Vanderbilt U.
15. Alfred Blalock, "Talk," History of Medicine Collections, Vanderbilt U.
16. Mark Ravitch, *Papers of Alfred Blalock*, JHU Press, 1966, p. xxii.
17. William Longmire, *Alfred Blalock: His Life and Times*, p. 41.

CHAPTER SEVEN: OUTRACING DEATH

1. Tinsley Harrison, Talk, "Early Days," History of Medicine Collections, Vanderbilt U.
2. General Education Board, "Methods and Problems," Rockefeller Foundation, 1929, p. 1.
3. Mark Ravitch, *The Papers of Alfred Blalock*, JHU Press, 1966, p. xxii.
4. Rudolf Kampmeier, *Recollections: The Department of Medicine, Vanderbilt U. Dept. of Medicine, 1925-1959*, Vanderbilt U. Press, 1980.
5. Walter Merrill, "What's Past is Prologue," *Annals of Thoracic Surgery*, Dec. 1999, pp. 2366-2375.
6. Louis Rosenfeld, *Memoirs of A Surgical House Officer: Vanderbilt U. Hospital*, Vanderbilt U. Press, 1991, p. 59.
7. Alfred Blalock, "A Mechanism and Treatment of Experimental Shock, 1: Shock Following Hemorrhage," *Arch Surgery*, 1927, 15 (5), pp. 762-798.
8. Barney Brooks notation, Vanderbilt U. Surgery Dept., "Surgery Budget 1927-1928," History of Medicine Collections, Vanderbilt U.

Endnotes

9. Alfred Blalock, "Mechanisms and Treatment of Experimental Shock," *Archives of Surgery*, 1927.
10. James Pittman, *Tinsley Harrison, MD: Teacher of Medicine*, NewSouth Books, 1991, p. 134.
11. Alfred Blalock, "Letter to Walter Dandy," Dec. 28, 1927, History of Medicine Collections, Vanderbilt U.
12. Alfred Blalock, "Letter to Barney Brooks," July 20, 1927, History of Medicine Collections, Vanderbilt U.
13. Bruce Murray, "Letter to Alfred Blalock," Dec. 15, 1945, History of Medicine Collections, Vanderbilt U.; George Zuidema, "Alfred Blalock, Norman Bethune and the Bethune Murals," *Surgery*, 130(5), 2001.
14. Vanderbilt U. Surgery Dept., "Surgery Budget, 1927–1928," History of Medicine Collections, Vanderbilt U.
15. Mao Tse-Tung, "In Memory of Mao Tse-Tung," *Selected Works of Mao Tse-Tung*, Dec. 21, 1939. http://www.marxists.org/reference/arcgive/mao/selected-works/vol-2mswv225.htlmb; Jean Deslauriers and Denis Goulet, The Medical Life of Henry Norman Bethune," *Canadian Respiratory J*, Nov.–Dec. 2015, pp. 32–42.
16. George Zuidema, "Alfred Blalock, Norman Bethune and the Bethune Murals," *Surgery*, 130(5), 2001, p. 866; Larry Stephenson, "Blalock-Bethune Connection," *Cardiothoracic Surgery*, pp. 882–889, 2001.
17. General Education Board, "Letter to Alfred Blalock," Rockefeller Foundation, Oct. 30, 1951, History of Medicine Collections, Vanderbilt U.
18. Harrison, Tinsley, "Letter to Alfred Blalock," Apr. 27, 1927, History of Medicine Collections, Vanderbilt U.
19. James Pittman, *Tinsley Harrison, MD: Teacher of Medicine*, NewSouth Books, 1991, p. 111; William Longmire, *Alfred Blalock: His Life and Times*, p. 46.
20. Mark Dewey, Ugo Schagen, Wolfgang Eckhart and Eva Schonenberer, "Erst Ferdinand Sauerbruch and His Ambiguous Role in the Period of National Socialism," *Annals of Surgery*, Aug. 2006, p. 315.
21. Barney Brooks, "Budget Surgery, 1929–1930," History of Medicine Collections, Vanderbilt U.
22. ___, "Letter to ASCS," Aug. 30, 1930, History of Medicine Collections, Vanderbilt U.
23. David Sabiston, "Alfred Blalock: The Man," Hopkins U. Chesney Archives.
24. Alfred Blalock, "Experimental Shock: The Cause of Low Blood Pressure Produced by Muscle Injury," *Archives of Surgery*, June 1930.
25. Atlantic (Ga.) *Journal*, "Miss O'Bryan," Oct. 28, 1930; Vivien Thomas, *Pioneering Research*, p. 18.
26. Ibid.
27. "Nashville Historic Research," *National Civic Design Center*, p. 14.
28. "Three Banks," *Nashville Tennessean*, Nov. 22, 1930.

29. Jessie Gladden, "Interview with Vivien Thomas," Feb. 1972, Maryland Room, Enoch Pratt Free Library, Special Collections, Baltimore, Maryland.

CHAPTER EIGHT: CAUGHT SHORT
1. "Nashville Historical Research," *National Civic Design Center*, p. 14.
2. Ray Hill, "Great Depression in Tennessee," *Nashville Focus*, 2016, p. 2.
3. Jay Gourney and Yip Harburg, "Brother, Can You Spare a Dime," Americana, Warner-Chappell Music, 1932. http://socialwelfare.library.vcu.edu/eras/great-depression/brother-can-you-spare-a dime.
4. Vivien Thomas, Unpublished MS deletions MMR, Mark M. Ravitch Collection, National Library of Medicine, NIH.
5. Mark Ravitch, "The Contributions of Alfred Blalock," *Hopkins Medical J.*, 1977, p. 58.
6. Vivien Thomas, *Pioneering Research*, p. 17.
7. Alex Haller, Interview with author, Glencoe. Maryland, July 30, 2014; R. Robinson Baker, Interview with author, Owing Mills, Maryland, June 22, 2017.
8. Vivien Thomas, Unpublished MS material, Johns Hopkins U. Chesney Archives.
9. Ibid.
10. Vivien Thomas, *Pioneering Research*, p. 25.
11. Ibid., p. 31.
12. Edward Halperin, "A Solitary Act in the Bell Building: Striking a Blow for Racial Desegregation at a Southern Medical School," *Pharos Alpha Omega Alpha Honorary Medical Society*, Spring: 71(2), 48–51, 2007.
13. Vivien Thomas, *Pioneering Research*, p. 28.
14. Alfred Blalock, "Letter of Recommendation for Standford Leeds," Surgery Papers, History of Medicine Collections, Vanderbilt U.
15. Peter Olch, Oral History Collections, "Stanford Leeds," Jan. 29, 1973. National Library of Medicine, NIH.
16. Vivien Thomas, *Pioneering Research*, p. 17.
17. "A Visit with Vivien Thomas," Oct. 28, 1974, p. 9, Johns Hopkins U. Chesney Archives.
18. Ibid.
19. United States Department of Commerce, Bureau of the Census. Nashville, Tennessee, 1920.
20. Vivien Thomas, *Pioneering Research*, p. 48.

CHAPTER NINE: THOMAS, BLALOCK AND HENRY FORD
1. Gwendolyn Clarke, Interview with author, White's Ford, Tennessee, July 17, 2017.

Endnotes

2. Vivien Thomas, *Pioneering Research*, p. 57.
3. Harold Norris, Interview with author, Baltimore, Maryland, July 30, 2014.
4. Theodosia Thomas Dullea, Conversations with author.
5. Vivien Thomas, *Pioneering Research*, p. 26.
6. Timothy Buchman, "Shock: Blalock and Cannon," *Archives of Surgery*, 2010.
7. Johns Hopkins U. Medical Institutes, "The Johns Hopkins Hospital Surgery Routine," 1937, History of Medicine Collections, Vanderbilt U.
8. Woove, "Letter to Alfred Blalock," July 14, 1931, Duke University Medical Center Archives.
9. Vivien Thomas, *Pioneering Research*, p. 38.
10. Roy McClure, "Letter to Alfred Blalock," Aug 24, 1937, Duke University Medical Center Archives.
11. Vivien Thomas, *Pioneering Research*, p. 38.
12. Beth Bates, *The Making of Detroit in The Age of Henry Ford*, University of North Carolina Press, 2012.
13. Diane Feely, "Black Workers, Fordism and the UAW," *Solidarity*, 2014. http://www.solidarity-us.org/atc/168/p4071.
14. Alfred Blalock, "Letter to Roy McClure," Sept. 29, 1937, Duke University Medical Center Archives.
15. Mark Ravitch, *The Papers of Alfred Blalock*, JHU Press, 1966, p. xxiii; Ralph Hruban. and Will Linder, *A Scientific Revolution: The Men and Women Who Reinvented American Medicine*, Pegasus Books, 2022, p. 245.
16. "Interview with Vivien Thomas," Oct. 2, 1976, Johns Hopkins U. Chesney Archives, 1961, p. 51.
17. Thomas Turner, *Heritage of Excellence*, Johns Hopkins University Press, 1974, p. 463.
18. Roy McClure, "Letter to Alfred Blalock," Aug 24, 1937, Duke U. Medical Center Archives.
19. The federal minimum wage was established in 1938 but the Michigan state's minimum wage was higher. Ford, that year, had established a minimum wage for its employees that was even greater than Michigan's, at a whopping sixty-two cents an hour. That same year, Thomas was earning $884 annually at Vanderbilt. Going to Detroit would have raised his salary to a minimum of $1,300 a year, which is 47 percentage points higher than his Vanderbilt salary.

CHAPTER TEN: O BROTHER, WHERE ART THOU?

1. Harold Norris, Interview with author, Baltimore, Maryland, July 30, 2014.

2. Walt Whitman, "I Hear America Singing," *The Complete Poems*, Penguin, p. 47.
3. Langston Hughes, "I, Too," *The Weary Blues*, Knopf, p. 25.
4. Alaine Locke, *The New Negro Aesthetic: Selected Writings*, Penguin, 2022.
5. Bruce Beezer, "Black Teachers' Salaries," *J of Negro Education*, 1986, p. 203.
6. Scott Baker, "Testing Equality," *History of Education Quarterly*, 1995, p. 50.
7. John Kirk, "The NAACP Campaign," *J of African American History*, 2009, p. 532.
8. Bruce Beezer, "Black Teachers' Salaries," *J of Negro Education*, 1986, pp. 201–202.
9. *Ibid.*, p. 204.
10. Scott Baker, "Testing Equality," p. 50.
11. John Kirk, "The NAACP Campaign," p. 534.
12. *Ibid.*, p. 532.
13. *Ibid.*, p. 535.
14. Sonya Ramsey, *Reading, Writing and Segregation: A Century of Black Women Teachers in Nashville*, University of Illinois Press, 2008, p. 47.
15. Thomas v. Hibbits, District Court, Tennessee, Nashville Division, July 28, 1942 (46 Federal Supplement 368).
16. Ramsey, *Reading, Writing and Segregation*, pp. 36–37.
17. *Ibid.*, p. 53.
18. *Ibid.*, p. 55.
19. *Ibid.*, p. 52.
20. *Ibid.*, p. 54.
21. Reavis Mitchell, Interview with author, Nashville, Tennessee, July 20, 2017; Kathy Bennett, "Lynching," *Tennessee Encyclopedia*; "Lynching by State and Race," Tuskegee University, http://archive.tuskegee.edu/repository/wp-content/uploads/2020/11/Lynchings-Stats-Year-Dates-Causes.pdf.
22. *Nashville Tennessean*, "Race Distinction Is Denied," Feb. 25, 1942.
23. *Nashville Tennessean*, "Negro Teacher's Charge Denied," May 21, 1941.
24. Bobby Lovett, *The Civil Rights Movement*, 2015, pp. 12–13.
25. Thomas v. Hibbits, District Court, Tennessee, Nashville Division, July 28, 1942 (46 Federal Supplement 368).
26. Sonya Ramsey, *Reading, Writing and Segregation*, p. 52.
27. *Ibid.*
28. "Thomas' Battle Pays Off," *The 780 Countdown* (Nashville, Tennessee), July 30, 1942.
29. Ramsey, *Reading, Writing and Segregation*, p. 53.
30. *Nashville Globe*, "Teacher Resigns," Oct 1, 1943.
31. *Ibid.*
32. "Thomas' Battle Pays Off," *The 780 Countdown*.

ENDNOTES

33. Benjamin Houston, *The Nashville Way*, 2012, pp. 36–37, 114, U. of Georgia Press.

CHAPTER ELEVEN: MOVING ON UP

1. Thomas Turner, *Heritage of Excellence: The Johns Hopkins Medical Institute*, Johns Hopkins University Press, 1974, p. 458.
2. R. Robinson Baker, Interview with author, Owings Mill, Aug. 17, 2017; Peter Olch, Oral History Collections, "Vivien Thomas," National Library of Medicine, NIH p. 33, April 20, 1967.
3. Kenneth Ludmerer, *Time to Heal*. Thomas Turner, *Heritage of Excellence*, p. 434–435. Alex Haller, Interview with author, Glencoe, Maryland, July 30, 2014. Alex Haller, "Letter to Rodgers," Feb. 5, 1971, Johns Hopkins U. Chesney Archives.
4. Thomas Turner, *Heritage of Excellence*, pp. 453–454.
5. *Ibid.*, pp. 458–459.
6. Vivien Thomas, *Pioneering Research*, p. 39.
7. *Ibid*, p. 38.
8. *Ibid.*, p. 42.
9. Reavis Mitchell, Interview with author, Nashville, Tennessee, July 17, 2020.
10. Program, Johns Hopkins U., "Dinner in Honor of Alfred Blalock," 1940, Duke U. Medical Center Archives.
11. Alfred Blalock, "Letter to Bowman," Feb. 1, 1941, Duke U. Medical Center Archives.
12. *Ibid.*
13. Vivien Thomas, Unpublished MS deletions MMR, Mark M. Ravitch Collection, National Library of Medicine, NIH.
14. *Ibid.*

CHAPTER TWELVE: MARYLAND, MY MARYLAND

1. The statue is a replica of the Church of Our Lady Carrera marble statue in Copenhagen, Denmark, called Christus, sculpted by Bertel Thorvalson. For whatever reason, Hopkins purchased a replica and renamed it Christ the Consolater. http://en.wikipedia.org/wiki/Christus; Nancy McCall, "The Statue of Christ the Consolator at the Johns Hopkins Hospital: Its Acquisition and Historic Origins," *Johns Hopkins Medical Journal*, 151 (1) July 1982, 11–19.
2. Vivien Thomas, *Pioneering Research*, p. 54.
3. *Ibid.*, pp. 54–55.
4. *Ibid.*, p. 55–56.
5. *Ibid.*, p. 56.
6. *Ibid.*, p. 57.

7. Levi Watkins, Interview with author, Baltimore, Maryland, August 22 and Sept. 14, 2014.
8. Harold Norris, Interview with author, Baltimore, Maryland, July 30, 2014.
9. "State Song of Maryland," http://sos.maryland.gov/mdkids/Pages/StateSong.aspx.
10. Antero Pietila, *Not in My Neighborhood: How Bigotry Shaped a Great American City*, Chicago, Illinois: Ivan R. Dee, 2010, pp. v–vi.
11. Antero Pietila, *The Ghosts of Johns Hopkins: The Life and Legacy that Shaped an American City*, Roman & Littlefield. 2018, p. x.
12. Pietila, *Not in My Neighborhood*, pp. 61–74.
13. W. Edward Orser, *Blockbusting in Baltimore*, U. Press of Kentucky, 1994, p. 18.
14. Ibid., p. 89. And Bernie Berkowitz, Interview with author, Miami Beach, Florida, Feb. 22, 2018.
15. Ibid., p. 172–173.
16. Ibid., p. 180.
17. Pietila, *Not in My Neighborhood*, p. 80.

CHAPTER THIRTEEN: PUTTING UP AND DOING WITHOUT

1. Spark Media, *Partners of the Heart*, PBS, 2004.
2. Antero Pietila, *Not in My Neighborhood*, p. 89.
3. Alfred Blalock, "Letter to Alan Chesney," Dec. 16, 1942, Johns Hopkins U. Chesney Archives. For those interested in symbolic interactions, see Erving Goffman, "On Cooling the Mark Out," *Psychiatry: Journal of Interpersonal Relations*, 1952, 15(4), pp. 451–463.
4. Peter Olch, Oral History Collections, "Interview with Vivien Thomas," April 20, 1967, National Library of Medicine, NIH.
5. "A Visit with Vivien Thomas," Oct. 28, 1974, Johns Hopkins U. Chesney Archives; Vivien Thomas, *Pioneering Research*, p. 60.
6. Ibid.
7. Ibid.
8. Vivien Thomas, *Pioneering Research*, p. 60.
9. Vivien Thomas, Unpublished MS material, Johns Hopkins U. Chesney Archives.
10. John Cameron, Interview with author, Baltimore, Maryland, March 16, 2015.
11. Vivien Thomas, *Pioneering Research*, p. 58.
12. Harold Norris, Interview with author, Baltimore, Maryland, July 30, 2014.
13. Vivien Thomas, Unpublished MS material, Johns Hopkins U. Chesney Archives.

14. Harold Norris, Interview with author.
15. Vivien Thomas, Unpublished MS material, Johns Hopkins U. Chesney Archives.
16. *Ibid.*
17. *Ibid.*
18. *Ibid.*
19. *Ibid.*
20. *Ibid.*
21. *Ibid.*
22. Theodosia Thomas Dullea, Conversations with author, telephone.
23. *Ibid.*
24. Harold Norris, Interview with author, Baltimore, Maryland, July 30, 2014.
25. *Ibid;* Marcia Rasberry Smith, Interview with author, telephone, Aug. 19, 2018; Ursula Rasberry-Dikhoffe, Interview with author, telephone, Aug. 15, 2016.
26. Vivien Thomas, Unpublished MS material, Johns Hopkins U. Chesney Archives.
27. Alfred Blalock, "Letter to Alan Chesney," Duke U. Medical Center Archives.
28. "A Visit with Vivien Thomas," Oct. 28, 1974, Johns Hopkins U. Chesney Archives.
29. Vivien Thomas, *Pioneering Research,* p. 65.
30. Alfred Blalock, "Letter to Alan Chesney," Dec. 23, 1942, Johns Hopkins U. Chesney Archives; William Fox, *Dandy of Johns Hopkins,* Williams and Wilkins, Baltimore, 1984., p. 270.
31. Thomas Turner, *Heritage of Excellence,* p. 413; Fox, *Dandy of Johns Hopkins.*
32. Alfred Blalock, "Letter to Alan Chesney," Dec. 16, 1942, Johns Hopkins U. Chesney Archives.
33. Alfred Blalock, "Letter to Alan Chesney," Oct. 28, 1943, Johns Hopkins U. Chesney Archives. For those interested in symbolic interactions, see Erving Goffman, "On Cooling the Mark Out," *Psychiatry: Journal of Interpersonal Relations,* 1952, 15(4), pp. 451-463.
34. Alfred Blalock, "Letter to Alan Chesney," Dec. 16, 1942, Johns Hopkins U. Chesney Archives.
35. Alfred Blalock, "Letter to Chesapeake & Potomac Telephone Co.," Aug. 14, 1945, Duke U. Medical Center Archives.
36. Alfred Blalock, "Letter to Chesapeake & Potomac Telephone Co.," Feb. 2, 1953, Duke U. Medical Center Archives.

CHAPTER FOURTEEN: HOPING TO DO GOOD

1. Antero Pietila, *The Ghosts of Johns Hopkins: The Life and Legacy that Shaped an American City*, Roman & Littlefield. 2018, pp. 3–23.
2. Ibid.
3. Martha Jones, "Hard History," http://hardhistoriesjhu.substack.com/p/owner-yes-enslaver-certainly; Sydney Van Morgan, et al., "Seeking the Truth: Johns Hopkins and Slavery," paper presentation, 2021; Jennifer Shuessler, "Johns Hopkins's Feet of Clay," *New York Times*, Dec. 10, 2020.
4. *New York Tribune*, Jan. 8, 1974.
5. Ibid.
6. Winchester, "Late Johns Hopkins's Will," *Baltimore Afro American*, June 13, 1925.
7. Ibid.
8. Ibid.
9. Leslie Makau, "Johns Hopkins and The Feminist Legacy," *Am. J of Clinical Medicine*, 20012, p. 123.
10. David Smith, *Here Lies Jim Crow*, 2012, p. 126.
11. Antero Pietila, *The Ghosts of Johns Hopkins*.
12. *Baltimore Afro American*, "The Ironclad Will," Jan. 23, 1960.
13. "The History of African Americans@JHU." http://www.11af1.jhu.edu.chronology/2010/html.
14. Alexis Fitts, "Medicine's On-going Race Problem," March 22, 2016, *Undark*.
15. W.E.B. Du Bois, "Negroes in College," *Nation*, April, 1926; "Johns Hopkins Leads in Race Prejudice," March 20, 1926, *Baltimore Afro American*.
16. William Rodriguez and Robert Garcia, *First, Do No Harm*, Am J Public Health, 103(12), Dec. 2013, p. 43.
17. William Jarrett, "Raising the Bar," U. of North Carolina Proceedings, Baylor U., 2011, p. 1.
18. Ibid.
19. Leslie Makau, *Johns Hopkins*, p. 1.
20. William Jarrett, *"Raising the Bar,"* 2001.
21. "Black Medical Pioneers, Part I," J. of the National Medicine Association, pp. 632–637.
22. Ibid.
23. Mat Edelson, "Homing in on Diversity," *Medicine*, Johns Hopkins U., 2018.
24. Levi Watkins, Interview with author, Baltimore, Maryland, August 22 and Sept. 14, 2014.
25. *Baltimore Afro American*, p. 34, circa 1870.

Endnotes

26. Vivien Thomas, Unpublished MS material, Johns Hopkins U. Chesney Archives.

CHAPTER FIFTEEN: IT'S WAR!

1. "Radio Reports Japan's Attack on Pearl Harbor," Modesto, California, Radio Museum. https://www.youtube.com/watch?v=6muWK4VMbEI.
2. "This is No Joke: This Is War," Michigan St. U. https://twitter.com/NewsHour/status/1600493581797625857.
3. "As Pearl Harbor Happened." http://dodgers.mlblogs.com/as-pearl-harbor-happened-the-dodgers-played-the-giants.
4. The football team was renamed the Washington Commanders in 2022. http://www.cnn.com/2022/02/02/us/washington-football-team-name/index.html.
5. "Pearl Harbor at Griffith Stadium," Mark Jones, "boundary Stones," WETA (Washington, DC). http://blogs.weta.org/boundrystone/2016/12/07/pearl-harbor-griffith-stadium.
6. Alfred Blalock, *Principles of Surgical Care, Shock and Other Problems*, Mosby, 1940.
7. Robert Hardaway, "Wound Shock: A History of Its Study and Treatment by Military Surgeons," *Military Medicine*, 169, 4:265, 2004.
8. Anastasia K. Lundquist, *Out for Blood: The Pursuit of Life for the Wounded on the Fighting Fronts of World War II*, CreateSpace Publishing., 2014, p. 260.
9. "Pearl Harbor Medical Activities," Naval History and Heritage Command, 1941. http://www.history.navy.mil/research/library/online-reading-room/title-list-alphabetically/p/pearl-harbor-navy-medical-activities.html.
10. Gwenneth R. Milbrath, "Grace Under Fire: The Army Nurses of Pearl Harbor," *US Army Medical Department J*, 2016, (3–16), 1941. pp. 112–117; http://pearlharborwarbirds.com/pearl-harbor-nurses; "Pearl Harbor As Remembered by the Nurses Who Were There." http://www.army.mil/article/179038/the_pearl_harbor_attack_as_remembered_by_the_nurses_who_were_there.
11. "Thomas S. Green, Maj. Gen." *Judge Advocate Journal*, 1945.
12. Thomas Helling, *Desperate Surgery in the Pacific War: Doctors and Damage Control for Pacific Wounded, 1941–1945*, 2017.
13. Gwenneth Milbrath, "Grace Under Fire," 1941, *US Army Medical Department J*, 2016, (3–16), 1941, pp. 112–117.
14. "What Happened" http://www.iwm.org.uk/history/what-happened-at-pearl-harbor. And "Pearl Harbor Navy Medical Activities," http://www.history.Navy/mil/research/library/online-reading-room/title-list-alphabetically/p/pearl-harbor-navy-medical-activities.

15. "16 Days to Die at Pearl Harbor." http://www.seattletimes.com/nation-world/16-days-to-die-at-pearl-harbor-families-werent-told-about-sailors-trapped-inside-sunken-battleship/; "Never Forgot the Smell of Death." http://www.spokesman.com/stories/2016/dec/04/ray-daves-a-sailor-at-pearl-harbor-never-forgot-the resources/research starters/research-starters-us-military-numbers.
16. Ralph E. Pottker, Cdr., USNR, Conversations, Highland Park, Illinois and Southern Pines, North Carolina.
17. "Research Starters: US Military by The Numbers," National World War II Museum. http://www.nationalww2museum.org.students-teacher/student.
18. Stephen Ambrose and C. Sulzberger, *The American Heritage History of World War II*, American Heritage, 1997, p. 421.
19. Ronald Takaki, *Double Victory: A Multicultural History of America in World War II*, Little, Brown and Company, 2000, p. 362.
20. In recognition of his heroism, The USS Doris Miller, a supercarrier CVN 81, described as "the most powerful and lethal warship ever," will be laid down in 2026 and commissioned in 2030. Thomas W. Cutrer and T. Michael Parrish, Oct. 31, 2019. "USS West Virginia's Action Report," Naval History and Heritage Command, *Navy Times*, 2015.
21. "He Fought—Keeps Mop," *Pittsburgh Courier*, July 25, 1942; Thomas Cutter and Michael Parrish, "How Dorrie Miller's Bravery Helped Fight Racism," *World War II Magazine*, Oct. 31, 2019; Paul Murray, "Blacks and the Draft: A History of Institutional Racism," *Journal of Black Studies*, 2:1, September 1971, pp. 57–76.
22. Thomas Turner, *Heritage of Excellence: The Johns Hopkins Medical Institute*, Johns Hopkins U. Press, 1974, p. 433.
23. Vivien Thomas, Unpublished MS material, Johns Hopkins U. Chesney Archives.
24. William P. Longmire, Jr., *Alfred Blalock: His Life and Times*, self-published, 1991, p. 90.
25. Mark M. Ravitch, *Papers of Alfred Blalock*, JHU Press, 1966, pp. xxxv.
26. Alexander Haller, Interview with author, Glencoe, Maryland, July 30, 2014.
27. "A Visit with Vivien Thomas," 1974, Johns Hopkins U. Chesney Archives.
28. Alfred Blalock, "Utilization of Oxygen by the Brain in Toxic Shock," *Archives of Surgery*, 1941.
29. ___, *Principles of Surgical Care, Shock and Other Problems*, Mosby, 1940.
30. Alfred Blalock, "Utilization of Oxygen by the Brain in Toxic Shock," *Archives of Surgery*, 1941.
31. Alex Haller, Interview with author. Glencoe, Maryland, July 30, 2014.
32. Vivien Thomas, *Pioneering Research*, p. 77.

ENDNOTES

CHAPTER SIXTEEN: BLALOCK, THOMAS AND CHARLES DREW
1. Mead Schaeffer, "He gave his blood. Will you give yours?" American Red Cross, National Library of Medicine, NIH. http://collections.nim.nih.gov/catalog/nlmuid-101452787-img.
2. Olga S. Pottker, Conversations with author, Highland Park, Illinois and Southern Pines, North Carolina.
3. "Charles R. Drew," American Chemical Society. http://www.acs.org/education/whatischemistry/african-americans-in-sciences/charles-richard-drew.html.
4. James, Rawn, *The Double V: How Wars, Protest and Harry Truman Desegregated America's Military*, Bloomsbury Press, 2014, p. 138.
5. Anastasia Kirby Lindquist, *Out for Blood*, 1981, pp. x–xii.
6. ___, "During World War II, Plasma Saved Lives," Defense Media Network. http://www.defensemedianetwork.com/stories/world-war-ii-plasma-saved-lives/.
7. ___, *Out for Blood*, pp. x–xi.
8. *Ibid*; James Rawn, *Double V*, 2014, p. 138. More information on plasma in the Pacific Theater can be found in "The US Navy Medical Department at War 1941-1945," Bureau of Medicine and Surgery, Navy Dept., 1946.
9. "World War II Statistics," National World War II Museum. http://www.secondworldwarhistory.com/world-war-2-statistics.asp.
10. *Ibid; The German Medical Establishment*, AMEDD Center of History and Heritage, US Army Center of Military History, National World War II Museum. http://achh.army.mil/history/book-wwii-medsvcsinmedtrnmnrthrtrs-appendices-appd.

CHAPTER SEVENTEEN: A WOMAN OF VALOR
1. Mary Allen Engle, *Helen Brooke Taussig: Living Legend in Cardiology*, 1985, p. 372.
2. *Ibid.*
3. Peter D. Olch, Oral History Collections, "Adventures in Medical Research: A. McGehee Harvey," 1981, National Library of Medicine, NIH.
4. Sherwin B. Nuland, *Doctors of Medicine: The Biography of Medicine*, Vintage, 1995, p. 434.
5. William N. Evans, "The Relationship Between Maude Abbott and Helen Brooke Taussig," *Cardiology of the Young*, 2008, pp. 559–560.
6. Helen Taussig, "On the Evolution of Our Knowledge of Congenital Malformations of the Heart," *Circulation*, vol. 31, no. 5, 1965, p. 770.
7. Marshall L. Jacobs, and Jeffrey P. Jacobs, "The Early History of Surgery for Patients with Tetralogy of Fallot." *Cardiology of the Young*, 18:3 (2008): 8–11; Catherine Neill and Edward P. Clark, "Tetralogy of Fallot: The First

Three Hundred Years," *Texas Heart Institute Journal*, 21, 1994 272–279; Joanne P. Starr, "Tetralogy of Fallot: Yesterday and Today," *World Journal of Surgery*, 29 (November 2009): 658–668.
8. Ibid.
9. Catherine Neil, *The Developing Heart: A History of Pediatric Cardiology*, Springer, 1995.
10. Samuel G. Gross, *Biographical Memoirs*, National Academies Press, 1995.
11. H. Bill, ed., "William E. Ladd, MD: Great Pioneer of North American Pediatric Surgery," in Peter Paul Rickham, ed., *Historical Aspects of Pediatric Surgery*, Springer, 1986.
12. Ibid.
13. Joyce Baldwin, *To Heal the Heart of a Child*, 1992, p. 55.
14. Ibid.
15. Ibid.
16. Vivien Thomas, *Pioneering Research*, p. 70.
17. Helen Taussig, "On the Evolution of Our Knowledge of Congenital Malformations," *Circulation*, 965, vol. 31, no. 5, 1965.
18. Ibid.
19. Vivien Thomas, *Pioneering Research*, pp. 80–82.
20. Ibid.

CHAPTER EIGHTEEN: THOMAS DECODES THE BLUE BABIES
1. Vivien Thomas, *Pioneering Research*, p. 81.
2. Ibid., p. 82.
3. Vivien Thomas, Unpublished MS material, Johns Hopkins U. Chesney Archives.
4. Vivien Thomas, *Pioneering Research*, p. 107.
5. Peter D. Olch, Oral History Collections, "Interview with Henry Bahnson," National Library of Medicine, NIH.
6. See Harry Minetree, *Cooley: The Career of a Great Heart Surgeon, 1973*; Cooley, Interview with author, telephone, March 23, 2016; Peter Olch, Oral History Collections, "Interview with Firor," National Library of Medicine, NIH, Feb. 9, Feb. 28 and March 21, 1967; Vivien Thomas, "Unpublished MS," Johns Hopkins U. Chesney Archives.
7. Vivien Thomas, *Pioneering Research*, p. 81.
8. Gwendolyn Clark, Interview with author, White's Ford, Tennessee, July 17, 2017.
9. See Alfred Blalock, "Letters to Mrs. George Blalock," Nov 7, 1952 and Nov. 3, 1954, History of Medicine Collections, Vanderbilt U.
10. Rowena Spencer, "Letter to Thomas," 1982, Johns Hopkins U. Chesney Archives.

Endnotes

11. Douglas Slatter, *Textbook of Small Animal Surgery*, W.B. Saunders, 2003; K. Lee Lerner, "Scientific Thought," *Biomedicine and Health*, pp. 468–481.
12. Vivien Thomas, *Pioneering Research*, p. 84.
13. Ibid., pp. 84–86.
14. David Cooper, *Open Heart*, p. 46.
15. Catherine Neil, *The Developing Heart*, p. 58.
16. Vivien Thomas, *Pioneering Research*, p. 90.
17. Ibid., p. 89.
18. Ibid., p. 89.

CHAPTER NINETEEN: A BLACK MAN, A BLUE BABY AND THE DAWN OF HEART SURGERY

1. Joyce Baldwin, *To Heal the Heart of a Child*, 1992, p. 61.
2. Ibid.
3. William P. Longmire, Jr., *Alfred Blalock: His Life and Times*, Self-published, 1991, pp. 102–103.
4. Denton Cooley, "First Blalock-Taussig Shunt," *J. of Thoracic and Cardiovascular Surgery*, October 2010.
5. Lisa Yount, *Alfred Blalock, Helen Taussig and Vivien Thomas*, Chelsea House, 2012, p. 55.
6. G. Reeves and Mark F. Newman, "Mark Harmel: Portrait of an Anesthesiology Pioneer," *Anesthesia and Analgesia*, 2016 Feb; 122(2)539-4.1; "Life Stories: Medical Skill and Compassion Marked Merel Harmel's Career," *News & Observer* (Raleigh, S.C.), March 6, 2023.
7. Vivien Thomas, *Pioneering Research*, p. 92.
8. Ibid.
9. Catherine Neill, *The Developing Heart: A History of Cardiac Surgery*, Springer, 1995, p. 55.
10. Vivien Thomas, *Pioneering Research*, p. 92.
11. Stephan Timmermans, "A Black Technician and Blue Babies." *Social Studies of Science*; 33:2 (April 2003): pp. 197–229.
12. Alex Haller, Interview with author, Glencoe, Maryland, July 30, 2014.
13. Vivien Thomas, *Pioneering Research*, p. 92; Clara Belle Puryear, "Letter to Vivien Thomas," Feb. 16, 1982, Johns Hopkins U. Chesney Archives.
14. Vivien Thomas, *Pioneering Research*, p. 92.
15. Stephan Timmermans, "A Black Technician and Blue Babies," *Social Studies of Science*, pp. 197–229.
16. Mary Allen Engle, "Helen Brooke Taussig: Living Legend in Cardiology," *Clinical Cardiology*, 1985.
17. Thomas Morris, *The Matter of the Heart: A History of the Heart in Eleven Operations*, St. Martin's Press, 2017.
18. Vivien Thomas, *Pioneering Research*, p. 95.

19. Joyce Baldwin, *To Heal the Heart of a Child*, 1992, p. 62.
20. Lisa Yount, *Alfred Blalock, Helen Taussig and Vivien Thomas*, pp. 57–58.

CHAPTER TWENTY: A VACATION, AT LONG LAST

1. Vivien Thomas, *Pioneering Research*, p. 130.
2. Victor Hugo Green, *Negro Motorist Green Book*, 1936 annually through 1966, Green Publishers.
3. Theodosia Thomas Dullea, Conversations with author.
4. Vivien Thomas, *Pioneering Research*, p. 141.
5. Theodosia Thomas Dullea, Conversations with author; Vivien Thomas, *Pioneering Research*, p. 130.
6. Vivien Thomas, Unpublished manuscript material, Johns Hopkins U. Chesney Archives.
7. Ibid.
8. Harold Norris, Interview with author, Baltimore, Maryland, July 30, 2014.
9. Vivien Thomas, *Pioneering Research*, p. 131.
10. William S. Stoney, *Pioneers of Cardiac Surgery*, Vanderbilt U. Press, 2008, p. 41.
11. Keiffer, "Letter to Cooley," April 17, 1972, Archives and Special Collections, U of Pittsburgh.
12. Vivien Thomas, *Pioneering Research*, p. 43.
13. Ira Katznelson, *When Affirmative Action Was White: An Untold History of Racial Inequality in Twentieth-century America*, W.W. Norton, 2006; Hillary Herbold, "Never a Level Playing-Field: Blacks and the GI Bill," *J. of Blacks in Higher Education*, Winter 1994; Shannon Luders-Manuel, "The Inequality Hidden Within the Race-Neutral GI Bill," Sept. 18, 2017, JSTOR, http://jstor.or/the-inequality-hidden-within-the-race-neutral-g-i-bill; Mathew Delmont, *Half American: The Epic Story of African Americans Fighting World War II at Home and Abroad*, Viking, 2022, pp. 268–270; National Bureau of Economic Research, "The GI Bill, World War II and the Education of Black Americans," The *Digest*, Dec. 2002.
14. Hillary Herbold, "Never a Level Playing-Field: Blacks and the GI Bill," *J. of Blacks in Higher Education*, Winter 1994; Shannon Luders-Manuel, "The Inequality Hidden Within the Race-Neutral GI Bill," Sept. 26, 2017, JSTOR. http://jstor.or/the-inequality-hidden-within-the-race-neutral-g-i-bill.
15. Gwendolyn Clarke, Interview with author, White's Creek, Tennessee, July 17, 2017.
16. Vivien Thomas, *Pioneering Research*, p. 136.
17. Gwendolyn Clarke, Interview with author, White's Creek, Tennessee, July 17, 2017.

ENDNOTES

18. Alex Haller, Interview with author, Glencoe, Maryland, July 30, 2014.
19. *Ibid.*
20. Jack Zimmerman, Interview with Andrew S. Fishel, telephone, August 2, 2018.
21. R. Robertson Baker, Interview with author, Owings Mill, Maryland, July 17, 2017.
22. Gwendolyn Clarke, Interview with author, White's Creek, Tennessee, July 17, 2017; Vivien Thomas, *Pioneering Research,* p. 131.

CHAPTER TWENTY-ONE: CLASH OF THE TITANS

1. Peter D. Olch, Oral History Collections, "Interview with Warfield Firor," Feb. 9 and 27, March 21, 1967, National Library of Medicine, NIH.
2. William N. Evans, "Clifton B. Leech: First Director of the Pediatric Cardiac Clinic at the Johns Hopkins U.," *Cardiology of the Young*, Sept. 26, 2008. William Evans, "The Relationship Between Maude Abbott and Helen Taussig: Connecting the Historical Dots," *Cardiology in the Young*, December 2008, 18(6), 2012, pp. 557–564.
3. Peter D. Olch, Oral History Collections, "Interview with Warfield Firor," Feb. 9, Feb. 28, March 21, 1967, National Library of Medicine, NIH.
4. Vivien Thomas, *Pioneering Research*, p. 98.
5. Austin Lamont, "Letter to Ravitch," Nov. 1, 1965, Mark Ravitch Files, National Library of Medicine, NIH.
6. Peter Olch, Oral History Collections, "Interview with Warfield Firor," Feb. 9, Feb. 8, and March 21, 1967, National Library of Medicine, NIH.
7. See William Longmire, *Alfred Blalock: His Life and Times*, 1991, 1999, p. 114. Lisa Yount, *Alfred Blalock, Helen Taussig and Vivien Thomas, Mending Children's Hearts,* Trailblazers in Science and Technology, Chelsea House, 2012, pp. 57–58.
8. Helen Taussig, "The Development of the Blalock-Taussig Operation and Its Results Twenty Years Later," *American Philosophical Society*, Nov. 1976, p. 120.
9. Alfred Blalock and Helen Taussig, "Surgical Treatments of Malformations of the Heart in Which There Is Pulmonary Stenosis or Pulmonary Atresia," *J. of the American Medical Association*, May 19, 1945.
10. *LIFE,* "Blue Baby Research," March 14, 1949.
11. *TIME,* "Medicine: Blue Babies," Dec. 31, 1945.
12. Richard Bing, "Recollections of An Eyewitness," *Perspectives in Biology and Medicine,* Winter 1996; "The Johns Hopkins: the Blalock–Taussig Era," *Indian Journal of Thoracic and Cardiovascular Surgery*, 6 (1989–1990): 78–81.
13. WMAR Baltimore radio, "A Will from Within," video recording, 1976, National Library of Medicine, NIH.

14. Rosalie S. Sauber, "Memories of Hospital Work in Wartime," Letters to Editor, *Baltimore Sun*. June 7, 1997.
15. "Fund Being Raised for 'Blue Baby' by Salisbury Post of Legionnaires" The *Charlotte* (North Carolina) *Observer*, Feb. 9, 1946.
16. Nat Kantar and James Davis, "Blue Baby Saved by Rare Surgery," *NY Daily News*, Dec. 13, 1948.
17. "Blue Baby Faces Surgery," *Norfolk* (Virginia) *Ledger Dispatch*, Dec. 15, 1945; "Hundreds Await Blue Baby Surgery, 2 Years Old Today," The *Brattleboro* (Vermont) *Reformer*, Nov. 29, 1946.
18. "Hundreds Await Blue Baby Surgery," The *Brattleboro* (Vermont) *Reformer*, Nov. 1946.
19. Alex Haller, Interview with author, Glencoe, Maryland, July 30, 2014.
20. Peter D. Olch, Oral History Collections, "Interview with Warfield Firor," National Library of Medicine, NIH.
21. Ibid.
22. W. E. B. Du Bois, *The Souls of Black Folks*, Penguin Books, p. 12.
23. "First Closed-Circuit Televised Blue Baby Surgery at JHU," Photo, 1947 (item 145872), Johns Hopkins U. Chesney Archives; Paul Murray, "Blacks and the Draft: A History of Institutional Racism," *Journal of Black Studies*, 2:1, September 1971, pp. 57–76.

CHAPTER TWENTY-TWO: THE BLUE BABY TOUR
1. Mark Ravitch, *Papers of Alfred Blalock*, JHU Press, 1966, p. xlviii.
2. Alex Haller, Interview with author, Glencoe, Maryland, July 30, 2014.
3. Thomas Morris, *A History of the Heart*, 2017, p. 35.
4. Harry Minetree, *Cooley: The Career of a Great Heart Surgeon*, 1973, p. 105.
5. "A Will from Within," WMAR-TV, Baltimore, 1976, National Library of Medicine, NIH.
6. "Gifts to Be Used at the Discretion of Dr. Alfred Blalock," Multiple years, Duke U. Medical Center Archives.
7. Yes, Hopkins medical had a Public Affairs office as noted in Thomas Turner's *Heritage of Excellence: The Johns Hopkins Medical Institute*, Johns Hopkins U. Press, 1974. The quote is from: Vivien Thomas, *Pioneering Research*, p. 101.
8. *Fort Worth* (Texas) *Star-Telegram*, Dec. 14, 1945.
9. Alfred Blalock, "Letter to Helen Taussig," March 21, 1947, Duke U. Medical Center Archives.
10. Helen Taussig, "Letter to Alfred Blalock," Nov. 21, 1947. Duke U. Medical Center Archives.
11. William Longmire, *Alfred Blalock: His Life and Times*, 1991, p. 115, April 15, 1997.

ENDNOTES

12. William Clifford Roberts, "Denton A. Cooley," *Am. J. of Cardiology*, pp. 1080–1081.

CHAPTER TWENTY-THREE: THE EVERLASTING SALARY ISSUE

1. Vivien Thomas, Unpublished MS material, Johns Hopkins U. Chesney Archives.
2. Vivien Thomas, *Pioneering Research*, p. 131.
3. See, for example, Robert Margo, "Explaining Black-White Wage Convergence, 1940–1950," *ILR Review*, Sage, 1995, pp, 470–481.
4. "Salary Trends, Federal Classified Employees, 1939–1964," Bulletin No. 144, Bureau of Labor Statistics, US Dept. of Labor, May 1965.
5. Gordon Fisher, "From Hunter to Orshansky: An Overview of (Unofficial) Poverty Lines in the United States from 1904 to 1965," Office of the Assistant Secretary for Planning and Evaluation, US Department of Health & Human Services, March 1994. http://aspe.hhs.gov/hunter-orshansky-overview-unofficial-poverty-lines-united-states-1904-1965-summary.
6. Vivien Thomas, Unpublished MS material, Johns Hopkins U. Chesney Archives.
7. Vivien Thomas, *Pioneering Research*, p. 19.
8. *Ibid.*, p. 131.
9. *Ibid.*, p. 136.
10. *Ibid.*, p. 131.
11. *Ibid.* p. 132.
12. Alfred Blalock, "Speech," circa 1945, Johns Hopkins U. Chesney Archives; Alex Haller, Interview with author, Glencoe, Maryland July 30, 2014.
13. Alex Haller, Interview with author, Glencoe, Maryland, July 30, 2014.
14. Johns Hopkins Medical Institute, "Surgical Department Budget, Private Patients," Duke U. Medical Center Archives.
15. *Ibid.*
16. *Ibid.*
17. See Vivien Thomas, *Pioneering Research*, p. 135; Stephan Timmermans, "A Black Technician and Blue Babies," *Social Studies of Science*; 33:2 (April 2003): pp. 197–229.
18. Vivien Thomas, "Letter to Mark Ravitch," Dec. 1981, Johns Hopkins U. Chesney Archives.
19. Vivien Thomas, Unpublished MS deletions M.M.R., Mark M. Ravitch Collection, National Library of Medicine, NIH.
20. Vivien Thomas, *Pioneering Research*, p. 135.
21. *Ibid.*
22. *Ibid.*
23. *Ibid.*

24. *Ibid.*
25. Vivien Thomas, Unpublished MS delections M.M.R., Mark Ravitch Collection, National Library of Medicine, NIH.

CHAPTER TWENTY-FOUR HOPKINS'S GREATEST SURGEON?

1. Denton Cooley, "The First Blalock-Taussig Shunt," *J of Thoracic and Cardiovascular Surgery,* Oct. 2010, p. 751.
2. William N. Evans, "The Blalock-Taussig Shunt: The Social History of An Eponym," *Cardiology of the Young,* 19 (2009): 119–128.
3. Vivien Thomas, *Pioneering Research,* pp. 105–106.
4. Vivien Thomas, Unpublished MS material, Johns Hopkins U. Chesney Archives.
5. *Ibid.*
6. Denton Cooley, Interview with author, telephone, March 23, 2016.
7. *Ibid.*
8. *Johns Hopkins University Magazine,* Feb. 1986, p. 60.
9. Peter Olch, Oral History Collections, "Interview with Richard Te Linde," National Library of Medicine, NIH.
10. ___, "Interview with Henry Bahnson," National Library of Medicine, NIH.
11. *Ibid.*
12. Vivien Thomas, Unpublished MS material, Johns Hopkins U. Chesney Archives.
13. *Ibid.*
14. *Ibid.*
15. Theodosia Thomas Dullea, Conversations with author. Gwendolyn Clarke, Interview with author, Whites Creek, Tennessee, July 17, 2017; Vivien Thomas, Unpublished MS material, Johns Hopkins U. Chesney Archives.
16. *Ibid.*
17. Koko Eaton, Interview with author, St. Petersburg, Florida, April 27, 2018.
18. Peter Olch, Oral History Collections, "Interview with Stanford Leeds," Jan. 29, 1973 National Library of Medicine, NIH.
19. Daniel Munoz and James Dale, *Alpha Doc: The Making of a Cardiologist,* 2015, p. 200.
20. William Stone, *Pioneers of Cardiac Surgery,* 2008, p. 41.
21. Walter Merrill, Interview with author, Nashville, July 17, 2017; "Alfred Blalock, MD" http://vumc.org/thoracicsurgerydept/alfred-blalock-md; William Longmire, *Alfred Blalock: His Life and Times,* 1991, p. 89; Vivien Thomas, *Pioneering Research,* p. 121; Rowena Spencer, "Letter to Vivien Thomas," 1982, Johns Hopkins U. Chesney Archives.

ENDNOTES

22. Thomas Turner, *Heritage of Excellence,* 1974, p. 461.
23. Vivien Thomas, *Pioneering Research,* p. 113.
24. Alfred Blalock, "Letter to William K. Rappleye," Jan. 23, 1946, Duke U. Medical Center Archives.
25. *Ibid.*
26. Peter Olch, Oral History Collections, "Interview with Stanford Leeds," Jan. 29, 1973, National Library of Medicine, NIH.
27. ___, Oral History Collections, "Interview with Warfield Firor," National Library of Medicine, NIH.
28. Sadie Dandy, "Letter to Alfred Blalock," Dec. 17, 1950, Duke U. Medical Center Archives.
29. The Nobel Prize, "Nomination Data Base." www.nobelprize.org.

CHAPTER TWENTY-FIVE: THEFT AND DECEPTION

1. Vivien Thomas, *Pioneering Research,* p. 95.
2. Jack Zimmerman, Interview with Andrew S, Fishel, telephone, Aug. 2, 2018.
3. Michael Szynabski, Sheila Moore, Stacy Kitzmire, and Amndeep Goyal, "Transposition of the Great Arteries," *StatsPearl,* Jan. 15, 2003.
4. TOF cite: http://www.hopkinsmedicine.org/health/conditions-and-diseases/tetralogy-of-fallottof#:~:text=Tetralogy%20of%20Fallot%20(TOF)%20is,in%20the%20US%20each%20year, 2024. TGA cite: http://www.hopkinsmedicine.org/health/conditions-and-diseases/transposition-of-the-great-arteries-tga, 2024.
5. William Cornell, Robert Maxwell, J. Alex Haller and David Sabiston, "Results of the Blalock-Hanlon Operation in 90 Patients," Forty-sixth Annual Meeting of the American Assoc. for Thoracic Surgery, May 16–18, 1966; Marathe and Talwar, "Surgery for Transposition of Great Arteries: A Historical Perspective," *Annals of Pediatric Cardiology,* 8:122–128, 2015.
6. M. Booth and G. Gordon, "Interview with Vivien Thomas," Feb. 10, 1976, Johns Hopkins U. Chesney Archives.
7. Vivien Thomas, *Pioneering Research,* p. 115.
8. *Ibid.,* pp. 115–117.
9. *Ibid.,* pp. 119–121.
10. *Ibid.,* p. 120.
11. *Ibid.*
12. *Ibid.*
13. *Ibid.,* p. 120–121.
14. *Ibid.,* pp. 121–123.
15. *Ibid.,* p. 122.
16. *Ibid;* Alex Haller, Interview with author, Glencoe, Maryland, July 30, 2014.

17. Vivien Thomas, *Pioneering Research*, p. 122.
18. M. Booth and G. Gordon, "Interview with Vivien Thomas," Feb. 10, 1976, Johns Hopkins U. Chesney Archives.
19. Ibid; Vivien Thomas, *Pioneering Research*, p. 122.
20. Vivien Thomas, *Pioneering Research*, p. 123.
21. Ibid., p. 124; Vivien Thomas, Unpublished MS material, Johns Hopkins U. Chesney Archives.
22. Vivien Thomas, Unpublished MS material, Johns Hopkins U. Chesney Archives.
23. Dan (Dandy) Blalock, Email to author, June 9, 2017.
24. Vivien Thomas, Unpublished MS material, Johns Hopkins U. Chesney Archives.
25. Vivien Thomas, *Pioneering Research*, p. 126.
26. Ibid., pp. 126–129.
27. Alfred Blalock and C. Rollins Hanlon, "Interatrial Septal Defects," *Surgery, Gynecology & Obstetrics*, 87:183, Aug. 1948.
28. C. Rollins Hanlon, T. Johns and Vivien Thomas, "An Apparatus for Anesthesia in Experimental Thoracic Surgery," *J of Thoracic Surgery*, 19(6):887, June 1950.
29. Vivien Thomas, Unpublished MS material, Johns Hopkins U. Chesney Archives.
30. Alex Haller, Interview with author, Glencoe, Maryland, July 30, 2014; Walter Merrill, Interview with author, Nashville, July 17, 2017.
31. Alfred Blalock and C. Rollins Hanlon, "The Surgical Treatment of Complete Transposition of the Aorta and the Pulmonary Artery," *Surgery, Gynecology & Obstetrics*, 90:1, Jan. 1950.
32. Clarence Weldon, "The Blalock-Hanlon Operation," *The Annals of Thoracic Surgery*, Apr. 1987, 43(4):448–449.
33. Denton Cooley, Interview with author, March 23, 2016. Lukman Faniyi, "Vivien Thomas: The Unnamed Father of Atrial Septostomy," *J of Am C of Surg*, 233:6, Aug. 2021.
34. Don Nakayama, Ed., "Vivien Thomas: Surgical Researcher and Innovator," *Black Surgeons and Surgery in America*, American College of Surgeons, 2021, p. 241.
35. Supreet Marathe and Sachin Talwar, "Surgery for the Transposition of Great Arteries: A Historical Perspective," *Ann Pediatr Cardiol*, May–Aug. 2015, pp. 122–128.
36. Suraj Nagre, "Historical Evolution of Surgery for Transposition of Great Arteries," *J Cardiovasc Med Cardiol*, 3(1), 26–29; Micheal Szymanski et al., "Transposition of the Great Arteries" *StatPearls*, Jan. 15, 2023. See also William Cornell, et al., "Results of the Blalock-Hanlon Operation in 90 Patient with Transposition of the Great Arteries," Read at the Forty-sixth Annual Meeting of the Am Asoc for Thorac Surg, May 16–18, 1966;

Daniella Caudle, "Transposition of the Great Arteries," *Embryo Project Encyclopedia,* Arizona State U., 2002; John Ochsner, et al., "Treatment of Complete Transposition of the Great Vessels with the Blalock-Hanlon Procedure," *Circulation,* July 1961, pp. 51–57.
37. C. Rollins Hanlon, T Johns, and Vivien Thomas, "An Apparatus for Anesthesia in Experimental Thoracic Surgery," *J of Thoracic Surgery,* 19 (6):887, June 1950.
38. Mark Ravitch, "Letter to Vivien Thomas," circa 1980s, Mark M. Ravitch Collection, National Library of Medicine, NIH; Vivien Thomas, Unpublished MS material, Johns Hopkins U. Chesney Archives.

CHAPTER TWENTY-SIX: A LULU OF A MEETING
1. *Baltimore Sun,* "Mayor Signs Dog Measure," Dec. 18, 1949.
2. *Washington Post,* Nov. 30, 1953.
3. "Case for Vivisection," *Pageant* magazine, Jan. 1946. p. 125.
4. A.C. Ivy and A.F. Zobel, "Are Animal Experiments Needed?" *J. Am. Pharmacological Assoc.,* Sept. 1946, p. 203.
5. Earnest Goodpasture, "Letter to Alfred Blalock," April. 1, 1935, Duke U. Medical Archives.
6. ___ "Letter to Alfred Blalock", Jan. 7, 1935, Duke U. Medical Archives.
7. National Humane Education Association, "A Series of Experiments to Produce Fatal Shock," p. 2.
8. *Ibid.,* pp. 31–32.
9. "Dog Researcher Backers Jeered," *Baltimore Sun,* Nov. 17, 1949.
10. "Baltimore's Great Dog Controversy," *Johns Hopkins Magazine.*
11. Thomas Morris, The *Matter of the Heart: A History of the Heart in Eleven Operations,* 2017.
12. "Lack of Animals Slowing Research," *New York Times,* Nov. 7, 1949.
13. Alan Chesney, "Letter to Board of Estimates," Baltimore City, Nov. 16, 1949, Duke U. Medical Archives.
14. ___, "Letter to Board of Estimates," Baltimore City, Nov. 16, 1949; "Urgent, Confidential Memorandum to Professors," 1949, both in Duke U. Medical Archives.
15. "Dog Rescue Backers Jeered," *Baltimore Sun,* Nov. 17, 1949, Duke U. Medical Archives.
16. "Medical Students," *Nashville Tennessean,* June 21, 1929.
17. "Baltimore's Great Dog Controversy," *Johns Hopkins Magazine.*
18. Maryland Anti-vivisection Society, Advertisement, "Should Dogs and Cats be Cut Open?" *Baltimore Sun,* Sept. 29, 1949.
19. John Stewart, "None So Fine," Buffalo Society of Natural History, p. 3.
20. "Society Maps War on Dog Research," *Baltimore Sun,* Sept. 26, 1950.
21. "Funeral Set for Chesney," *Baltimore Sun,* Sept. 3, 1964.

22. "Program for Hearing Before the Board of Estimates," Baltimore City, Maryland, Nov. 16, 1949.
23. Pamela Gray, "Humans and Other Animals," *Johns Hopkins Magazine*, Oct. 1978.
24. "Aisle Splits the Factions," *Baltimore Sun*, Nov. 17, 1949.
25. "Council Passes Doctors' Dog Bill," *Baltimore Sun*, Dec. 16, 1949.
26. *Anna, Her Story*, JHU, School of Medicine, Stark Films, 1950.
27. Jack Zimmerman, Interview with Andrew Fishel, telephone, August 2, 2018.
28. Vivien Thomas, *Pioneering Research*, pp. 152–153; James E. Hague, "Dog Issues' Victories Teach Doctors New Tactics," *Washington Post*, Nov. 25, 1950.

CHAPTER TWENTY-SEVEN: TOO MUCH SOUTHERN COMFORT

1. Maryland Commission on Interracial Problems and Relations, *Annual Report of the Commission to the Governor and General Assembly of Maryland*, 1953, 1954, 1956, 1957, 1958, 1959, 1960, 1961, 1962, 1963, 1964, 1965, 1966, 1967, 1968.
2. Marcia Rasberry Smith, Interview with author, telephone, Aug. 19, 2018.
3. Vivien Thomas, Unpublished MS material, Johns Hopkins U. Chesney Archives.
4. *Ibid.*
5. Photograph of Alfred Blalock, Yousuf Karsh photo, Johns Hopkins U. Chesney Archives.
6. Signed copy of Blalock's *Principles of Surgical Care: Shock*, Mosby, 1940, "For Vivien Thomas," Johns Hopkins U. Chesney Archives.
7. John Cameron, Interview with author, Baltimore, Maryland, March 16, 2015.
8. C.R. Hatcher, "Profiles in Cardiology: Alfred Blalock," *Clinical Cardiology*, 1936, p. 173.
9. Alfred Blalock, "Letter to Mrs. G. Z. Blalock," Aug. 9, 1952, Duke U. Medical Archives.
10. Denton Cooley, Interview with author, telephone, March 23, 2016.
11. An extensive collection of about 400 revealing letters from Alfred Blalock to family members—his mother, brother, sisters, children—and to others can be found at Duke U. Medical Center Archives. E.g., Alfred Blalock, "Letter to Mrs. G.Z. Blalock," July 7 and Aug. 9, 1950.
12. William Longmire, *Alfred Blalock: His Life and Times*, 1991, p. 207.
13. Valerie Thomas Spann, Interview with author, telephone, Aug. 29, 2017.
14. Koco Eaton, Interview with author, St. Petersburg, Florida, April 27, 2018.

Endnotes

15. Vivien Thomas, "Letter to Buchholz," June 8, 1981, Johns Hopkins U. Chesney Archives.
16. Raymond Heimbecker, Vivien Thomas and Alfred Blalock, "Experimental Reversal of Capillary Blood Flow," *Circulation,* July 1951.
17. Vivien Thomas, "Letter to Ravitch," Dec. 1981, Johns Hopkins U. Chesney Archives.
18. Vivien Thomas, Unpublished MS deletions MMR, Mark M. Ravitch Collection, National Library of Medicine, NIH.
19. Alex Haller, Interview with author, Glencoe, Maryland, July 30, 2014; Haller, "Letter to Rodgers," Feb 5, 1971, Johns Hopkins U. Chesney Archives.
20. Smith, Donald, "Learning Canine Surgery with Vivien Thomas," *Perspectives in Veterinary Medicine,* Feb. 2, 2014.
21. *Ibid.*
22. *Ibid.*
23. "Doctor Blalock Returns Dogs' Favors, Operates on One," *Baltimore Sun,* Dec. 14, 1957.
24. Vivien Thomas, *Pioneering Research,* p. 207.
25. "Doctor Blalock," *Baltimore Sun,* Dec. 14.
26. "Medicine: Squeaky in Surgery," *TIME,* Dec. 23, 1957.

CHAPTER TWENTY-EIGHT: POWER MOVES

1. Allen Weise, *Heart to Heart,* Rutgers U. Press, 2002, p. 70.
2. Dan (Dandy) Blalock, E-mail to author, June 9, 2017.
3. William Longmire, *Alfred Blalock: His Life and Times,* 1991, p. 175.
4. Bruce Frye, "Ventricular Fibrillation and Defibrillation," *Circulation,* 1985.
5. Vivien Thomas, *Pioneering Research,* Fig. 44, p. 159.
6. See, e.g., Stephan Timmermans, "Closed Chest Cardiac Massage: The Emergence of a Discovery Trajectory," *Science, Tech & Human Values,* 1999.
7. Jerome Kay, "Letter to Vivien Thomas," April 11, 1980, Johns Hopkins U. Chesney Archives.
8. Mark Ravitch, "Letter to Vivien Thomas," June 24, 1982, Johns Hopkins U. Chesney Archives.
9. See William Kouwenhoven, "Cardiopulmonary Resuscitation," *JAMA,* Nov. 19, 1973; Kouwenhoven, James Jude and Guy Knickerbocker, "Closed-Chest Cardiac Massage," *JAMA,* July 9, 1960.
10. Jerome Kay and Vivien Thomas and Alfred Blalock, "The Experimental Production of High Interventricular Septal Defects," *Surg. Gynecol. Obstet.,* 96:529, May 1953.
11. Jerome Kay and Vivien Thomas, "The Experimental Production of Pulmonary Stenosis," *Archives of Surgery,* 69:646, Nov. 1954; __ "The

Experimental Production of Pulmonary Insufficiency," *Archives of Surgery*, 646, Nov. 1954.
12. Vivien Thomas, "Letter to Jerome Kay," April 1971, Johns Hopkins U. Chesney Archives.
13. "AMA Gold Medal Doctor: Alfred Blalock," Script, 1953, Johns Hopkins U. Chesney Archives.
14. Theodosia Dullea, Conversations with author, telephone.
15. Vivien Thomas, *Pioneering Research*, p. 180.
16. Ibid.
17. "A Visit with Vivien Thomas," 1974, Johns Hopkins U., Chesney Archives.
18. Vivien Thomas, *Pioneering Research*, p. 183.
19. Ibid., p. 181.

CHAPTER TWENTY-NINE: THE HEADACHE MAN

1. Vivien Thomas, *Pioneering Research*, p. 142.
2. Ibid., p. 139.
3. Ibid.
4. Ibid., p. 137.
5. Ibid., p. 140.
6. Ibid., p. 141.
7. Theodosia Dullea, Conversations with author.
8. Vivien Thomas, "Letter to IRS," April 1954, Johns Hopkins Chesney Archives.
9. Vivien Thomas, "Letter to DC Maldon," April 23, 1952, Johns Hopkins Chesney Archives.
10. "McDonald's Hourly Rate," 2023. http://www.payscale.com/researchj/YS/Employer-McDonald%27s-_Corporation/Hourly_Rate.
11. Jessie Gladden, "Interview with Vivien Thomas," Nov. 23, 1973, H. L. Mencken Room, Enoch Pratt Free Library Special Collections, Baltimore.
12. Theodosia Thomas Dullea, Conversations with author, telephone.
13. Vivien Thomas. Unpublished MS material, Johns Hopkins U. Chesney Archives.
14. Vivien Thomas, *Ibid*.
15. Jack Greenfield, Interview with Andrew S. Fishel, telephone, March 22, 2018.
16. Vivien Thomas, Unpublished MS deletions MMR, Mark M. Ravitch Collection, National Library of Medicine, NIH.
17. Ibid.
18. Vivien Thomas, *Pioneering Research*, p. 173.
19. Don K. Nakayama, Ed., *Black Surgeons and Surgery in America*, Am. College of Surgeons, 2021, p. 243.
20. "Headache Man Honored," Johns Hopkins *Dome*, March 1971.

Endnotes

21. Vivien Thomas, *Pioneering Research*, p. 186.
22. Alex Haller, Interview with author, Glencoe, Maryland, July 30, 2014.
23. *Ibid.*
24. Ralph Hruban. and Will Linder, *A Scientific Revolution: The Men and Women Who Reinvented American Medicine*, Pegasus Books, 2022, p. 257.
25. Lazar Zimmerman, Interview with author, telephone, March 23, 2018.
26. Rowena Spencer, *Partners of the Heart,* Transcript, PBS.

CHAPTER THIRTY: BLALOCK'S NADIR

1. William Longmire, *Alfred Blalock: His Life and Times,* 1991, p. 157.
2. Alfred Blalock, "Letter to Mrs. G.Z. Blalock," Aug. 9, 1952, Duke U. Medical Center Archives.
3. William Longmire, *Alfred Blalock: His Life and Times,* 1991, p. 159.
4. Peter Olch, Oral History Collections, "Interview with Warfield Firor," Feb. 9 and 28, March 21, 1967, National Library of Medicine, NIH.
5. William Longmire, *Alfred Blalock: His Life and Times,* 1991, p. 159.
6. Richard Te Linde, "Memories of Alfred Blalock," unpublished, Duke U. Medical Center Archives.
7. R. Robinson "Bricks" Baker, Interview with author, Owings Mill, Md., June 27, 2017.
8. Vivien Thomas, "Letter to Ransom Buchholz," Jan. 8, 1980, Johns Hopkins U. Chesney Archives.
9. Richard Te Linde, "Memories," Johns Hopkins U. Chesney Archives.
10. Vivien Thomas, Unpublished MS material, Johns Hopkins U. Chesney Archives.
11. *Ibid.*
12. *Ibid.*
13. Alfred Blalock, "Letter to Mrs. G, Z. Blalock," Feb 12, 1958, Duke U. Medical Center Archives.
14. Alfred Blalock, "Letter to Mrs. G. Z. Blalock," April 11, 1958, Duke U. Medical Center Archives.
15. Alfred Blalock, "Letter to Mrs. G.Z. Blalock," Nov. 8, 1958, Duke U. Medical Center Archives.
16. Alfred Blalock, "Letter to Mrs. G.Z. Blalock," Dec. 3, 1958, Duke U. Medical Center Archives.
17. Alfred Blalock, "Letter to Mrs. G.Z. Blalock," May 20, 1957, Duke U. Medical Center Archives.
18. William Longmire, *Alfred Blalock: His Life and Times,* p. 220.
19. Jack Zimmerman, Interview with author, telephone, August 2, 2018.
20. William Longmire, *Alfred Blalock: His Life and Times,* pp. 226–227.
21. *Ibid.,* p. 226.

22. Vivien Thomas, "Letter to Ravitch," March 8, 1981, Johns Hopkins U. Chesney Archives.

CHAPTER THIRTY-ONE: BETRAYAL AT THE SOUTHERN HOTEL

1. Truly Jackson, Interview with author, Nashville, Tennessee, July 19, 2017; "Interview with Lillian (Ootsie) Thomas," Civil Rights Collection, Nashville, Tennessee, Public Library.
2. Lazar Greenfield, Interview with Andrew S. Fishel, telephone, March 22, 2018.
3. Levi Watkins, Interviews with author, Baltimore, Maryland, Aug. 22 and Sept. 14, 2014.
4. "Guest Program, A Dinner in Honor of Alfred Blalock," Mark M. Ravitch Collection, National Library of Medicine, NIH.
5. Vivien Thomas, Unpublished MS material, Johns Hopkins U. Chesney Archives.
6. David Sabiston, "Untitled guest list," Duke U. Medical Center Archives.
7. Vivien Thomas, Unpublished MS material, Johns Hopkins U. Chesney Archives.
8. Harold Norris, Interview with author, Baltimore, Maryland, July 30, 2014; Levi Watkins, Interviews with author, Aug. 22 and Sept. 14, 2014.
9. See Maryland Commission on Interracial Problems and Relations, "Annual Report of the Commission to the Governor and General Assembly of Maryland," 1953; 1955, p.14; 1956, pp. 19–20; 1957, pp. 14–15; 1958, pp. 12–13; 1960, pp. 12–17; 1962, pp. 13–14, p. 19; Frederick Rasmussen, "'Toward Equality' Pamphlet Took the Place of the State's Race Relations," *Baltimore Sun*, Feb. 5, 2011; Fraser Smith, *Here Lies Jim Crow, Civil Rights in Maryland*, 2012; L.H. Foster, "Race Relations in the South: 1960" *J. of Negro Education*, Spring 1961; "Baltimore Hotel Ease Racial Bias," *Washington Post*, Dec. 10, 1964.
10. Mark Ravitch, "Note attached on Southern Hotel Party program," Mark M. Ravitch Collection, National Library of Medicine, NIH.
11. Ibid; Mark Ravitch, "Letter to A. McGeHee Harvey," Jan 6, 1986, Johns Hopkins U. Chesney Archives.
12. Mark Ravitch, "Note Attached on Southern Hotel Party program," Mark M. Ravitch Collection, National Library of Medicine, NIH.
13. Mark Ravitch, "Guest Program," Mark M. Ravitch Collection, National Library of Medicine, NIH.
14. Vivien Thomas, Unpublished MS material, Johns Hopkins U. Chesney Archives.
15. Ibid.
16. Ibid.

Endnotes

17. Southern Hotel, Dinner Menu, "Alfred Blalock, MD Celebration," April 2, 1960, Duke U. Medical School Archives.
18. Vivien Thomas, Unpublished MS material, Johns Hopkins U. Chesney Archives.
19. Ibid.
20. Ibid.
21. "Photographs, Dinner at the Southern Hotel," 1960, Duke U. Medical Center Archives.
22. Mark Ravitch, "Letter to Harvey," Jan. 6, 1986, Johns Hopkins Chesney Archives.
23. Ibid.

CHAPTER THIRTY-TWO: SHATTERED ILLUSIONS

1. Alfred Blalock, "Prepared Remarks of Dr. Alfred Blalock at a Dinner Given in His Honor at the Southern Hotel," April 2, 1960; "Typed Transcript, Videotape and Audiotape," of Blalock's comments, all at Duke U. Medical Archives. Please note that Thomas's unpublished MS says that Kouwenhoven had told him that Blalock had acknowledged Thomas. However, neither the video or the audio recordings of Blalock's comments include a mention of either Thomas or Taussig, nor does the typed transcript of the remarks Blalock made that night. Thomas eventually learned and repeated to his wife that he was not thanked by Blalock, as his son-in-law, Harold Norris, reported to this author. (Endnote 6, below). Later, Thomas learned that Blalock's prepared comments prior to the dinner had included a reference to him and Taussig.
2. Vivien Thomas, Unpublished MS material, Johns Hopkins Chesney Archives.
3. Ibid.
4. Ibid.
5. Ibid.
6. Harold Norris, Interview with author, Baltimore, Maryland.
7. Vivien Thomas, Unpublished MS material, Johns Hopkins Chesney Archives.
8. Ibid.
9. Ibid.
10. Ibid.
11. Ibid.
12. Jewell Chambers, "Baltimore Hotel Begins Road Home", *Baltimore Afro American,* April 30, 1960.
13. "Baltimore Landmark to Be Home for Aged," *Washington Post,* Dec. 10, 1964.

14. Frederick Rasmusen, "Southern Hotel Finally to Fall." *Baltimore Sun*, June 5, 1999; Jacque Kelly, "Downtown Hotel's Obituary Being Written," *Baltimore Sun*, Oct. 10, 1998.
15. Harold Norris, Interview with author, Baltimore, Maryland, July 20, 2013.
16. *Ibid.*

CHAPTER THIRTY-THREE: THE END OF AN ERA
1. R. Robinson "Bricks" Baker, Interview with author, Owings Mill, Md., June 27, 2017; Alex Haller, Interview with author, Glencoe, Maryland, July 30, 2014.
2. Neil Grauer, "George Zuidema, Who Transformed Johns Hopkins Surgery Dept., Dies." http://www.hopkinsmedicine.org/news/articles/george-zuidema-who-transformed-johns-hopkin-surgery-department-revitalized-university-of-michigan-medical-center-dies.
3. R. Robinson "Bricks" Baker, Interview with author, Owing Mills, Md., June 22, 2017; Alex Haller, Interview with author, Glencoe, Maryland, July 30, 2014.
4. Vivien Thomas, *Pioneering Research*, p. 209.
5. *Ibid.*, p. 210.
6. Gwendolyn Clarke, Interview with author, White's Ford Creek, Tennessee, July 17, 2017.
7. George Zuidema, Interview with author, telephone, June 15, 2015.
8. R. Robinson "Bricks" Baker, Interview with author, Owing Mills, Maryland, June 22, 2017.
9. George Zuidema, Interview with author, telephone, June 15, 2015.
10. Vivien Thomas, *Pioneering Research*, pp. 210–211.
11. Gwendolyn Manlove Clarke, Interview with author, White's Ford Creek, Tennessee, July 17, 2017.
12. James Isaacs, "Letter to Mark Ravitch," Sept. 11, 1981, Mark M. Ravitch Collection, National Library of Medicine, NIH. See also James Isaacs, "My View of Alfred Blalock, 1945 to 1965," Johns Hopkins U. Chesney Archives.
13. John Cameron, Interview with author, Baltimore, Maryland, March 16, 2015.
14. Jean Queen, Interview with Andrew S. Fishel, telephone, March 29, 2018.
15. Anonymous quotation at request of interviewee, Interview with author.
16. R. Robinson "Bricks" Baker, Interview with author, Owing Mills, Maryland, June 22, 2017.
17. Jean Queen, Interview with Andrew S. Fishel, telephone, March 29, 2018.
18. Gwendolyn Clark, Interview with author; R. Robinson "Bricks" Baker, Interview with author, Owing Mills, Maryland, June 22, 2017.

Endnotes

19. Alfred Blalock, "Letter to Edward Blalock," July 10, 1964, Duke U. Medical Center Archives.
20. Vivien Thomas, "Letter to Buchholz," Jan. 8, 1980, Duke U. Medical Center Archives.
21. Mark Ravitch, *Papers of Alfred Blalock,* JHU Press, 1966, p. lxvi.
22. Alex Haller, Interview with author, Glencoe, Maryland, July 30, 2014; Robinson Baker, Interview with author, Owing Mills, Maryland, June 22, 2017.
23. Ibid.
24. Vivien Thomas, *Pioneering Research,* p. 214.
25. William Longmire, "Letter to Old Hands Club Members," Sept. 25, 1964, Mark R. Ravitch Collection, National Library of Medicine, NIH.
26. Robert D. Bloodwell, "Letter to Denton Cooley," Apr. 27, 1972, National Library of Medicine, NIH.
27. Collection of condolence letters to Mrs. Alice Blalock, Duke U. Medical Center Archives.
28. "30 Receive Freedom Medal at the White House; They are Praised by Johnson as He Confers the Highest Civilian Recognition, *New York Times,* Sept. 15, 1964; "Dr. Alfred Blalock Dead at 65; Developed Blue Baby Surgery; Ex-Department Head at Johns Hopkins; Performed Pioneer Surgery There in 1944," *New York Times,* Sept. 16, 1964.

CHAPTER THIRTY-FOUR: TOKEN RECOGNITION

1. Alex Haller, Interview with author, Glencoe, Maryland, July 30, 2014; William Stoney, *Pioneers of Cardiac Surgery,* 2008, pp. 208 and 265.
2. Alex Haller, Interview with author, Glencoe, Maryland, July 30, 2014.
3. Vivien Thomas, Unpublished MS material, Johns Hopkins U. Chesney Archives.
4. Jewell Chambers, "Baltimore Begins Road Back," *Baltimore Afro American,* Apr. 13, 1968.
5. John Cameron, Interview with author, Baltimore, Maryland, March 16, 2015.
6. Vivien Thomas, Unpublished MS material, Johns Hopkins U. Chesney Archives.
7. Ibid.
8. Ibid.
9. Gwendolyn Clarke, Interview with author, White's Ford Creek, Tennessee, July 17, 2017.
10. Bob Gee, "Letter to Jessie Gladden," May 8, 1972, H. L. Mencken Room, Enoch Pratt Free Library Special Collections, Baltimore, Maryland.
11. Alex Haller, "Letter to Medical Dean," Feb. 5, 1971, Johns Hopkins U. Chesney Archives.

12. *Ibid.*
13. George Zuidema, Interview with author, telephone, June 15, 2015.
14. *Ibid.* And Chester Hampton, "MD Aide," *Washington Post*, April 1, 1971.
15. Vivien Thomas, *Pioneering Research*, p. 219.
16. Jean Queen, Interview with Andrew Fishel, telephone, March 29, 2018.
17. "Presentation of a Portrait of Vivien Thomas," Feb. 27, 1971, Johns Hopkins U. Chesney Archives; Rollins Hanlon, Thomas Johns and Vivien Thomas, "An Apparatus for Anesthesia in Experimental Surgery," *J. of Thoracic Surgery*, 19(6), p. 847, June 1950.
18. *Ibid.*
19. *Ibid.*
20. *Ibid.*
21. *Ibid.*
22. Vivien Thomas, Unpublished MS material, Johns Hopkins U. Chesney Archives.
23. Richard Shackelford, "Letter to Vivien Thomas," Feb. 28, 1971, Johns Hopkins U. Chesney Archives.
24. Vivien Thomas, *Pioneering Research*, p. 220.
25. Johns Hopkins Medical Institutes, Press Release, Feb. 26, 1971, Johns Hopkins U. Chesney Archives.
26. Vivien Thomas, *Pioneering Research*, p. 221.
27. *Ibid.*
28. *Ibid*, p. 220.
29. Jean Queen, Interview with Andrew Fishel, telephone, March 29, 2018.
30. Vivien Thomas, "Letter to Lillian (Ootsie) Thomas," March 2, 1971, Civil Rights Collection, Nashville Public Library.
31. *Ibid.*
32. Levi Watkins, Interviews with author, Baltimore, Maryland, Aug. 2. and Sept. 14, 2014.
33. *Ibid.*
34. *Ibid.*
35. Johns Hopkins University, *A Crisis in Medical Education SOS*, 1974, Johns Hopkins U. Chesney Archives.

CHAPTER THIRTY-FIVE: VIVIEN THOMAS, LLD
1. Alex Haller, Interview with author, Glencoe, Maryland, July 30, 2014.
2. Vivien Thomas, *Pioneering Research*, p. 225.
3. George Callcott, Interview with author, telephone, May 1, 2017; Alex Dragt, "Letter to Claude Kacser," Feb. 25, 1976, Maryland Room Archives, U. of Maryland.
4. Vivien Thomas, *Pioneering Research*, pp. 226–227.
5. *Ibid.*, pp. 226–227.

Endnotes

6. George Callcott, Interview with author. telephone, May 1, 2017.
7. Ibid.
8. Vivien Thomas, *Pioneering Research*, p. 227.
9. Ibid., p. 228.
10. Ibid., p. 225.
11. Ibid.
12. Interview with George Zuidema, telephone, June 15, 2015.
13. Ibid.
14. Vivien Thomas, Unpublished MS material, Johns Hopkins U. Chesney Archives.
15. Ibid.
16. Harold Norris, Interview with author, Baltimore, Maryland, Aug. 21, 2014.
17. Ibid.
18. Vivien Thomas, Unpublished MS material, Johns Hopkins U. Chesney Archives.
19. Joyce Baldwin, *To Heal the Heart of a Child,* p. 114.
20. Lillian (Ootsie) Thomas, Interview, May 3, 2005, "Civil Rights Collections," Nashville Public Library; Truly Jackson, Interview with author, Nashville, Tennessee, July 19, 2017.
21. Ibid.
22. "Citation, Eisenhower Medal, Helen Brooke Taussig," Johns Hopkins U. Chesney Archives.
23. "Citation, Conferring of Honorary Degree, Vivien Thomas," Johns Hopkins U. Chesney Archives; Thomas, Unpublished MS material, Johns Hopkins U. Chesney Archives.
24. Vivien Thomas, *Pioneering Research,* p. 229.
25. ___, "Letter to George Zuidema," July 2, 1976, Johns Hopkins U. Chesney Archives.
26. ___, *Pioneering Research*, pp 231–232.
27. ___, Unpublished MS material, Johns Hopkins U. Chesney Archives.
28. George Zuidema, Interview with author, telephone, June 15, 2017.
29. Ibid.
30. Jean Queen, Interview with Andrew Fishel, telephone, March 29, 2018.
31. Vivien Thomas, Unpublished MS material, Johns Hopkins U. Chesney Archives.
32. Richard Ross, "Letter to Vivien Thomas," Jan. 26, 1977, Johns Hopkins U. Chesney Archives.
33. Jean Queen, Interview with Andrew Fishel, telephone, March 29, 2018.

CHAPTER THIRTY-SIX: PIONEERING RESEARCH IN SURGICAL SHOCK AND CARDIOVASCULAR SURGERY

1. Vivien Thomas, Unpublished MS material, Johns Hopkins U. Chesney Archives.
2. Vivien Thomas, "Letter to Mark Ravitch," Sept. 24, 1982, Johns Hopkins U. Chesney Archives.
3. Vivien Thomas, "Draft letter to Mark Ravitch," Johns Hopkins U. Chesney Archives.
4. Ibid.
5. Vivien Thomas, "Handwritten Speech to Provident Hospital," Nov. 15, 1981, Johns Hopkins U. Chesney Archives.
6. Ibid.
7. Thomas Turner, "Letter to Vivien Thomas," Dec. 18, 1981, Johns Hopkins U. Chesney Archives.
8. Vivien Thomas, *Pioneering Research in Surgical Shock and Cardiovascular Surgery: Vivien Thomas and His Work with Alfred Blalock*, U. of Pennsylvania Press, 1985.
9. James Labosier, "Mark Ravitch," *Circulating Now*, Oct. 1976.
10. Vivien Thomas, *Pioneering Research*, p. 117.
11. Theodosia Thomas Dullea, Conversations with author, telephone.
12. Ursula Rasberry-Dijkhoffz, Interview with author, telephone and emails; Marcia Rasberry Smith, Interview with author, telephone, Aug. 19, 2018 and emails; "Meet Dr. Vivien Thomas's Granddaughter—Marcia Rasberry Smith." http://www.spreaker.com/user/kimjacobsthebalancedoctor/meet-dr-vivien-thomas-granddaughter-marcia-rasberry-smith, March 21, 2022.
13. Koco Eaton, Interview with author, St. Petersburg, Florida, April 27, 2018.
14. Levi Watkins, Interviews with author, Baltimore, Maryland, Aug. 22 and Sept. 14, 2014.
15. Vivien Thomas, "Letter to Mark Ravitch," Oct 2. 1980, Johns Hopkins U. Chesney Archives.
16. Mark Ravitch, "Letter to Vivien Thomas," Oct. 16, 1980, Johns Hopkins U. Chesney Archives.
17. Vivien Thomas, Unpublished MS material, Johns Hopkins U. Chesney Archives.
18. Mark Ravitch, "The Blood Bank of Johns Hopkins University," *JAMA*, July 20, 1940, p. 171.
19. M. Booth and G. Gordon, "Interview with Vivien Thomas," Feb. 10, 1976, Johns Hopkins U. Chesney Archives.
20. Vivien Thomas, Unpublished MS material, Johns Hopkins U. Chesney Archives.
21. Ibid.

Endnotes

22. *Ibid.*
23. *Ibid.*
24. International Committee of Medical Journal Editors, "Defining the Role of Authors and Contributors," 2023. http://www.icmje.org.
25. Baerlocher, T. Guatam, G..Tomlinson and A. Detsky, "The Meaning of Author Order in Medical Research." *J. of Investigative Medicine,* 2007, May; 55(4): pp 174–180.
26. Vivien Thomas, "Letter to C. Rollins Hanlon," Oct. 4, 1974, Johns Hopkins U. Chesney Archives.
27. Mark Ravitch, "Letter to Thomas," April 23, 1979, Johns Hopkins U. Chesney Archives.
28. See Rollins Hanlon, "Letter(s) to Vivien Thomas," Oct. 9, 1974, and Nov. 11,1974 and Dec. 11, 1974, National Library of Medicine, NIH.
29. Vivien Thomas, Unpublished MS material, Johns Hopkins U. Chesney Archives.
30. Vivien Thomas, Letter to Mark Ravitch, Dec. 1981, Johns Hopkins U. Chesney Archives; "Letter to Mark Ravitch," Sept. 24, 1982, Johns Hopkins U. Chesney Archives.
31. Denton Cooley, "Letter to Corrine Hammett," Feb. 17, 1971, Johns Hopkins U. Chesney Archives; Denton Cooley, Interview by author, telephone, March 23, 2016; Minetree, *Cooley: The Career of a Great Heart Surgeon,* 1973.
32. Jerome Kay, "Letter to Vivien Thomas," Sept. 15, 1980, Johns Hopkins U. Chesney Archives.
33. Rowena Spencer, "Letter to Vivien Thomas," Johns Hopkins U. Chesney Archives; Alex Haller, Interview with author, Glencoe, Md., July 30, 2014.
34. William Evans, "The Arterial Switch Operation Before Jantene," *J. of Pediatric Cardiology,* 30 (2009): 119–124, 2009.
35. C. Rollins Hanlon, "Ethical Principles for Everyone in Health Care," *Journal of the American College of Surgeons,* 219 (4), 2000, p. 72.
36. Vivien Thomas, "Draft Letter to Rollins Hanlon," Oct. 20, 1975, Johns Hopkins U. Chesney Archives.
37. Vivien Thomas, "Letter to Mark Ravitch," March 15, 1982, Johns Hopkins U. Chesney Archives.
38. *Ibid.*
39. Vivien Thomas, "Draft letter to Mark Ravitch," Johns Hopkins U. Chesney Archives.
40. *Ibid.*
41. Mark Ravitch, "Letter to Vivien Thomas," Dec. 2, 1981, Johns Hopkins U. Chesney Archives.
42. Theodosia Thomas Dullea, Conversations with author; Valeria Thomas Spann, "Interview with author, telephone, Aug. 29, 2017.

43. Wendy Harris (JHU Press), "Letter to Vivien Thomas," May 5, 1983, National Library of Medicine, NIH.
44. Harold Norris, Interview with author, Baltimore, Maryland, Aug. 21, 2014.
45. Thomas Rotell, "Letter to Ravitch," May 16, 1985, Mark M. Ravitch Collection, National Library of Medicine, NIH.
46. Mark Ravitch, "Letter to Richard Ross," May 23, 1985, Mark M. Ravitch Collection, National Library of Medicine, NIH.
47. Nancy McCall, "Memo to Harvey and Ross," March 28, 1984, Mark M. Ravich Collection, National Library of Medicine, NIH.
48. Richard Ross, "Letter to Thomas Rotell," June 7, 1985; Chuba, "Letter to Thomas Rotell", June 26, 1985. Both Mark M. Ravitch Collection, National Library of Medicine, NIH.
49. Thomas Rotell, "Letter to Ravitch," June 10, 1985, Mark M. Ravitch Collection, National Library of Medicine, NIH.

CHAPTER THIRTY-SEVEN: STONY SILENCE

1. John Cameron, Interview with author, Baltimore, Maryland, March 16, 2015.
2. *Ibid.*
3. *Ibid.*
4. *Ibid.*
5. *Ibid.*
6. Mark Ravitch, "Letter to Ransome Buchholz," Nov. 5, 1985, History of Medicine Collections, Vanderbilt U.
7. "Memorial Service for Vivien T. Thomas," Madison Avenue Presbyterian Church (Baltimore, Maryland), Johns Hopkins U. Chesney Archives.
8. Jean Queen, Interview with author, telephone, March 29, 2018.
9. Levi Watkins, Interviews with author, Baltimore, Maryland, Aug. 22 and Sept. 14, 2014.
10. Helen Taussig, "Letter to Clara Thomas," Feb. 20, 1986, Johns Hopkins U. Chesney Archives.
11. JHMI News Release, "Vivien Thomas, Hopkins's Pioneer Surgical Technical, Dies," Nov. 26, 1985. http://hub.jhu.edu/2019/11/26/blue-baby-operation.
12. *Ibid.* In 2023, Vanderbilt U. mentioned Thomas's creation of the transposition surgery in its "Medical Scientist Training Program" website http://medschool.vanderbilt.edu/mstp/person/vivien-t-thomas/ Whereas Hopkins's Vivien Thomas Scholars website only mentions his blue baby work http://hub.jhu.edu/2023/08/23/vivien-thomas-scholars-johns-hopkins-second-cohort/.
13. William Glenn, "Book Review," *New England J. of Medicine,* July 6, 1986.

Endnotes

14. American Medical Writers Association, 1986. http://www.amwa.org/page/past_awards.
15. George Zuidema, Interview with author, telephone, June 15, 2015.
16. John Cameron, Interview with author, Baltimore, Maryland, March 16, 2015.
17. Mark Ravitch, "Letter to Thomas Rotell," June 23, 1986, Mark M. Ravitch Collection, National Library of Medicine, NIH.
18. Fry, "Book Review," *JHU Bulletin,* History of Medicine, Jan. 23, 1986, Johns Hopkins U. Chesney Archives.
19. Program, "Symposium in Honor of Alfred Blalock," 1991, Johns Hopkins U. Chesney Archives.
20. Program, "A Celebration: Fiftieth Anniversary of the Blalock-Taussig Shunt," 1995, Johns Hopkins U. Chesney Archives.
21. Judith Minkove, "Johns Hopkins Celebrates 75 Years Since Historic Blue Baby Operation," HUB, Nov. 26, 2019. http://hub.jhu.edu/2019/11/26/blue-baby-operation/.
22. The sister magazines gave the feature different titles. Katie McCabe, "A Legend of the Heart," *Baltimore* magazine, June 1989 and "Like Something the Lord Made," *Washingtonian* magazine, August 1989.
23. National Magazine Awards, "National Magazine Award for Feature Writing," 1990. http://en.wikipedia.org/wiki/National_Magazine_Awards.
24. Public Broadcasting Station, *American Experience,* "Partners of the Heart," Season 15, Episode 8, 2003.
25. Greg Rienza, "Partners of the Heart: PBS to Tell the Story of Two Blue Baby Pioneers," The Johns Hopkins University *Gazette,* Jan. 13, 2003.
26. HBO, *Something the Lord Made,* 2004.
27. Several Hopkins physicians told the author that Johns Hopkins has never given an honorary MD degree because doing so would not be allowed, yet Thomas's colleague William B. Kouerhoven received an honorary MD degree in 1969 and Ralph Gibson received an honorary MD degree in 1972.
28. Theodosia Thomas Dullea, Conversations with author, telephone. Aug. 19, 2018; Levi Watkins, Interviews with author, Baltimore, Maryland, August 22 and Sept. 14, 2014; Harold Norris, Interview with author, Baltimore, Maryland, Aug. 21, 2014.
29. Marcia Rasberry Smith, Interview with author, telephone and e-mail.
30. Theodosia Thomas Dullea, Conversations with author, telephone; Harold Norris, Interview with author, Aug. 21, 2014.
31. Nancy McCall, "Letter to Mark Ravitch," Jan. 1986, Mark M. Ravitch Collection, National Library of Medicine, NIH.
32. Theodosia Thomas Dullea, Conversations with author.

CHAPTER THIRTY-EIGHT: UNSUNG HERO

1. Koco Eaton, Interview with author, St. Petersburg, Florida, April 27, 2018.
2. There are a number of professional surgery groups. Presidents of the American College of Surgeons include William P. Longmire, H. William Scott Jr., William Muller Jr., David C. Sabiston, James V. Maloney Jr., C. Rollins Hanlon, Mark M. Ravitch, Henry T. Bahnson, and Frank C. Spencer. Presidents of the American Surgical Association included John L. Cameron and Lazar Greenfield. Also see Walter Merrill, "What's Past is Prologue," *Annals of Thoracic Surgery*, Dec. 1999, pp. 2366–2375.
3. Rollins Hanlon, Alfred Blalock and Vivien Thomas, "An Apparatus for Anesthesia in Experimental Thoracic Surgery, *J. of Thoracic Surgery*, 19 (6):887, June 1950; R. Heimbecker, Vivien Thomas and Alfred Blalock, "Experimental Reversal of the Capillary Blood Flow," *Circulation*, 4:116, July 1951; Jerome Kay, Vivien Thomas and Alfred Blalock, "The Experimental Production of High Interventricular Septal Defects," *Surgery, Gyn and Ob*, 96: 529, May 1953; Jerome Kay and Vivien Thomas, "The Experimental Production of Pulmonary Insufficiency," *Arch Sur*, 69: 646, November 1954; Jerome Kay and Vivien Thomas, "Experimental Production of Pulmonary Stenosis; Physiological and Pathological Study, *AMA Arch Surg*, 69: pp. 651–656; A. Pollock and Vivien Thomas, "Replacement of a Tricuspid Valve Cusp in Dogs," *Surgery, Gyn and Ob*, 103: 731, Dec. 1956; J. Miller and Vivien Thomas, "The Use of Oxidized Regenerated Cellulose as a Hemostatic Agent in Dogs," *Exp Med Surg*, Rockefeller Institute, 19: pp. 192–195, 1961; M. Bush, Daniel Pieroni, Dawn Goodman, Robert White, Vivien Thomas, and A. James, "Tetralogy of Fallot in Cats," *J. of the Am. Veterinary Med. Assoc*, 1972.
4. Yancy, Clyde, MD "On Why Renaming the Blalock-Taussif Shunt Matters." *AMA Moving Medicine Series*, Feb. 28, 2022; "The Blalock Taussig Shunt: The Social History of an Eponym," *Cardiology of the Young*, 19 (2009): 119–128; Thomas Brogan, George Alfieris, "Has the Time Come to Rename the Blalock-Taussig Shunt?", *Pediatr Crit Care Med*, 2003, p. 450; Denton Cooley, "In Pursuit of an Eponym," *Tex Heart Inst J.*, 2004, p. 117–118; Natalia Ceneda, Salvatore Giordano, G. Biondi-Zoccai, M. Bernardi, "Vivien T. Thomas, The Pioneering Lab Assistant Who Revolutionized Congenital Heart Disease Surgery," *Hearts, Vessels and Transplantation*, July 2023.
5. "Cardiac Procedure Renamed at SickKids in Honour of Surgical Pioneer Vivien Thomas," Jan. 31, 2023. http://www.sickkids.ca/er/news/archive/2023/cardiac-procedure-renamed-at-sickkids-in-honor-of-vivien-thomas/.

6. John Cameron, Interview with author, Baltimore, Maryland, March 16, 2015.
7. Koco Eaton, Interview with author, St. Petersburg, Florida, April 22, 2018.
8. Theodosia Thomas Dullea, Conversations with author.
9. Koco Eaton, Interview with author, St. Petersburg, Florida, April 22, 2018.
10. Vivien Thomas, "Unsung Hero" speech, Provident Hospital, Baltimore, Maryland, Johns Hopkins U. Chesney Archives.
11. Koco Eaton, Interview with author, St. Petersburg, Florida, April 22, 2018.
12. "Meet Vivien Thomas's Granddaughter—Marcia Rasberry Smith," March 21, 2022. http://www.speaker.com/user/kimjacobsthebalanceddoctor/meet-dr-vivien-thomas. granddaughter-rasberry-smith; Marcia Rasberry Smith, Interview with author, Aug. 19, 2018.
13. Valeria Thomas Spann, Interview with author, telephone, Aug. 29, 2017.
14. Harold Norris, Interview with author, Baltimore, Maryland, Aug. 21, 2014.
15. Robert Higgins, Interview with author, Baltimore, Maryland, June 28, 2018.
16. Ibid.
17. Ibid.
18. Vivien Thomas, "Unsung Hero Speech," Provident Hospital, Johns Hopkins U. Chesney Archives.
19. Vivien Thomas, "Dr. Coffee, Mr. Chairman" speech, Johns Hopkins U. Chesney Archives.
20. Vivien Thomas, "Letter to Alex Haller," Sept. 12, 1975, Johns Hopkins U. Chesney Archives.
21. Vivien Thomas, *Pioneering Research*, p. 220.
22. Levi Watkins, Interviews with author, Baltimore, Maryland, August 22 and Sept. 14, 2014.
23. Ibid.

SOURCES

Archives and Libraries

- *Columbia University Medical Center Archives*
  Thanks to Stephen Novak.

- *Duke University Medical Center Library and Archives*
  Alfred Blalock Collection and David Sabiston Collection.
  Thank you to Rebecca Williams.

- *Enoch Pratt Free Library, City of Baltimore Public Libraries, Special Collections*
  Vivien Thomas Collection.
  Thanks to Mike Donnelly.

- *Fisk University, Special Collections*
  Thanks to DeLisa Harris.

- *Henry Ford Health System, Sladen Libraries, Conrad R. Lam Archives*
  Thanks to Julia Pope.

- *Johns Hopkins University, Sheridan Libraries, Special Collections*
  Thanks to James Stimpert.

- *Johns Hopkins University Medicine, Alan Mason Chesney Medical Archives*
  Vivien T. Thomas Collection
  Alfred Blalock Collection
  Helen Brooke Taussig Collection
  Mark Ravitch Collection
  Thanks to Andy Harrison, Timothy Wisniewski, and Nancy McCall.

- *Meharry Medical College, Library Archives Department*
  Thanks to Christyne Douglas and to Sandra Parham.
- *Nashville Public Library, Special Collections, Civil Rights*
- *National Institutes of Health, National Library of Medicine, History of Medicine Division*
  Oral History Collection and Mark Ravitch Collection
  Thank you to John Rees and Jeremy Withnell.
- *Pearl High School Museum and Archives (Nashville, Tenn.)*
  Thank you to Melvin Black.
- *Rockefeller Archive Center, Sleepy Hollow, NY*
  Thanks to Monica Blank.
- *Tennessee State Library and Archives*
  Pearl High School Microfilm
- *Tennessee State University, Library Archives*
- *University of Maryland, Hornbake Library, Maryland Room Archives*
  Commission on Interracial Problems and Relations Collection
  Thanks to Jennifer G. Edison.
- *University of Pennsylvania, University Archives*
  Thanks to Timothy Horning.
- *University of Pennsylvania Press*
  Thanks to Laura Waldron.
- *University of Pittsburgh, Archives and Special Collections*
  Thanks to Laura Brooks.
- *University of Virginia, Claude Moore Health Sciences Library, Historical Collection Archives*
  William H. Muller Collection.
  Thanks to Daniel Cavanaugh.
- *Vanderbilt University, History of Medicine Collections*
  Vivien T. Thomas Collection and Alfred Blalock Collection.
  Thank you to James Thweatt.

Sources

Interview List

Baker, R. Robinson, MD "Bricks" Baker worked on and off with Vivien Thomas from the mid-fifties as a Hopkins medical student to the early sixties, when he became chief resident in surgery. He was named surgeon emeritus and had been director of its breast clinic. His vast knowledge of the Hopkins institutions also derives from his mother, who was a nurse at Hopkins, and his father, who was its vice president for Finance. He was married to a descendant of Johns Hopkins, Jean Hogarth Harvey, who was the Elizabeth Todd Professor of History at Goucher College.

Berkowitz, Bernie. The deputy director of City Planning for Baltimore City, he also served as the president of the Baltimore Economic Development Corporation and was president of the Black/Jewish Forum of Baltimore, Inc. There are few people who know both the white and the Black communities of Baltimore as well as he.

Black, Melvin. He is a former student and teacher at Pearl High School, the award-winning high school from which Vivien Thomas received his diploma. He is the founder and director of the Pearl High School Museum and Archives in Nashville.

Callcott, George, PhD Professor of History emeritus at the University of Maryland, Prof. Callcott also served as its vice chancellor for Academic Affairs, which is when he approached Vivien Thomas about the University of Maryland's awarding of an honorary DSc to Thomas.

Cameron, John, MD Studied and worked with Thomas and Blalock from 1960 until their retirement. In 1984, became surgeon in chief, JHU Medical School and Hospital, a position he held for nineteen years. He is a thoracic surgeon and Hopkins's Alfred Blalock Scholar.

Clarke, Gwendolyn Manlove. As the daughter of Charles Manlove, Vivien Thomas's best friend, she was extremely close to Clara and Vivien Thomas and lived with the Thomases in their Baltimore house when she was doing course work for a master's degree at Hopkins University. Many nights after dinner, Thomas talked candidly to her about his experiences at Hopkins and Vanderbilt universities with Alfred Blalock.

Cooley, Denton, MD He studied and worked with Thomas and Blalock. He was the best-known heart surgeon of his time and was the first to implant a totally artificial heart in a human being. He was the founder and surgeon-in-chief of the Texas Heart Institute in Dallas, where he worked until a few days before his death at age ninety-six. He also was an authentic friend of Vivien Thomas.

Dullea, Theodosia Thomas Rasberry The younger daughter of Clara and Vivien Thomas, she was very helpful in our conversations about growing up with Vivien and Clara Thomas and about her parents' experiences and points of view.

Eaton, Koco (Katuelle), MD A cousin of Vivien Thomas who lived near Baltimore, he graduated from the Johns Hopkins Medical School after Thomas had retired. He holds several patents and heads the practice, Eaton Orthopedics in St. Petersburg, Florida. He is also the orthopedic surgeon for the Tampa Bay Rays. He considers Vivien Thomas to have been his mentor, both professionally and personally.

Greenfield, Lazar J., MD (Jack) The former surgery chair at the Medical College of Virginia, he trained at Hopkins in general and thoracic surgery from 1958 to 1966, which meant that he knew Thomas and Blalock at a later time than most surgeons interviewed here.

Haller, J. Alex Jr., MD The surgeon studied and worked with Blalock and Thomas at JHU Medical School and Hospital from 1958 until Thomas's retirement in 1978. He was also friends with both men and was instrumental in having Thomas's photo painted and hung. He established the nation's first Regional Trauma Center at Hopkins Hospital and was also Hopkins Children's Hospital surgeon-in-charge, JHU Hospital, 1964–1997. He was the subject of C-SPAN's *Emergency Services* in 1993 and PBS's *Operation Lifeline* in 1978, and he served as a consultant to PBS's *American Experience* "Partners of the Heart" in 2003 as well as HBO's television movie, *Something the Lord Made*, in 2004.

Haller, Emily, MD Also a Hopkins physician, she knew Vivien Thomas from 1959 until his death.

Higgins, Robert, MD As the surgery chief at Johns Hopkins Medical Institute in 2015, Higgins became the first Black person to head any department at Johns Hopkins. Dr. Higgins is now president and chief academic officer at Rush University in Chicago. He studied with Hank

Sources

Bahnson at the University Hospitals of Pittsburgh and feels a close connection to Thomas because Bahnson had been trained by Thomas and Blalock.

Jackson, Truly. She married "Little Harold" Thomas, Vivien Thomas's nephew through his younger sister Melba. Jackson knew the entire Thomas family in Nashville and was particularly close with Lillian "Ootsie" Thomas, a Nashville civil rights leader, and Ootsie's husband, Harold Thomas, a Nashville civil rights leader who won equal pay for Black and white teachers in the city.

Merrill, Walter, MD One of Thomas's and Blalock's outstanding surgery students, he was a professor of cardiac surgery and chief of staff at the Vanderbilt University Hospital and was elected to the American Board of Thoracic Surgery. He was also chief of surgical services at the Veteran Affairs National Center.

Mitchell, Reavis, PhD He was a professor of sociology at Fisk University and its dean of the School of Humanities and Behavioral Social Sciences. He and his family knew Vivien Thomas and the entire Thomas family. He was an active Nashville community member, a much-published writer, and a consultant to WTVF in Nashville.

Norris, Harold. He was the son-in-law of Vivien Thomas whom he first met in 1948 when he began dating his daughter, Olga Thomas. They were married from 1955 until their deaths in 2020. The former US Air Force officer was also a Social Security administrator, a Baltimore County Election Assistant Chief Judge, and the managing director, Horizons Group, LTD. He was a consultant to the HBO movie *Something the Lord Made* and to PBS's *American Experience*.

Queen, Jean. She was hired by Vivien Thomas to be the supply manager in his laboratory. With Thomas as her mentor, she became a surgical technician at Hopkins and succeeded Thomas as lab supervisor. The two became good friends as well.

Rasberry-Dijkhoffz, Ursula. She is a granddaughter of the Thomases, having lived with Clara and Vivien Thomas for several years as a child. Her grandparents never spoke about her grandfather's work. She is a businesswoman in St. Maarten.

Smith, Marcia Rasberry. She, with her sister Ursula, lived with her mother and her grandparents, Clara and Vivien Thomas, for a few years during her parents' divorce. She and her sister Ursula had no idea of their grandfather's medical achievements while he was alive.

Spann, Valeria Thomas. The niece of Vivien Thomas, she and her mother remained friends with the Thomas family for years after her mother had divorced Harold Thomas. Ms. Spann was a social worker in New York City and helped comment on Thomas's book manuscript for *Pioneering Research.*

Watkins, Levi, MD This writer interviewed him twice, with the third interview forfeited because of his untimely death at age seventy in 2015. Watkins had studied under Vivien Thomas as JHU Medical School resident and worked with him from 1970 until Thomas's death in 1985. The Thomas family requested him to give Vivien Thomas's eulogy. Watkins considered Thomas a close friend and mentor. He was also the associate dean of Diversity at JHU Medical School and was the first surgeon to implant a human automatic cardiac defibrillator, for which Thomas assisted during its research stage. In 2023, Hopkins renamed its outpatient center the Levi Watkins, Jr., MD Outpatient Center.

Zimmerman, Jack McKay, MD He was a surgeon who studied and worked with Thomas and Blalock from 1949 to 1959 while he trained as a thoracic surgeon and began his lifelong interest in surgical palliation. A graduate of JHU Medical School, he was appointed chief resident surgeon and later held the position of associate professor.

Zuidema, George, MD He was a surgeon who studied and worked with Thomas and Blalock beginning in 1949. Upon Blalock's retirement in 1964, he became surgeon in chief at JHU Medical School and Hospital and was Thomas's supervisor. He was the first surgery chief at Hopkins to be interested about Thomas's status; he arranged to have his portrait hung, to award him the honorary LLD, and to promote him to the rank of instructor of Surgery. In 1984, he left Hopkins to become vice provost of Medical Affairs at the University of Michigan and retired in 1994 as professor emeritus of Surgery, University of Michigan.

ACKNOWLEDGMENTS

Vivien Thomas encompasses new stories and previously undisclosed truths that derive from original research. Incredible anecdotes were told to me by the older surgeons who had actually trained under Vivien Thomas and Alfred Blalock at both the Vanderbilt and Johns Hopkins Universities. I was the last writer to interview five of these late surgeons and hear their eloquent tales. I thank them—R. Robinson Baker, Alex Haller (and Emily Haller, MD), Denton Cooley, Jack Zimmerman, George Zuidema, and Levi Watkins, and their families.

I also spoke at length with Walter Merrill, who hospitably answered my questions and showed me the sites at Vanderbilt where Thomas and Blalock had worked. The three men who were former surgery chiefs at Hopkins generously gave me time to talk about the trio of Vivien Thomas, Alfred Blalock, and Johns Hopkins University: they are John Cameron, Robert Higgins, and the late George Zuidema.

A hearty thank you also extends to Vivien and Clara Thomas's relatives, whom I interviewed: their daughter, Theodosia Thomas Rasberry Dullea, and Theodosia's daughters, Ursula D. Rasberry-Dijkhoffz and Marcia T. Rasberry Smith. My interactions with Mrs. Dullea were conversational in nature. I also talked Vivien Thomas's son-in-law, Harold Norris, who provided perspectives on the family, Johns Hopkins University, and the city of Baltimore. Thanks to Valeria Thomas Spann, Vivien Thomas's niece, who added a social worker's insight to her thoughts.

Many thanks, also, to Koco Eaton, a Thomas cousin, who is a Hopkins-trained surgeon himself. Thank you to Truly Jackson, who had married the Thomases' nephew "Little Harold" Thomas and gave me a lively description of "Little Harold" and of Oatsie Thomas, Vivien Thomas's sister-in-law. In the Alfred Blalock family, his son, Dan Blalock, shared his insights in an email.

Vivien Thomas had many friends and colleagues: among them, I interviewed his best friend's daughter, the late Gwyneth Manlove Clark, and his Hopkins lab colleague, Jean Queen. Clark had lived with Clara and Vivien Thomas while she was a graduate student at Hopkins and generously shared her experiences and thoughts with me. My thanks also extend to the people who provided firsthand information about the social and family background of Mr. Thomas and his hometown, Nashville, as well as what his life was like as a Black man in Baltimore. They were the late Reavis Mitchell, PhD, Bernie Berkowitz, and Melvin Black. Additionally, George Callcott, PhD explained Vivien Thomas's honorary DSc degree offer from the University of Maryland. Alex Dragt, PhD, Professor Emeritus of Physics at the University of Maryland, explained his motivation for nominating Mr. Thomas for an honorary Doctor of Science degree from that university.

At home, I must thank my sister, Mary Hélène Pottker Rosenbaum, the writer and editor who painfully corrected my mishmash of semi-colons and colons, and who always provided the word that I wanted to use but couldn't quite remember what it was. She has been the first editor of all my books and I appreciate her excellent work. My daughters, Tracy Pottker-Fishel and Carrie Gene Kennedy, gave continual support and they both assisted in obtaining hard-to-find research material that I needed. Their husbands, Scott Bernstein and Riley Kennedy, offered warm reassurances when I was discouraged. My grandchildren, Parker Bryce Bernstein, Logan Andrew Kennedy, and Dylan Eugene Kennedy, all love stories and reading, which keeps each and every writer working at their desks. The comments of my husband, Andrew S. Fishel, were insightful, his suggestions about organization were useful, and the aid he offered when we travelled for my research and interviews were crucial. My friends consoled me when I became frustrated: some of them

ACKNOWLEDGMENTS

are Cathy O'Donnell, M Kathleen McCulloch, Judy Pomeranz, Eleanor Baker, the late great Mary Ann Elliott, Lilliann Zamora, Steven Brady, David Berkowitz, and Armita and Rudy Watson. Justin McArthur provided support and friendship, as always. And many thanks to David Wogahn for shepherding this MS to print. The index was created by the capable Catherine A. Barr. My friend Mark Woodland, MD who is Associate Dean Policy/Advocacy at Drexel University School of Medicine, the chair of the Pennsylvania State Medical Board, and a member of the Board of Directors of the Federation of State Medical Boards, took time to read and comment on the chapter describing the TOF babies. Any mistakes in this Vivien Thomas biography remain mine.

In my earlier eight books, I unfortunately neglected to thank the late Mrs. Inger Boye, the extraordinary children's librarian at the Highland Park (Ill.) Public Library for whom the Children's Room, with its blazing fireplace, is now named. With her kind assistance, I was able to explore all its wonderful children's titles and, when I was ten years old, she marched me into the adult section and told its librarian to issue an adult card that gave me access to every book in the library. People are often asked to name the teacher who most inspired them, but I always say my greatest encouragement came from a very special librarian, Inger Boyer.

And thank you to all readers around the world. As the Baltimore writer John Waters has said, "It wasn't until I started reading and found books they wouldn't let us read in school that I discovered you could be insane and happy and have a good life without being like anyone else."

ABOUT JAN POTTKER

This is Jan Pottker's ninth book. She has worked as research chief and analyst at the Office for Civil Rights at both the former US Department of Health, Education and Welfare as well as at the US Department of Education. Her experiences provide a depth of understanding of the discrimination Vivien Thomas faced at the universities and hospitals where he was employed. Pottker has appeared on hundreds of radio and television shows, including *Inside Edition* and *Biography*, and has talked about her books on more than forty international cruise ships. She has also given many hundreds of talks before business and community groups as well as speaking to the National Archives, the Smithsonian Institution, and several presidential libraries. She earned a PhD from Columbia University.

BIBLIOGRAPHY

For full bibliography,
please contact the author at
VivienThomasBook.com

INDEX

"Thomas" refers to Vivien Thomas
"Blalock" refers to Alfred Blalock
"p" before a page number refers to a picture

A
Abbot, Maude, 119, 120
Abernathy, Ralph, 245
Alabama State College, 245
Alan Mason Chesney Medical
　Archives, 255, 258, 261, 263, 270
AMA (American Medical
　Association), 115, 210, 276
Ambrose, Stephen E., 109
American Board of Thoracic Surgery,
　328
American College of Surgeons, 195,
　259–260
American Heart Association, 276
American Medical Association
　(AMA), 115, 210, 276
American Medical Writers
　Association, 266
American Society of Clinical Surgery,
　54
animal rights, 31, p152, 196, 198–201.
　see also dogs
Anna (dog), 133, p149, 201
Anna, Her Story (film), 201
AP (Associated Press), 167–168

Archives of Surgery, 210
Arizona, USS, 108
Associated Press (AP), 167–168
Association of Black Cardiologists,
　276
Atlanta Loan and Banking Company,
　40
Atrial Septal Defect (ASD). *see*
　Transposition of the Great Arteries
　(TGA)

B
Bahnson, Henry "Hank"
　Bahnson, Louise, p150
　Blalock—homage visit, 238
　Blalock—insecurity, 183
　Blalock—Southern Hotel party,
　　223, 224, 226–228, 230
　Blalock—talent scouting, 184
　Royal Tour, p150, 172
　University of Pittsburgh, 238, 277,
　　327–328
Bahnson, Louise, p150
Baker, R. Robinson "Bricks," 235, 326

Baltimore
  animal rights, 152, 196, 198–201
  Baltimore (magazine), 268
  Baltimore Afro American, 102, 105, 232
  Baltimore and Ohio railroad, 101, 103
  Baltimore Dog Referendum, 201
  Baltimore Economic Development Corporation, 326
  Baltimore riot of 1861, 90
  Baltimore Sun, 91–92, 196, 200
  Berkowitz, Bernie, 91, 326
  Bethlehem Steel, 93
  Black/Jewish Forum of Baltimore, Inc., 326
  blockbusting, 91
  Board of Estimates, 198
  Breckinridge, John C., 90
  Chesapeake and Potomac Telephone Company, 98–99
  City Planning, 326
  civic unrest, 90–91, 240–241
  civil rights movement, 202, 225, 232, 240–241
  Diggs, Louis, 91
  Fifteenth Amendment, 90
  Fourteenth Amendment, 90
  Gray, Freddie, 90
  Hopkins, Johns, 100–103, 105
  Johns Hopkins Colored Orphanage Asylum, 101, 102
  Johns Hopkins University. *see* Johns Hopkins University
  Key, Francis Scott, 224
  Lincoln, Abraham, 90
  Maritime Engineers Beneficial Association, 232
  "Maryland, My Maryland" (state song), 90
  Maryland Club, 242
  Maryland National Guard, 240–241
  Morgan State University, 163–164, 177, 205, 256
  Negro removal program, 90–91
  News-Post, 196
  Orser, Edward, 91
  Provident Hospital, 246, 255
  race discrimination, 87, 89, 90–91, 93, 98–99, 224–225, 227
  Southern Hotel, 224–225, 226, 227, 232–233, 268
  University of Maryland, 198, 248–249, 250, 326
  Vivien T. Thomas Medical Arts Academy, 275
  Washington, George, 224
  World War II, 91–92
Baltimore (magazine), 268
Baltimore Afro American, 102, 105, 232
Baltimore and Ohio railroad, 101, 103
Baltimore Dog Referendum, 201
Baltimore Economic Development Corporation, 326
Baltimore Sun, 91–92, 196, 200
Bass, Novella, 82
Beard, Joseph W., 61–62
Berger, Olive, 3, 137, 167, 194
Berkowitz, Bernie, 91, 326
Bethlehem Steel, 93
Bethune, Henry Norman, 52–53
Bethune, Norman, 52
Bing, Richard, 168, 182
Black, Melvin, 16, 326

Black/Jewish Forum of Baltimore, Inc., 326
Blalock, Aaron O., 40
Blalock, Alfred C., 40
Blalock, Alfred Dandy, 23, 68, 128
Blalock, Alfred—character & characteristics
  accent, 45
  aging fears, 207
  alcoholism, 64, 128, 204, 218, 219, 220–221, 237
  ambitions, 69–70, 184–185
  argumentative, 218–219
  Bahnson, Henry "Hank," 183
  Brooks, Barney, 52, 53
  car, 53
  charisma, 46
  colas, 59, 171
  Cooley, Denton, 110–111, 127, 174–175, 184
  crocheting, 52
  dating, 45, 46, 52, 55
  Famous Blalock O.R. Sayings, 183
  Grebel, Frances Wolff, 184
  Haller, J. Alex, 216
  Harrison, Tinsley, 45, 46, 51, 53, 60, 61
  health, 47, 51–54, 68, 84, 109, 207, 218, 229, 235, 237–239
  insecurity, 127, 183, 187
  Leeds (Levy), Stanford, 184, 185
  liar, 69, 71–72
  Longmire, William P., 207, 218, 220
  mechanical skills, 184
  narcissism, 166–167
  passive-aggressive, 113
  physical characteristics, 22, 46
  race discrimination, 112–113, 129, p153, 162–163, 176–178, 179–180, 225, 230–232
  religion discrimination, 50, 52
  research process, 60
  Sabiston, David, 184
  scouting talent, 110–111, 184
  self-confidence, 50
  sex discrimination, 166–167, 174–175
  slide rule, 61
  smoking, 52, 171
  Southern viewpoint, 43, 63, 162, 184
  student, 46
  studious, 46
  supervisory skills, 60–61
  surgical skills, 60, 127, 182, 216
  Taussig, Helen, 239
  Te Lind, Richard, 183
  teacher, 184
  temper, 64
  tennis, 41, 45
  theoretical work skills, 127
  Thomas—alcoholism, 219, 237
  whiskey, 59
Blalock, Alfred—events
  American Society of Clinical Surgery, 54
  animal rights, 31
  Bahnson, Henry "Hank," 223, 224, 226–228, 230, 238
  Baltimore move, 86–87
  Bethune, Henry Norman, 52
  birth, 39
  Brooks, Barney, 30, 48, 53, 54, 70
  capillary circulation, 204–205
  cardiac arrest. *see* cardiac arrest

Blalock, Alfred cont'd
Chesapeake and Potomac Telephone Company, 98–99
Circulation, 204–205
Columbia University job offer, 184–185
death, 238–239
Distinguished Service Award, 226, 229
fatherhood, 68
Georgia Military College, 43
Grebel, Frances Wolff, 85, 98
Guilford house sale, 220
Hanlon, C. Rollins, 238, 267
Harrison, Tinsley, 229
Heimbecker, Raymond, 204–205
Henry Ford Hospital job offer, 69–72
homage final visit, 238
house purchase, 86–87
hypertension, 63–64
Johns Hopkins University School of Medicine—academic papers credit, 162
Johns Hopkins University School of Medicine—admission, 43–44
Johns Hopkins University School of Medicine—anniversary (75th) party, 237
Johns Hopkins University School of Medicine—assistant dispensary urologist, 46
Johns Hopkins University School of Medicine—assistant resident surgeon, 46
Johns Hopkins University School of Medicine—Distinguished Service Award, 226, 229
Johns Hopkins University School of Medicine—extern in urology, 46
Johns Hopkins University School of Medicine—graduation, 30, 46
Johns Hopkins University School of Medicine—new dog lab, 216–217
Johns Hopkins University School of Medicine—publish studies, 47
Johns Hopkins University School of Medicine—salary, 184–186
Johns Hopkins University School of Medicine—science building name, 237
Johns Hopkins University School of Medicine—Southern Hotel party, p153, 223–230
Johns Hopkins University School of Medicine—Student Army Training Corps, 45
Johns Hopkins University School of Medicine—student bookstore, 45
Johns Hopkins University School of Medicine—surgery chair fight, 234
Johns Hopkins University School of Medicine—surgery chief, 84–85
Johns Hopkins University School of Medicine—Symposium in Honor of Alfred Blalock, 267
Johns Hopkins University School of Medicine—welcome party, 86
Jonesboro, move to, 41
Longmire, William P., 220, 238
marriage to Alice Waters, 220
marriage to Mary O'Bryan, 55
McClure, Roy B., 69–70, 70–71, 71–72

Morrow, A. Glenn, 223, 224, 226, 228
O'Bryan, Mrs. moves in, 129
Old Hands Club, 238, 239
Park, Edwards A., 123
Peter Bent Brigham Hospital, 47
Physiological Laboratories (UK), 54
Principles of Surgical Care: Shock and Other Problems (book), 84–85
published papers, 84–85, 123, 162, 204–205
Rappleye, Willard C., 185
Ravitch, Mark, 71, 223, 225–226, 228, 236, 238, 239
retirement, 235
Rockefeller General Education Board (GEB), 53
Sabiston, David, 223, 225–226, 228, 234
Sauerbruch, Ferdinand, 54
Southern Hotel party, p153, 223–230
Student Army Training Corp, 45
summer house rental, 96–97
surgeons' Chicago meeting (1934), 68–69
Symposium in Honor of Alfred Blalock, 267
Tetralogy of Fallot (TOF) blue babies. *see* Tetralogy of Fallot (TOF) blue babies
Thomas—Chesapeake and Potomac Telephone Company, 98–99
Thomas—Henry Ford Hospital discrimination lie, 71–72
Thomas—introduction to guests in lab, 188
Thomas—job interview, 21–25
Thomas—job title for, 36, 37
Thomas—Johns Hopkins University campus tour, 88–89
Thomas—recognition denied, 257–258, 258–259, 272
Thomas—repents lack of support for, 238
Thomas—salary for, 23–24, 34–38, 97–98, 162, 176–178, 179–180, 213
Thomas—Southern Hotel party, 223–224, 225–226, 226–228, 231–232
Thomas—surprise house visit, 98
Thomas—visit to Gibson Island, 220–221
Transposition of the Great Arteries (TGA). *see* Transposition of the Great Arteries (TGA)
traumatic shock. *see* traumatic shock
Trudeau Sanatorium, 51–53
University of Georgia, 43
University of Louisville job offer, 69
Vanderbilt University— departure, 86
Vanderbilt University—American Society of Clinical Surgery, 54
Vanderbilt University—assistant professor, 50–51
Vanderbilt University—associate professor of surgery, 54
Vanderbilt University—chief resident surgeon, 52

Blalock, Alfred cont'd
  Vanderbilt University—full
    professor, 70–71
  Vanderbilt University—move to, 48
  World War II. *see* traumatic shock
  Zimmerman, Jack McKay, 220
  Zuidema, George, 234
Blalock, Alfred—family & friends
  Atlanta Loan and Banking
    Company, 40
  Blalock, Aaron O., 40
  Blalock, Alfred C., 40
  Blalock, Alfred Dandy (son), 23,
    68, 128
  Blalock (birth name Waters), Alice,
    220, 221, 237
  Blalock, Edgar (brother), 41
  Blalock, Elizabeth (sister), 41
  Blalock, Eugene M., 40
  Blalock, George (father), 39–40,
    41, 43
  Blalock, Georgia (sister), 41
  Blalock, Martha (Mattie) (mother),
    39
  Blalock (birth name O'Bryan),
    Mary. *see* Blalock (birth name
    O'Bryan), Mary
  Blalock, Mary Elizabeth
    (daughter), 68, 128
  Blalock, Mary (sister), 41
  Blalock, William, 40
  Blalock, William Rice (son), 68,
    128
  Blalock, Zadock (grandfather), 40,
    42
  Blalock plantation, 39–40, 42–43
  Civil War, 42
  Fulton National Bank, 40
  Harrison, Tinsley. *see* Harrison,
    Tinsley
  lineage, 39–40
  Moore, Joe, 40
  O'Bryan, Mrs. (mother-in-law), 55,
    129
  wealth, 42
  Blalock (birth name Waters), Alice,
    220, 221, 237
  Blalock, Edgar, 41
  Blalock, Elizabeth, 41
  Blalock, Eugene M., 40
  Blalock, George, 39–40, 41, 43
  Blalock, Georgia, 41
  Blalock, Martha (Mattie), 39
  Blalock (birth name O'Bryan), Mary
    alcoholism, 68, 128, 203–204, 219,
      220
    alone, 96, 220
    Baltimore move, 86–87
    Blalock—absences, 128
    Cooley, Denton, 204
    death, 220
    Guilford house sale, 220
    health, 204, 219
    Karsh portrait, 203
    Longmire, William P., 204
    marriage, 55, 203–204
    O'Bryan, Mrs. moves in, 129
    Royal Tour, p150
    sense of humor, 96
    servants, 97
    summer house rental, 96–97
  Blalock, Mary (Alfred's sister), 41
  Blalock, Mary Elizabeth (Alfred's
    daughter), 68, 128
  Blalock, William, 40
  Blalock, William Rice, 68, 128
  Blalock, Zadock, 40, 42

Blalock Clamp, 131, 169
Blalock-Hanlon procedure. *see*
  Transposition of the Great Arteries
  (TGA)
Blalock-Taussig shunt. *see* Tetralogy
  of Fallot (TOF) blue babies
blockbusting, 91
blood banks, 102, 115, 258
blood drives, 114–115, 115–116
Bloomberg Philanthropies, 276
blue babies. *see* Tetralogy of Fallot
  (TOF) blue babies
Body, Issaac, 23, 24
Bond, Julian, 16
Boston University, 119
Bowman, Isaiah, 87, 185
Bowman-Gray medical college, 86
Breckinridge, John C., 90
Brimmer, Andrew F., 249
Brinkley, David, 222
Brock, Russell, 188
Brooks, Barney
  Blalock—American Society of
    Clinical Surgery, 54
  Blalock—Cannon challenge, 30
  Blalock—full professor, 70
  Blalock—health, 52, 53
  Blalock—Rockefeller General
    Education Board (GEB), 53
  Blalock—Vanderbilt University
    move, 48
  Leeds (Levy), Stanford, 63
  Thomas—dismissal, 85–86, 235
  Thomas—salary, 35–36, 36–37,
    37–38
"Brother, Can You Spare a Dime?"
  (song), 58
Burton, Harold, 205–206

C

Caldwell & Co., 55
Calhoun (birth name Thomas), Olga
  (sister)
  birth, 11
  career, 64–65
  Henry Ford Hospital, 70
  marriage & nursing, 17–18
  preschool & kindergarten, 13–14
  Tennessee State University, 19
Callcott, George H., 248, 249, 326
Cameron, John L., 236, 264–265,
  266–267, 273
Cannon, Walter, 29–30, 68–69
capillary circulation, 204–205
cardiac arrest
  cardiopulmonary resuscitation
    (CPR), 6, p154, 209–210
  causes of, 208
  Consolidated Edison Electric
    Company, 208
  defibrillator, 209, 209–210, 214–215
  defibrillator, implantable cardiac
    (ICD), 6, 246
  Edison, Thomas, 208
  electric jolt, 208–209
  Jude, James R., 209
  Kay, Jerome, 208, 209, 209–210
  Knickerbocker, G. Guy, p154, 209,
    209–210
  Kouwenhoven, William B., p154,
    208, 209, 209–210, 230
  Mount Sinai Hospital, 246
  Ravitch, Mark, 210
  television, 208
  Thomas—cardiopulmonary
    resuscitation (CPR), 6, 209–210
  Thomas—contributions overview,
    6, 272

cardiac arrest *cont'd*
  Thomas—defibrillator, 209, 209–210, 214–215
  Thomas—dogs, 209, 246
  Thomas—implantable cardiac defibrillator (ICD), 6, 246
  Thomas—recognition denied, 209–210
  Thomas—recognition given, 210
  Watkins, Levi, 6, 246, 329
cardiac catheterization, 168, 182
cardiopulmonary resuscitation (CPR), 6, p154, 209–210
Carnegie endowment, 12
Case Western Reserve University, 207
Casper, Alfred, 216
Cavagnaro, Louise, 237
Chesapeake and Potomac Telephone Company, 98–99
Chesney, Alan, 103–104, 198, 200
Chit Chat Farms, 237
Chrysler, 70
Circulation, 204–205
civil rights movement. *see also* race discrimination
  Abernathy, Ralph, 245
  Baker, R. Robinson "Bricks," 235
  Baltimore, 202, 225, 232, 240–241
  Bass, Novella, 82
  Bond, Julian, 16
  Brinkley, David, 222
  Carnegie endowment, 12
  Cronkite, Walter, 222
  Davies, Elmer, 78, 79, 82
  Du Bois, W.E.B., 75
  education system, 76–78, 78–83
  equal protections, 77
  Faubus, Orval, 222

Fifteenth Amendment, 90
Ford Motor Company, 70
Fourteenth Amendment, 90
Greenfield, Lazar J. "Jack," 223
Harlem, 75, 76
Harrison, Tinsley, 50
Hopkins, Johns, 101
Hughes, Langston, 76
"I, Too" (poem), 76
John D. Rockefeller General Education Board (GEB), 15
Johns Hopkins University, 223, 235, 240–241
Julius Rosenwald Fund, 15–16
King, Martin Luther, Jr., 240, 245
Little Rock Nine, 222
Locke, Alain, 76
Looby, Alexander, 78, 79, 83
Lynn, William S., 62
Madry, Sadie, 82
Marshall, Thurgood, 77, 78, 79, 81–82
Mitchell, Reavis, 11–12, 80–81
Montgomery Bus Boycott, 245
NAACP, 12, 73–74, 75–78, 78–82
Nashville, 73–74, 78–83
Parks, Rosa, 74
Pearl High School, 222
Pittsburgh Courier, 77
Quakers, 15
Ramsey, Sonya, 80
Renaissance, 75–76
sit-ins, 222
Southern Hotel, 232–233
Talented Tenth, 75
Thomas, Harold (brother), 72–73, 78–83, 187, 328
Thomas, Lillian "Ootsie" Dunn, 222, 328

347

Thomas—washrooms, 274–275
Watkins, Levi, 245
Williams, Juan, 77
women's rights, 104
Civil War, 9, 28, 39–40, 42, 89–90, 101
Clarke, Gwendolyn Manlove, 236, 241, 326
Claudius Galen of Pergamon, 27
collapse therapy (pneumothorax treatment), 54
colleges. *see* universities & colleges
Columbia University, 7, 115, 184–185, 257
Congressional Black Caucus foundation, 276
Consolidated Edison Electric Company, 208
Cooley, Denton
   Blalock (birth name O'Bryan), Mary, 204
   Blalock—insecurity, 127
   Blalock—scouting talent, 110–111, 184
   Blalock—sex discrimination, 174–175
   Blalock—surgical skills, 127
   heart transplant, 207, 326
   tennis, 172
   Tetralogy of Fallot (TOF) blue babies surgery, 3, 136–137
   Texas Heart Institute, 326–327
   Thomas—condolence note, 266
   Thomas—friendship, 327
   Thomas—instructor, 217
   Thomas—portrait, 242
   Thomas—surgical skills, 182–183
   Thomas—Transposition of the Great Arteries (TGA), 194, 260

traumatic shock, 110–111, 127
CPR (cardiopulmonary resuscitation), 6, p154, 209–210
Crile, George Washington, 28–29
A Crisis in Medical Education SOS (film), 246–247
Cronkite, Walter, 222
Crosby, Bing, 58
C-SPAN, 327
Cushing, Harvey W., 46–47, 47

D

Dandy, Sadie, 185–186
Dandy, Walter E., 23, 51, 68, 98, 162, 185–186
Dartmouth College, 277
Davies, Elmer, 78, 79, 82
Def, Mos, 269–270
defibrillator, 209, 209–210, 214–215
defibrillator, implantable cardiac (ICD), 6, 246
Delano, Victor, 109
Devereux, James, 199
Diggs, Louis, 91
Distinguished Service Award, 226, 229
dogs
   animal rights, 31, p152, 196, 198–201
   Anna (dog), 133, p149, 201
   Anna, Her Story (film), 201
   Baltimore, p152, 196, 198–201
   Baltimore Dog Referendum, 201
   Baltimore Sun, 196
   Blalock—advocate for, 196–197, 198
   cardiac arrest, p154, 209, 246
   Chesney, Alan, 198, 200
   Devereux, James, 199
   Hearst, William Randolph, 196
   hypertension, 63–64

dogs   cont'd
  Johns Hopkins University—Stark
    Films, 201
  Johns Hopkins University—
    suppliers, 198
  medical schools, 197–198, 200
  military, 199, 199–200
  Nashville, 196–197
  new lab building, 216–217
  News-Post, 196
  pounds, 197, 198, 200
  Sister Jessica, 200
  Society to Prevent Cruelty to
    Animals (S.P.C.A.), p152, 197,
    198, 200
  Stark Films, 201
  Taussig, Helen, 200
  Tetralogy of Fallot (TOF) blue
    babies, 126, 129–130, 131–133,
    200, 201
  Thomas—anonymity, 197
  Transposition of the Great Arteries
    (TGA), 189, 190–192
  traumatic shock, 5, 30–32, 33–34,
    62–63, 108, 110, 111, 112, 123–124
  University of Maryland, 198
  Vanderbilt University, 197
  Washington, D.C., 198
  Washington Post, 196
Drake, 15
Drew, Charles, 115–116
Drew, Thomas, 275
Du Bois, W.E.B., 12, 13–14, 75, 103,
  170
Duke University, 61–62, 238
Dullea (birth name Thomas),
  Theodosia (daughter)
  birth, 67
  business school, 256

  divorce, 256
  family, p145, 327
  hospital equipment reproduction,
    214, 215
  *Pioneering Research in Surgical
    Shock and Cardiovascular Surgery:
    Vivien Thomas and His Work with
    Alfred Blalock* (book), 261
  Rasberry-Dijkhoffz, Ursula
    (daughter), 256–257, 269–270,
    328
  Smith (birth name Rasberry),
    Marcia (daughter), 256–257,
    269–270, 274, 329
  Thomas—portrait, 243
  Thomas—resilience, 273
  Thomas—visit to lab, 211
  vacation to Nashville, Tennessee,
    159–160
Duncan, George W., 85, 111–112,
  125–126

E

Eaton, Koco (Katuelle), 183–184, 257,
  273, 327
Eaton Orthopedics, 327
Edison, Thomas, 208
Emergency Services (television
  program), 327
"Experimental Shock: The Cause of
  the Low Blood Pressure Produced
  by Muscle Injury," 54–55

F

Fallot, Étienne-Louis Arthur, 119–120
Famous Blalock O.R. Sayings, 183
Faubus, Orval, 222
Fifteenth Amendment, 90
"fight or flight," 29
Firor, Warfield, 185

Fisk College Training School, 13–14
Fisk University
  Carnegie endowment, 12
  Du Bois, W.E.B., 12, 13–14
  Fisk College Training School, 13–14, 14
  Fisk University Place, 13
  John D. Rockefeller General Education Board (GEB), 12
  Locke, Alain, 76
  Mitchell, Reavis, 11–12, 328
  Thomas—carpentry work, 18, 19, 24
Fisk University Place, 13
Flanders, Leonard (father-in-law), 65
Flanders, Mary Gross (mother-in-law), 65
Ford, Edsel, 70
Ford, Henry, 70
Ford Motor Company, 70
Fourteenth Amendment, 90
Freeman, Morgan, 268
Fulton National Bank, 40

G

Gamble, Robert, 104
Garrett, Mary Elizabeth, 103, 178
Gazette, 268
Gee, Bob, 240, 241
General Motors, 70
Georgia Military College, 43
GI Bill, 163
Gilman, Daniel Coit, 104
GlaxoSmithKline, 276
Gone with the Wind, 41–42, 63
Goucher College, 46, 326
Gray, Freddie, 90
Great Depression, 19–20, 55–56, 57–58

Grebel, Frances Wolff, 85, 98, 184, 215, 242
Green, Thomas, 108
Green Book, 159, 160
Greenfield, Lazar J. "Jack," 217, 223, 327
Gross, Robert, 121–122
Gross, Samuel D., 28
The Gross Clinic, 28
Gwinn, Mary Mackell, 103

H

Haller, Emily, 327
Haller, J. Alex
  Blalock—surgical skills, 216
  C-SPAN, 327
  Emergency Services (television program), 327
  HBO, 327
  Johns Hopkins University—Regional Trauma Center, 327
  Operation Lifeline (television program), 327
  "Partners of the Heart" (television documentary), 327
  PBS (Public Broadcast System), 327
  Royal Tour, 172
  Something the Lord Made (television movie), 327
  Thomas—bartending, 164
  Thomas—BS degree, 248
  Thomas—instructor, 217
  Thomas—portrait, 240, 241–242, 327
  Thomas—surgical skills, 112
  Thomas—Transposition of the Great Arteries (TGA), 260
Halsted, William S., 44

Hanlon, C. Rollins
 American College of Surgeons, 195, 259–260
 Blalock—homage visit, 238
 Blalock—scouting talent, 110–111, 184
 Blalock—Symposium in Honor of Alfred Blalock, 267
 "Interatrial Septal Defects," 193
 photo, p154
 positive pressure anesthesia machines, 195
 published papers, 193, 194, 195
 Saint Louis University, 195, 238
 "The Surgical Treatment of Complete Transposition of the Aorta and the Pulmonary Artery," 194
 Thomas—handwritten notes, 193, 195, 259–261
 Thomas—portrait, 242–243
 Thomas—recognition denied, 195, 243, 259–260
 Thomas—recognition given, 195, 242–243
 Transposition of the Great Arteries (TGA), 193, 194, 195, 259–261
Harlem, 75, 76
Harmel, Merel, 3, 137, 139, 140
Harriet Lane Home for Invalid Children, 119, 135
Harrison, Groce, 45
Harrison, Tinsley
 Blalock—accent, 45
 Blalock—dating, 46
 Blalock—friendship, 46, 49, 50
 Blalock—health, 51, 53
 Blalock—research process, 60
 Blalock—slide rule, 61
 Blalock—Southern Hotel party, 229
 Blalock—studious, 46
 Blalock—surgical skills, 60
 Bowman-Gray medical college, 86
 ghostwriting, 51
 Harrison, Groce, 45
 heart failure research, 50
 Peter Bent Brigham Hospital, 46–47
 studious, 45
 Timms, Minnie Mae, 36, 259
 University of Michigan, 45
 Vanderbilt University, 36, 48, 49, 86
Harvard University
 Cushing, Harvey W., 46–47, 47
 Gross, Robert, 121–122
 Harvard Hospital Unit, 29
 heart surgery, 121–122
 Ladd, William E., 121–122
 sex discrimination, 118–119
 Taussig, Frank William, 118
 Taussig, Helen, 118–119
 Watkins, Levi, 245–246
Harvey, Jean Hogarth, 326
Harvey, William, 27
HBO, 269, 270, 327, 328
Hearst, William Randolph, 196
Heimbecker, Raymond, 204–205
Henry Ford Hospital, 69–72
Hibbitts, Louis H., 78, 81
Higgins, Robert S., 276–277, 327–328
Hippocrates, 27
Hitler, Adolf, 1
Hopkins, Johns, 100–103, 105
Howard University, 15, 116
Hughes, Langston, 76
Hunter, John, 89
hypertension, 63–64

hypotrophy, 210

I

"I, Too" (poem), 76
"I Hear America Singing" (poem), 75–76
ICD (implantable cardiac defibrillator), 6, 246
Indiana University, 236
Institute for Technical Skills (UK), 276
"Interatrial Septal Defects," 193
International Committee of Medical Journal Editors, 259
Isaacs, James P., 236

J

Jackson, Truly, 251, 328
Jefferson Medical College, 28
J.J. Deknatel & Son, 169
John D. Rockefeller General Education Board (GEB), 12, 15, 35, 37, 49, 53
Johns Hopkins Colored Orphan Asylum, 101, 102
The Johns Hopkins Magazine, 182–183
Johns Hopkins University
  Alan Mason Chesney Medical Archives, 255, 258, 261, 263, 270
  anniversary (75th) party, 237
  Bahnson, Henry "Hank," 184
  Baker, R. Robinson "Bricks," 235, 326
  Bing, Richard, 168, 182
  Blalock, Alfred. *see* Blalock, Alfred—events
  Blalock, George, 41
  blood banks, 102, 258
  Bloomberg Philanthropies, 276
  bookstore, 267

Bowman, Isaiah, 87, 185
Cameron, John L., 264, 266–267, 273
cardiac arrest. *see* cardiac arrest
cardiac catheterization, 168, 182
Cavagnaro, Louise, 237
Chesney, Alan, 103–104, 198, 200
civil rights movement, 223, 240–241
condition of buildings, 88–89
Cooley, Denton. *see* Cooley, Denton
A Crisis in Medical Education SOS (film), 246–247
Dandy, Walter E., 23, 51, 68, 98, 162, 185–186
the doghouse, 89
dogs. *see* dogs
Du Bois, W.E.B., 103
Duncan, George W., 85
Financial Four, 103–104
Firor, Warfield, 185
founding, 44, 100, 101–103
Founding Four, 103
Gamble, Robert, 104
Garrett, Mary Elizabeth, 103
Gazette, 268
Gilman, Daniel Coit, 104
Gwinn, Mary Mackell, 103
Haller, J. Alex, 327
Halsted, William S., 44
Hanlon, C. Rollins. *see* Hanlon, C. Rollins
Harriet Lane Home for Invalid Children, 119, 135
Harrison, Groce, 45
Higgins, Robert S., 276–277, 327–328
Hopkins, Johns, 100, 103, 105

Johns Hopkins University cont'd
  Hunter, John, 89
  Hunterian doghouse, 216
  "The Johns Hopkins Hospital Surgical Routine" (publication), 69
  The Johns Hopkins Magazine, 182–183
  Johns Hopkins University Press, 262
  Kelly, Howard, 44
  King, Elizabeth Tabor, 103
  Levi Watkins, Jr. MD Outpatient Center, 329
  Longmire, William P. *see* Longmire, William P.
  Maryland National Guard, 240–241
  Mayo, Julius, 211–212
  McCall, Nancy, 263, 270
  Merrill, Walter, 184
  Milton S. Eisenhower Medal for Distinguished Service, 251
  mop and bucket squad, 95
  Muller, Steven, p155
  neighborhood of, 88
  new dog lab, 216–217
  Nobel prize Blalock wish, 186
  Old Hands Club, 238, 239, 240, 241–242, 258
  Osler, William, 44, 45, 103
  Park, Edwards A., 119, 166
  parties, 164
  the plantation, 105
  Poth, Edgar, 94
  Quakers, 100
  race discrimination, 86, 93, 94–95, 97–98, 102, 102–103, 104–105, 164, 170, 211, 211–212, 223, 226, 241–242, 246–247, 251–252, 261, 268
  Ravitch, Mark. *see* Ravitch, Mark
  Regional Trauma Center, 327
  research, focus on, 44–45
  Ross, Richard S., 251, 263
  Sabiston, David. *see* Sabiston, David
  salaries for lab workers, 211, 212
  sex discrimination, 102–103, 104, 119, 166–167, 172–173
  Sherwood, Elizabeth "The King," 136
  Something the Lord Made (television movie), 269–270, 327, 328
  Spencer, Rowena, 129
  Squeaky (dog) story, 206
  student body, 45
  surgery chair, 234
  Symposium in Honor of Alfred Blalock, 267
  Taussig, Helen. *see* Tetralogy of Fallot (TOF) blue babies
  Taussig, Helen—admission, 119
  Taussig, Helen—house purchase, 251
  Taussig, Helen—Milton S. Eisenhower Medal for Distinguished Service, 251
  Taussig, Helen—photo portrait, 203
  Taussig, Helen—promotion, 251
  Tetralogy of Fallot (TOF) blue babies. *see* Tetralogy of Fallot (TOF) blue babies
  Thomas, M. Carey, 103, 104
  Thomas, Vivien. *see* Thomas, Vivien—events: Johns Hopkins University to death

Transposition of the Great Arteries (TGA). *see* Transposition of the Great Arteries (TGA)
traumatic shock. *see* traumatic shock
Turner, Thomas, 71, 255
Vivien T. Thomas College Advisory Program, 275
Vivien T. Thomas Fund, 275–276
"Vivien Thomas, Hopkins Pioneer Surgical Technician, Dies" (newspaper article), 266
Vivien Thomas Scholars Initiative, 276
Watkins, Levi, 89, 105, 223, 245–246, 329
Welch, William H., 44
Woolfe, Harvey, p155
World War II, 110
Zuidema, George. *see* Zuidema, George
Johns Hopkins University Press, 262
Johnson, Lyndon B., 239
Jones, William O., 130, 131
Journal of the American Medical Association, 167
journals. *see* magazines & journals
Jude, James R., 209
Julius Rosenwald Fund, 15–16

K

Karsh, Yousef, 202–203
Kay, Jerome, 208, 209, 209–210, 260
Kelly, Howard, 44
Key, Francis Scott, 224
Kimmel, Billy, 272
Kimmel, Jimmy, 272
King, Elizabeth Tabor, 103
King, Martin Luther, Jr., 240, 245

Knickerbocker, G. Guy, p154, 209, 209–210
Kouwenhoven, William B., p154, 208, 209, 209–210, 230

L

Ladd, William E., 121–122
Lake Providence, 9–10, p143
Lamont, Austin, 3, 137, 166–167
Le Dran, Henri-François, 27
"Leaves of Grass" (poem), 75
Leeds (Levy), Stanford, 63–64, 123–124, 184, 185
LIFE, 168
Life Along The Mississippi, 10
Limpert, Jack, 268
Lincoln, Abraham, 90
Lincoln University, 16
Little Rock Nine, 222
Locke, Alain, 76
Longmire, William P.
  Blalock (birth name O'Bryan), Mary, 204
  Blalock—aging fears, 207
  Blalock—alcoholism, 218
  Blalock—Guilford house sale, 220
  Blalock—homage visit, 238
  Blalock—talent scouting, 110–111, 184
  Taussig, Helen, 174
  Tetralogy of Fallot (TOF) blue babies surgery, 3, 136–137, 139, 141
  Thomas—portrait, 242
  Thomas—Tetralogy of Fallot (TOF) blue babies. *see* Tetralogy of Fallot (TOF) blue babies
Looby, Alexander, 78, 79, 83
lynchings, 80–81
Lynn, William S., 62

M

Madry, Sadie, 82
magazines & journals
  Archives of Surgery, 210
  Baltimore (magazine), 268
  Circulation, 204–205
  Gazette, 268
  International Committee of Medical Journal Editors, 259
  The Johns Hopkins Magazine, 182–183
  Journal of the American Medical Association, 167
  LIFE, 168
  New England Journal of Medicine, 266
  Surgery, Gynecology and Obstetrics, 210
  TIME, 168, 206
  Washingtonian, 268
Manlove, Andrew, p144
Manlove, Charles
  bullies scuffle, 20
  job search for Thomas, 20–22
  photo, p156
  Vanderbilt University lab assistant, 20–21
Marathe, Supreet, 194–195
Maritime Engineers Beneficial Association, 232
Marshall, Thurgood, 77, 78, 79, 81–82
"Maryland, My Maryland" (state song), 90
Maryland Club, 242
Maryland National Guard, 240–241
Mayo, Julius, 211–212
McCabe, Katie, 268, 269
McCall, Nancy, 263, 270
McClure, Roy B., 69–70, 70–71, 71–72
McGill University (Canada), 115
"Mechanism and Treatment of Experimental Shock: Shock Following Hemorrhage," 51
Medical College of Virginia, 327
Meharry Medical College
  Black middle class, 12, 13, 15
  costs for, 18
  Vivien Thomas Endowed Scholarship, 276
Merrill, Walter, 184, 328
Metropolitan Nashville Teachers Association, 78
Miller, Dorrie (Doris), 109–110
Milton S. Eisenhower Medal for Distinguished Service, 251
Mississippi River, 10
Mitchell, Charlotte, 3, 137
Mitchell, Margaret, 41–42, 63
Mitchell, Reavis, 12, 80–81, 328
Montgomery Bus Boycott, 245
Moore, Joe, 40
Morgan College, 163–164
Morgan State University, 163–164, 177, 205, 256
Morrow, A. Glenn, 215–216, 223, 224, 226, 228
Mount Sinai Hospital, 210, 246
Muller, Steven, p155
Murray Baumgartner, 169

N

NAACP, 12, 73–74, 75–78, 78–82
Nashville
  animal rights, 196–197
  Athens of the South, 12
  Black Mecca, 12
  Black middle class, 11–13

civil rights movement, 73–74, 78–83
drought, 57
education system, 11, 15–16, 73–74, 78–83
Fisk University. *see* Fisk University
Great Depression, 57
Hibbitts, Louis H., 78, 81
John D. Rockefeller General Education Board (GEB), 15
Julius Rosenwald Fund, 15–16
Meharry Medical College. *see* Meharry Medical College
Metropolitan Nashville Teachers Association, 78
Nashville Banner, 13
Nashville Black City Business Directory (book), 13
Nashville Globe, 82–83
Pearl High School, 15, 16–17, p143, 222, 273, 326
Pearl High School Museum and Archives, 16, 326
Quakers, 15
race discrimination, 13, 14, 15–16, 21, 73–74
Ryman Auditorium (Mother Church of Country Music), 17
sex discrimination, 80
The Tennessean, 13
Tennessee State University (TSU), 12, 18, 245
Thomas v. Hibbitts et al, 78–83
United Methodist Church, 14
Vanderbilt University. *see* Vanderbilt University
Nashville Banner, 13
Nashville Black City Business Directory (book), 13

Nashville Globe, 82–83
National Heart Institute (National Institutes of Health), 215–216
National Medical Association, 276
National Research Council, 107, 108–109, 114
Native Americans, 40
Negro removal program, 90–91
Nembutal, 63
New England Journal of Medicine, 266
New York Tribune, 101
newspapers
  Baltimore Afro American, 102, 105, 232
  Baltimore Sun, 91–92, 196, 200
  Nashville Banner, 13
  Nashville Globe, 82–83
  New York Tribune, 101
  News-Post, 196
  Pittsburgh Courier, 77, 110
  The Tennessean, 13
  Washington Post, 196
News-Post, 196
Nokawama, Dan, 194
Norris (birth name Thomas), Olga (daughter)
  birth, 67
  family photo, p145
  marriage, 328
  Morgan State University, 256
  Norris, Nena, 256–257
  Thomas—portrait, 243
  vacation to Nashville, Tennessee, 159–160
Norris, Harold (son-in-law), 250, 262, 274, 328
Norris, Nena (granddaughter), 256–257

O

O'Bryan, Mrs., 55, 129
Office of Scientific Research and Development, 107, 168
Old Hands Club, 238, 239, 240, 241–242
Operation Lifeline (television program), 327
Orser, Edward, 91
Osler, William, 44, 45, 103

P

Panic of 1893, 103
Park, Edwards A., 119, 123, 166–167, 174
Parks, Rosa, 74
"Partners of the Heart" (television documentary), 268–269, 327, 328
Patton, George S., 116–117
PBS (Public Broadcast System), 268–269, 327, 328
Pearl Harbor attack, 106–107, 115
Pearl High School, 15, 16–17, p143, 222, 273, 326
Pearl High School Museum and Archives, 16, 326
Peoples Savings and Loan, 55
Peter Bent Brigham Hospital, 46–47, 47
Physiological Laboratories (UK), 54
Pioneering Research in Surgical Shock and Cardiovascular Surgery: Vivien Thomas and His Work with Alfred Blalock (book), p157, 254–255, 255–256, 257–259, 264–265, 266–267, 269, 329
Pittsburgh Courier, 77, 110
positive pressure anesthesia machines, 214
Posthumous Scroll of Merit, 276
Poth, Edgar, 94
Pottker, Jan, 7–8, 335
Presidential Medal of Freedom, 239
Principles of Surgical Care: Shock and Other Problems (book), 84–85
Provident Hospital, 246, 255
pulmonary stenosis, 210
Puryear, Clara Belle, 4, 112, 132, 137, 174
Pyle, Ernie, 116

Q

Quakers, 15, 100
Queen, Jean, 236–237, 252, 265, 328

R

race discrimination. *see also* civil rights movement; Civil War; religion discrimination; sex discrimination
  Ambrose, Stephen E., 109
  Baltimore, 87, 89, 90–91, 93, 98–99, 224–225, 227
  Baltimore Afro American, 102
  Baltimore Sun, 91–92
  Beard, Joseph W., 61–62
  Bethlehem Steel, 93
  Blalock, Alfred, 112–113, 129, p153, 162–163, 167, 176–178, 179–180, 225, 230–232
  blockbusting, 91
  Chesapeake and Potomac Telephone Company, 98–99
  Chrysler, 70
  Du Bois, W.E.B., 103
  Duke University, 61–62
  education system, 15–16, 73–74, 76
  Ford, Henry, 70
  Ford Motor Company, 70
  General Motors, 70

GI Bill, 163
Gone with the Wind, 41–42, 63
Gray, Freddie, 90
Great Depression, 57
Green Book, 159, 160
Henry Ford Hospital, 71–72
Hopkins, Johns, 100
housing—Baltimore, 87, 89, 90–91, 93, 96
housing-Lake Providence, 9–10
housing—Nashville, 12–13
incognegro, 170
Johns Hopkins Colored Orphanage Asylum, 101, 102
Johns Hopkins University, 86, 93, 94–95, 97–98, 102, 102–103, 104–105, 164, 170, 211, 211–212, 223, 226, 241–242, 246–247, 251–252, 261, 268
Lake Providence, 9–10
lynchings, 80–81
Maryland Club, 242
medical supply company, 213
military, 109–110
Miller, Dorrie (Doris), 109–110
Mitchell, Margaret, 41–42, 63
Nashville, 13, 14, 15–16, 21, 73–74
Negro removal program, 90–91
Pioneering Research in Surgical Shock and Cardiovascular Surgery: Vivien Thomas and His Work with Alfred Blalock (book), 257–259, 261
Pittsburgh Courier, 110
Southern Hotel, 224, 225, 232–233, 268
Thomas—portrait, 241–242
University of Alabama, 245

Vanderbilt University, 20–21, 35, 36, 37, 49, 85–86, 235, 245
Watkins, Levi, 89, 105, 223, 245
World War II, 91–92, 109
racism. see race discrimination
Radcliffe College, 118
Ramsey, Sonya, 80
Rappleye, Willard C., 185
Rasberry-Dijkhoffz, Ursula (granddaughter), 256–257, 269–270, 328
Ravitch, Mark
  Blalock—condolence notes, 239
  Blalock—Henry Ford Hospital, 71
  Blalock—homage visit, 238
  Blalock—Southern Hotel party, 223, 225–226, 228, 236
  Johns Hopkins University—blood bank segregation, 258
  Mount Sinai Hospital, 210
  Thomas—cardiopulmonary resuscitation (CPR), 210
  Thomas—friendship, 254–255
  Thomas—handwritten notes, 259–260
  Thomas—health, 264
  Thomas—Pioneering Research in Surgical Shock and Cardiovascular Surgery: Vivien Thomas and His Work with Alfred Blalock (book), 255, 255–256, 257, 258, 261–263, 264–265, 267
  Thomas—portrait, 242
  Thomas—published papers, 205
University of Pittsburgh, 254
Red Cross, 107–108, 114–115, 115–116
religion discrimination, 50, 52, 63. see also race discrimination; sex discrimination

Renaissance, 75–76
Rickman, Alan, 269
Riva-Rocci, Scipione, 28
Robert Garrett Foundation, 178
Robinson, Dean, 50–51
Rockefeller General Education Board (GEB), 37, 49, 53
Roosevelt, Franklin Delano, 1
Ross, Richard S., 251, 263
Rotell, Thomas, 262, 263
Royal College of Surgeons (UK), 172
Royal Tour, p150, 171–172
Rush University, 277, 327
Ryman Auditorium (Mother Church of Country Music), 17

S

Sabiston, David
   Blalock—homage visit, 238
   Blalock—scouting talent, 184
   Blalock—Southern Hotel party, 223, 225–226, 228
   Blalock—surgery chair fight, 234
   Duke University, 238
   Thomas—portrait, 242
Saint Louis University, 195, 238
Satterfield, Thomas, 130, 190–191
Sauerbruch, Ferdinand, 54
Saxon, Eileen, 1–5, 134–141, 167–168, 267
Schlossberg, Leon, 262
Scruggs, Afi-Odelia E., 15
segregation. *see* race discrimination
septal defects, 210
sex discrimination, 104, 118–119, 166–167, 172–173, 174–175. *see also* race discrimination; religion discrimination
Shackelford, Richard, 230, 243, 254
sharecropping, 9, 10, 42–43

Sherwood, Elizabeth "The King," 136
shockless surgery, 28–29
Sister Jessica, 200
sit-ins, 222
slavery, 9
slide rule, 61
Smith (birth name Rasberry), Marcia (granddaughter), 256–257, 269–270, 274, 329
Smith, Gardner, 206
Society of Thoracic Surgeons, 276
Society to Prevent Cruelty to Animals (S.P.C.A.), p152, 197, 198, 200
Solace, USS, 108
Something the Lord Made (television movie), 269–270, 327, 328
Southern Hotel, p153, 224–225, 226, 227, 232–233, 268
Spann (birth name Thomas), Valeria, 74, 261, 274, 329
S.P.C.A. (Society to Prevent Cruelty to Animals), p152, 197, 198, 200
Spencer, Rowena, 129, 190, 217, 260
Squeaky (dog) story, 206
Stark Films, 201
stock market crash of 1929. *see* Great Depression
Student Army Training Corp, 45
surgeries
   Blalock-Hanlon surgery. *see* Transposition of the Great Arteries (TGA)
   Blalock-Taussig shunt. *see* Tetralogy of Fallot (TOF) blue babies
   collapse therapy (pneumothorax treatment), 54
   shockless surgery, 28–29
Surgery, Gynecology and Obstetrics, 210

"The Surgical Treatment of Complete Transposition of the Aorta and the Pulmonary Artery," 194
"The Surgical Treatment of Malformations of the Heart in Which There Is Pulmonary Stenosis or Pulmonary Atresia," 167, 170
Symposium in Honor of Alfred Blalock, 267

T
Talented Tenth, 75
Talwar, Sachin, 194–195
Taussig, Frank William, 118
Taussig, Helen
  Abbot, Maude, 119
  animal rights, 200
  Blalock—demeanor towards, 127–128
  Boston University, 119
  congenital heart disorders expert, 119
  diagnostician, 3, 119
  Gross, Robert, 122
  Harriet Lane Home for Invalid Children, 119
  Harvard University, 118–119
  health, 118
  Johns Hopkins University—admission, 119
  Johns Hopkins University—house purchase, 251
  Johns Hopkins University—Milton S. Eisenhower Medal for Distinguished Service, 251
  Johns Hopkins University—photo portrait, 203
  Johns Hopkins University—promotion, 251
  Johnson, Lyndon B., 239
  Longmire, William P., 174
  Milton S. Eisenhower Medal for Distinguished Service, 251
  Park, Edwards A., 119, 123, 166–167, 174
  Presidential Medal of Freedom, 239
  Puryear, Clara Belle, 174
  Radcliffe College, 118
  sex discrimination, 119, 127, 166–167, 172–173, 202–203, 229–230, 239, 251
  Taussig, Frank William, 118
  Taussig, William, 118
  Tetralogy of Fallot (TOF) blue babies. see Tetralogy of Fallot (TOF) blue babies
  thalidomide, 239
  Thomas—condolence note, 266
  University of California, Berkeley, 118
Taussig, William, 118
Te Lind, Richard, 183
television, 208
The Tennessean, 13
Tennessee Agricultural & Industrial State College (Tennessee A & I). see Tennessee State University (TSU)
Tennessee State University (TSU), 12, 18, 245
Tetralogy of Fallot (TOF) blue babies
  Abbot, Maude, 120
  American Medical Association (AMA), 210
  animal rights, 200, 201
  Anna (dog), 133, p149, 201
  Anna, Her Story (film), 201

Tetralogy of Fallot cont'd
artificial breathing apparatus, 130
Associated Press (AP), 167–168
Bahnson, Henry "Hank," p150, 172
Berger, Olive, 3, 137, 167
Blalock Clamp, 131, 169, 271
Blalock—American Medical Association (AMA) award, 210
Blalock—Blalock-Taussig shunt, naming of, p148, 166–167
Blalock—Karsh party, 203
Blalock—*Legion d'honneur*, 172
Blalock—portrait, 202–203
Blalock—publications on, 167, 170
Blalock—Royal Tour, p150, 171–172
Blalock—Saxon surgery, 4, 136–140
Blalock—Saxon surgery preparations, 134–136
Blalock—surgeries, 136–140, p148, 167, 169, 170, 172, 183, 187
Blalock—Taussig, Helen feud, 166–167, 173–174
Blalock—Taussig meeting, 123
Blalock—Taussig shunt, naming of, 166–167
Blalock—"The Surgical Treatment of Malformations of the Heart in Which There Is Pulmonary Stenosis or Pulmonary Atresia," 167, 170
Blalock-Thomas-Taussig surgery renaming effort, 272
Blalock—Tribute to Alfred Blalock, 267
causes of, 2, 120–121, p147
A Celebration: 50th Anniversary of the Blalock-Taussig Shunt, 267
Cooley, Denton, 3, 136–137
Du Bois, W.E.B., 170

Fallot, Étienne-Louis Arthur, 119–120
Garrett, Mary Elizabeth, 178
Gross, Robert, 122
Haller, J. Alex, 172
Harmel, Merel, 3, 137, 139, 140
Harriet Lane Home for Invalid Children, 135
heart specimens, 126
J.J. Deknatel & Son, 169
Johns Hopkins University—A Celebration: 50th Anniversary of the Blalock-Taussig Shunt, 267
Johns Hopkins University—cash gifts, 173
Johns Hopkins University—fees collected, 168–169, 178–179
Johns Hopkins University—patient surge, 168–169
Johns Hopkins University—press release (1945), 1
Johns Hopkins University—press release (1971), 243
Johns Hopkins University—press release (2019), 267–268
Johns Hopkins University—"Vivien Thomas, Hopkins Pioneer Surgical Technician, Dies" (newspaper article), 266
Jones, William O., 130, 131
Journal of the American Medical Association, 167
Karsh, Yousef, 202–203
Kimmel, Billy, 272
Lamont, Austin, 3, 137, 166–167
Legion d'honneur, 172
LIFE, 168
Longmire, William P., 3, 136–137, 139, 141

Mitchell, Charlotte, 3, 137
Murray Baumgartner, 169
photos, 5, p148
Presidential Medal of Freedom, 239
publications on, 167, 170
pulmonary arteriovenous fistula, 132
Puryear, Clara Belle, 4, 132, 137
Robert Garrett Foundation, 178
Royal Tour, p150, 171–172
Satterfield, Thomas, 130
Saxon, Eileen, 1–5, 134–141, 167–168, 267
side-to-end-anastomosis, 133
surgeries—costs, 168–169
surgeries—first, 1–5, 134–141
surgeries—news coverage, 167–168, 173
surgeries—second & third, 167
surgeries—Vanderbilt University, 169
surgeries—wait times, 168–169
"The Surgical Treatment of Malformations of the Heart in Which There Is Pulmonary Stenosis or Pulmonary Atresia," 167, 170
symptoms of, 2, 120
Taussig, Helen—animal rights, 200
Taussig, Helen—Blalock and Thomas meeting, 123
Taussig, Helen—Blalock feud, 166–167, 173–174
Taussig, Helen—cyanosis calculations, 132
Taussig, Helen—Gross, Robert, 122
Taussig, Helen—heart specimens, 126

Taussig, Helen—interest in TOF, 3, 119–120
Taussig, Helen—photo portrait, 203
Taussig, Helen—Presidential Medal of Freedom, 239
Taussig, Helen—publications on, 167, 170
Taussig, Helen—Royal Tour, 171, 172–173
Taussig, Helen—Saxon, Eileen, 3, 134–135, 136, 139, 140, 140–141
Taussig, Helen—"The Surgical Treatment of Malformations of the Heart in Which There Is Pulmonary Stenosis or Pulmonary Atresia," 167, 170
Taussig, Helen—Tribute to Helen Taussig, 267
Taussig—*Legion d'honneur*, 172
Thomas—American Medical Association (AMA) award, 210
Thomas—artificial breathing apparatus, 130
Thomas—Blalock Clamp, 131, 169, 271
Thomas—contributions overview, 271
Thomas—counseling parents, 181–182
Thomas—cyanosis recreation, 131–132
Thomas—cyanosis reversal, 133
Thomas—dogs, 126, 129–130, 131–133, 200, 201
Thomas—Karsh party, 203
Thomas—needles, 130, 169

Tetralogy of Fallot cont'd
   Thomas—recognition denied, 2, p148, 170, 173, 210, 251–252, 267–268
   Thomas—recognition given, 243, 266
   Thomas—Saxon surgery, 4–5, 137–140
   Thomas—Saxon surgery preparations, 134–136
   Thomas—Taussig meeting, 123
   TIME, 168
   treatments for, 133
   Tribute to Alfred Blalock, 267
   Tribute to Helen Taussig, 267
   University of Toronto (Canada), 272
   Vanderbilt University, 169
   White, Shaun, 271–272
   Woods, Alan, 138
Texas Heart Institute, 326–327
TGA (Transposition of the Great Arteries). see Transposition of the Great Arteries (TGA)
thalidomide, 239
Thomas (birth name Flanders), Clara Beatrice (wife)
   Baltimore—fear of, 96
   Baltimore—move to, 90
   Blalock, Alfred—surprise house visit, 98
   catering, 164
   death, 270
   driving skills, 160
   Dullea (birth name Thomas), Theodosia (daughter). see Dullea (birth name Thomas), Theodosia (daughter)
   family photo, p145
   grit, 274
   health, 236
   homemaking skills, 65, 65–66, 96
   intelligence, 65
   Isaacs, James P., 236
   Norris (birth name Thomas), Olga (daughter). see Norris (birth name Thomas), Olga (daughter)
   Something the Lord Made (television movie), 269–270
   Southern Hotel party, 236
   Thomas—alcoholism, 204, 274
   Thomas—as "Mrs. Thomas," 65
   Thomas—book dedication, 263
   Thomas—courtship, 65
   Thomas—death, 265
   Thomas—long work days, 128
   Thomas—marriage, 65
   Thomas—portrait, p154, 243
   travel, 270
   vacation to Nashville, Tennessee, 159–162, 165
Thomas, Harold (brother)
   ambitions, 75, 76
   birth, 11
   civil rights movement, 72–73, 78–83, 187, 328
   college graduation, 64
   Collegiate Professional Certificate, 74
   divorce, 329
   Fisk University, 18, 19
   NAACP, 73–74, 78–83
   Nashville Globe, 82–83
   preschool & kindergarten, 13–14
   Spann (birth name Thomas), Valeria, 74, 261, 274, 329
   teacher, 73, 82–83

Thomas, Lillian "Ootsie" Dunn, 222, 244, 251, 328
Thomas, Lillian "Ootsie" Dunn, 222, 244, 251, 328
Thomas, M. Carey, 103, 104
Thomas, Maceo (brother), 11, 13, 18, 251
Thomas, Mary E. (mother)
  children, birth of, 11, 14
  children, teaching of, 17
  cooking, 14
  divorce, 58
  sewing, 14
  Tennessee, move to, 11, 13
  visit from Vivien and family, 160–161
Thomas, Melba (sister), 14
Thomas, Vivien—character & characteristics
  addiction center, 237
  alcoholism, 204, 219, 236–237, 274
  Blalock—alcoholism, 219
  Blalock—resentments towards, 257–259
  Burton, Harold, 205–206
  Cameron, John L., 236, 264–265
  carpentry, 17, 18, 34
  Casper, Alfred, 216
  Cavagnaro, Louise, 237
  civil rights movement, 274–275
  cooking, 87
  Cooley, Denton, 182–183, 217
  creativity, 127, 274
  depression, 274
  Dullea (birth name Thomas), Theodosia (daughter), 273
  Eaton, Koco (Katuelle), 183–184, 273
  exhaustion, 128, 181
  Haller, J. Alex, 112, 216, 217
  "headache man," 216
  health, 207, 257, 264–265
  humor, 274
  instructor, 217
  The Johns Hopkins Magazine, 182–183
  kindness, 274
  loneliness, 160–161
  mechanical skills, 127, 183–184
  Norris, Harold (son-in-law), 274
  passive-aggressive, 113
  patience, 73, 183, 211
  photos, p143, p144, p145, p148, p155, p156, p157
  physical characteristics, 16–17, 21
  portrait, p154
  potential, 62, 275
  Pottker, Jan, 7–8
  psychiatric care, 204
  Queen, Jean, 236–237
  Ravitch, Mark, 264
  religion, 14–15, 274
  resilience, 7, 113, 273, 274
  scouting talent, 211
  service, 15, 34
  Spann (birth name Thomas), Valeria, 274
  Spencer, Rowena, 217
  surgical skills, 5–6, 60, 111, 112, 138–140, 182–183, 191–192, 194, 205, 206, 216, 217, 266
  Tumulty, Philip, 264
  Watkins, Levi, 277
  work satisfaction, 277
  Zuidema, George, 237, 274
Thomas, Vivien—events:birth to Vanderbilt University
  birth, 9, 11

Thomas, Vivien   cont'd
  Blalock—job interview, 21–25
  bullies scuffle, 20
  Fisk University carpentry work, 18, 19, 24
  job search, 19–21
  Manlove, Charles, 20
  Pearl High School, 15, 16–17, p143
  preschool & kindergarten, 13–14, 14
  stock market crash of 1929, 19–20
  Tennessee, move to, 10, 13
  Tennessee State University (TSU), 18
Thomas, Vivien—events: Vanderbilt University to Johns Hopkins University
  bank failure, 56–57, 58
  Beard, Joseph W., 61, 62
  Blalock—Henry Ford Hospital discrimination lie, 71–72
  Blalock—marriage, 55
  Blalock—surgeons' meeting preparation, 68
  Brooks, Barney, 35–36, 36–37, 37–38, 85–86, 235
  Great Depression, 55–56, 57, 57–58
  house purchase, 67
  hypertension, 63–64
  Manlove, Andrew, p144
  Manlove, Charles, 20–22
  marriage to Clara Flanders, 65
  Peoples Savings and Loan, 55
  recognition denied, 5, 112
  recognition given, 110, 112
  slide rule, 61
  Thomas, Harold college graduation, 64
  traumatic shock. see traumatic shock
  Vanderbilt University—dismissal, 85–86, 235
  Vanderbilt University—first day at work, 26, 33
  Vanderbilt University—job title, 36, 37
  Vanderbilt University—lab technician, p144
  Vanderbilt University—resigned job, 35, 36, 64
  Vanderbilt University—salary, 23–24, 34–38, 97
Thomas, Vivien—events: Johns Hopkins University to death
  Alan Mason Chesney Medical Archives, 255, 261
  American Heart Association, 276
  American Medical Writers Association, 266
  Archives of Surgery, 210
  Association of Black Cardiologists, 276
  Baltimore (magazine), 268
  Baltimore—Chesapeake and Potomac Telephone Company, 98–99
  Baltimore—move to, 87, 89, 90, 97
  Blalock—Chesapeake and Potomac Telephone Company, 98–99
  Blalock—retirement, 235
  Blalock—Southern Hotel party, 223–224, 225–226, 226–228, 231–232
  Blalock—visit to Gibson Island, 220–221
  blood pressure experiment, 123–124

Bloomberg Philanthropies, 276
Brock, Russell, 188
BS degree proposed, 248
Callcott, George H., 248, 249, 326
Cameron, John L., 266–267, 273
capillary circulation, 204–205
cardiac arrest. *see* cardiac arrest
cardiac catheterization, 182
Casper, Alfred, 216
Chesapeake and Potomac Telephone Company, 98–99
Chit Chat Farms, 237
Circulation, 204–205
Clarke, Gwendolyn Manlove, 236
Congressional Black Caucus foundation, 276
Cooley, Denton, 242, 266
A Crisis in Medical Education SOS (film), 246–247
death, 263, 265
death—funeral service, 265–266
death—legacy, 275–277
death—obituaries, 266
Def, Mos, 269–270
DSc degree, 248–249, 250, 326
Eaton, Koco (Katuelle), 257
Freeman, Morgan, 268
funeral service, 265–266
Gee, Bob, 240, 241
GlaxoSmithKline, 276
Grebel, Frances Wolff, 215
Haller, J. Alex, 164, 217, 240, 241–242, 248, 327
Hanlon, C. Rollins, p154, 195, 242–243, 259–261
HBO, 269, 270, 327, 328
Heimbecker, Raymond— recognition given, 204–205

high school summer science program, 212, 275
hospital equipment reproduction, 214–215
house purchase, 202
hypotrophy, 210
Indiana University, 236
Institute for Technical Skills (UK), 276
job search, 236–237
Johns Hopkins University Press, 262
Johns Hopkins University—*A Crisis in Medical Education SOS* (film), 246–247
Johns Hopkins University—BS degree, 248
Johns Hopkins University—campus tour, 88–89
Johns Hopkins University— instructor, 252–253
Johns Hopkins University— instructs animal surgeries, 217, 272
Johns Hopkins University—lab coat incident, 95
Johns Hopkins University—lab organization, 94
Johns Hopkins University—lab personnel decisions, 211
Johns Hopkins University—LLD degree, p155, 249–250, 251–252, 266
Johns Hopkins University—master of the hounds, 205–206
Johns Hopkins University—medical supply salesman, 215
Johns Hopkins University—new dog lab, 216–217

Thomas, Vivien cont'd
Johns Hopkins University—
 pension, 235
Johns Hopkins University—
 portrait, p154, 240, 241–245, 327, 329
Johns Hopkins University—
 recognition denied, 206, 229–230, 241–242, 246–247, 262
Johns Hopkins University—
 recognition given, p155, 242–243, 249–250, 251–252, 252, 266
Johns Hopkins University—respect of colleagues, 95
Johns Hopkins University—salary, 93–94, 98, 160–161, 161, 162, 176–178, 179–180, 213, 214, 252–253
Johns Hopkins University—
 Squeaky incident, 206
Johns Hopkins University—"Vivien Thomas, Hopkins Pioneer Surgical Technician, Dies" (newspaper article), 266
Kay, Jerome, 210
Kouwenhoven, William B., 230
legacy, 275–277
Limpert, Jack, 268
LLD degree, p155, 249–250, 251–252, 266
Longmire, William P., 242
McCabe, Katie, 268, 269
McCall, Nancy, 263
medical supply company, 213
Meharry Medical College, 276
Morgan College, 163–164
Morgan State University, 205
Morrow, A. Glenn, 215–216
Muller, Steven, p155

National Heart Institute (National Institutes of Health), 215–216
National Medical Association, 276
New England Journal of Medicine, 266
Norris, Harold (son-in-law), 250, 262, 328
obituaries, 266
Old Hands Club, 240, 241–242
"Partners of the Heart" (television documentary), 268–269, 327, 328
PBS (Public Broadcast System), 268–269, 327, 328
pharmaceutical detail man, 214
Pioneering Research in Surgical Shock and Cardiovascular Surgery: Vivien Thomas and His Work with Alfred Blalock (book), p157, 254–255, 255–256, 257–259, 261–263, 264–265, 266–267, 269, 329
portrait, p154, 240, 241–245, 327, 329
positive pressure anesthesia machines, 214
positive pressure anesthesia machines—recognition given, 195
Posthumous Scroll of Merit, 276
Provident Hospital—recognition given, 255
published book, p157, 254–255, 255–256, 257–259, 261–263, 264–265
published papers, 204–205, 210, 272
pulmonary stenosis, 210
Queen, Jean, 252, 265, 328
Ravitch, Mark. *see* Ravitch, Mark

recognition denied, 2, 6, p148, 170, 173, 193–194, 195, 209–210, 210, 243, 251–252, 257–258, 258–259, 259–261, 267–268, 272
recognition given, 192, 210, 243, 260, 266
retirement, 253
Rickman, Alan, 269
Ross, Richard S., 251, 263
Rotell, Thomas, 262, 263
Sabiston, David, 242
Schlossberg, Leon, 262
septal defects, 210
Shackelford, Richard, 230, 243, 254
Smith, Gardner, 206
Society of Thoracic Surgeons, 276
Something the Lord Made (television movie), 269–270, 327, 328
Squeaky (dog) incident, 206
supplementary jobs—bartender, 164
supplementary jobs—handyman, 96
supplementary jobs—medical instruments, 214–215
supplementary jobs—salesman, 213
Surgery, Gynecology and Obstetrics, 210
Taussig, Helen, 266
Tennessee pioneer proclamation, 276
Tetralogy of Fallot (TOF) blue babies. *see* Tetralogy of Fallot (TOF) blue babies
Thomas, Lillian "Ootsie" Dunn, 244
Transposition of the Great Arteries (TGA). *see* Transposition of the Great Arteries (TGA)
Turner, Thomas, 255
Union, Gabrielle, 269
University of Maryland, 248–249, 250, 326
University of Pennsylvania Press, 262, 265, 267, 269
Unsung Hero award, 255
vacation to Nashville, Tennessee, 159–162, 164–165
Vanderbilt University—job, 236
Vanderbilt University—portrait, 276
Vanderbilt University—Vivien Thomas Award for Clinical Research, 276
Vanderbilt University—Vivien Thomas Medical Training Program, 276
Vanderbilt University—Vivien Thomas Way, 276
Vivien T. Thomas College Advisory Program, 275
Vivien T. Thomas Fund, 275–276
Vivien T. Thomas Medical Arts Academy, 275
Vivien Thomas Award for Clinical Research, 276
Vivien Thomas Endowed Scholarship, 276
Vivien Thomas High School Research Program, 275
Vivien Thomas Medical Training Program, 276
Vivien Thomas Scholars Initiative, 275–276

Thomas, Vivien cont'd
  Vivien Thomas Scholarship for Medical Science and Research, 276
  Vivien Thomas Technical Leadership program, 276
  Vivien Thomas Young Investigator award, 276
  Washingtonian, 268
  Watkins, Levi, 257, 265–266, 269, 277, 329
  Woolfe, Harvey, p155
  World War II. *see* traumatic shock
  Young, Ralph J., 214
  Zuidema, George, 237, 240, 242, 248, 249–250, 252, 266–267, 329
Thomas, Vivien—family & friends
  Calhoun (birth name Thomas), Olga (sister). *see* Calhoun (birth name Thomas), Olga (sister)
  Clarke, Gwendolyn Manlove, 236, 241, 326
  Cooley, Denton, 327
  Dullea (birth name Thomas), Theodosia (daughter). *see* Dullea (birth name Thomas), Theodosia (daughter)
  Eaton, Koco (Katuelle), 183–184, 257, 273, 327
  family photo, p145
  Flanders, Leonard (father-in-law), 65
  Flanders, Mary Gross (mother-in-law), 65
  Great Depression, 57–58
  Jackson, Truly, 251, 328
  Manlove, Charles, 20–22, p156
  Norris (birth name Thomas), Olga (daughter). *see* Norris (birth name Thomas), Olga (daughter)
  Norris, Harold (son-in-law), 250, 262, 274, 328
  Norris, Nena (granddaughter), 256–257
  Queen, Jean, 236–237, 252, 265, 328
  Rasberry-Dijkhoffz, Ursula (granddaughter), 256–257, 269–270, 328
  Ravitch, Mark, 254–255
  Smith (birth name Rasberry), Marcia (granddaughter), 256–257, 269–270, 274, 329
  Spann (birth name Thomas), Valeria, 74, 261, 274, 329
  Thomas (birth name Flanders), Clara Beatrice (wife). *see* Thomas (birth name Flanders), Clara Beatrice (wife)
  Thomas, Harold (brother). *see* Thomas, Harold (brother)
  Thomas, Lillian "Ootsie" Dunn, 222, 244, 251, 328
  Thomas, Maceo (brother), 11, 13, 18, 251
  Thomas, Mary E. (mother). *see* Thomas, Mary E. (mother)
  Thomas, Melba (sister), 14
  Thomas, William M. (father). *see* Thomas, William M. (father)
  Watkins, Levi, 245–246, 329
  Woods, Alan C., 138, 231–232
Thomas, William M. (father)
  carpentry, 10, 11, 17, 20, 57
  children, birth of, 11, 14
  children, teaching of, 17

divorce, 58
Great Depression, 57-58
housing contractor, 12-13
real estate investor, 12-13
Tennessee, move to, 11, 13
Thomas, Vivien—loan from, 57-58
Thomas v. Hibbitts et al, 78-83
TIME, 168
Timms, Minnie Mae, 36, 259
TOF (Tetralogy of Fallot) blue babies. *see* Tetralogy of Fallot (TOF) blue babies
Transposition of the Great Arteries (TGA)
   Berger, Olive, 194
   Blalock—dog autopsy, 191-192
   Blalock-Hanlon surgery, naming of, 193-194
   Blalock—publications on, 193, 194, 195
   Blalock—"The Surgical Treatment of Complete Transposition of the Aorta and the Pulmonary Artery," 194
   Blalock—Thomas meetings, 189-190
   causes of, p151, 188, 189
   Cooley, Denton, 194, 260
   Haller, J. Alex, 260
   Hanlon, C. Rollins, 193, 194, 195, 259-261
   "Interatrial Septal Defects," 193
   Johns Hopkins University—"Vivien Thomas, Hopkins Pioneer Surgical Technician, Dies" (newspaper article), 266
   Kay, Jerome, 260
   Marathe, Supreet, 194-195
   Nokawama, Dan, 194
   Satterfield, Thomas, 190-191
   Spencer, Rowena, 190, 260
   "The Surgical Treatment of Complete Transposition of the Aorta and the Pulmonary Artery," 194
   symptoms of, 188
   Talwar, Sachin, 194-195
   Thomas—Blalock meetings, 189-190
   Thomas—career contribution, 192-193, 194
   Thomas—clamp, 190, 192, 193
   Thomas—contributions overview, 5, 271
   Thomas—dogs, 189, 190-192
   Thomas—handwritten notes on, 195, 259-260
   Thomas—publications on, 195
   Thomas—recognition denied, 6, 193-194, 195, 243, 259-261, 272
   Thomas—recognition given, 192, 260, 266
   treatments for, 6, p151, 190-191, 195
   Weldon, Clarence, 194
traumatic shock
   Beard, Joseph W., 61-62
   Blalock—blood plasma transfusions, 115
   Blalock—career contribution, 192
   Blalock—dogs, 30, 31-32, 33-34, 62-63, 111
   Blalock—instructing Thomas, 30, 31-32
   Blalock—lab responsibilities, 58-59
   Blalock—National Research Council, 107, 108-109
   Blalock—Office of Scientific Research and Development, 107

traumatic shock cont'd
  Blalock—Pearl Harbor trip,
    107–108
  Blalock—publications on, 5, 23, 30,
    50–51, 54–55, 84–85, 111–112
  Blalock—research motivation, 27
  Blalock—research techniques, 50
  Blalock—shock manual, 107
  blood plasma, 114–115, 115–117,
    p146
  Cannon, Walter, 29–30, 68–69
  causes of, 26, 27, 28, 111
  Civil War, 28
  Claudius Galen of Pergamon, 27
  Cooley, Denton, 110–111, 127
  Crile, George Washington, 28–29
  defined, 26
  Duncan, George W., 111–112,
    125–126
  "Experimental Shock: The Cause
    of the Low Blood Pressure
    Produced by Muscle Injury,"
    54–55
  Gross, Samuel D., 28
  Hanlon, C. Rollins, 110–111
  Harvard Hospital Unit, 29
  Harvey, William, 27
  Hippocrates, 27
  history of, 27–30
  Johns Hopkins University—"The
    Johns Hopkins Hospital Surgical
    Routine" (publication), 69
  Le Dran, Henri-François, 27
  Leeds (Levy), Stanford, 123–124
  Longmire, William P., 110
  "Mechanism and Treatment of
    Experimental Shock: Shock
    Following Hemorrhage," 51
  National Research Council, 107,
    108–109, 114
  Nembutal, 63
  Office of Scientific Research and
    Development, 107, 168
  *Principles of Surgical Care: Shock
    and Other Problems* (book),
    84–85
  Puryear, Clara Belle, 112
  Riva-Rocci, Scipione, 28
  shock manual, 107
  Thomas—contributions overview,
    5, 271
  Thomas—dogs, 5, 30, 31–32, 33–34,
    62–63, 108, 110, 111, 112, 123–124
  Thomas—lab responsibilities,
    58–59, 62
  Thomas—Office of Scientific
    Research and Development, 168
  Thomas—recognition denied, 5, 112
  Thomas—recognition given, 110,
    112
  Traumatic Shock, 30
  treatments for, 54–55, 115, 116
  World War I, 29
  World War II—Blalock, 107–108,
    108–109, 127
  World War II—blood plasma,
    114–115, 115–117, p146
  World War II—London's Blitz, 111
  World War II—Patton, George S.,
    116–117
  World War II—Pyle, Ernie, 116
  World War II—Thomas, 86, 109,
    110, 168
Traumatic Shock, 30
Trudeau Sanatorium, 51–53
Tubman, Harriet, 90
Tumulty, Philip, 264

Turner, Thomas, 71, 255
Twain, Mark, 10

U

Union, Gabrielle, 269
United Methodist Church, 14
universities & colleges
   Alabama State College, 245
   Boston University, 119
   Bowman-Gray medical college, 86
   Case Western Reserve University, 207
   Columbia University, 7, 115, 184–185, 257
   Dartmouth College, 277
   Duke University, 61–62, 238
   Fisk University. *see* Fisk University
   Georgia Military College, 43
   Goucher College, 46, 326
   Harvard University. *see* Harvard University
   Howard University, 15, 116
   Indiana University, 236
   Jefferson Medical College, 28
   Johns Hopkins University School of Medicine. *see* Johns Hopkins University
   Lincoln University, 16
   McGill University (Canada), 115
   Medical College of Virginia, 327
   Meharry Medical College. *see* Meharry Medical College
   Morgan State University, 163–164, 177, 205, 256
   Radcliffe College, 118
   Royal College of Surgeons (UK), 172
   Rush University, 277, 327
   Saint Louis University, 195, 238
   Tennessee State University (TSU), 12, 18, 245
   University of Alabama, 245
   University of California, Berkeley, 118
   University of California, Los Angeles, 238
   University of Georgia, 43
   University of Louisville, 69
   University of Maryland, 198, 248–249, 250, 326
   University of Michigan, 45, 234, 264, 329
   University of Pittsburgh, 238, 254, 277, 327–328
   University of Toronto (Canada), 272
   Vanderbilt University. *see* Vanderbilt University
   Yale University, 104, 277
University of Alabama, 245
University of California, Berkeley, 118
University of California, Los Angeles, 238
University of Georgia, 43
University of Louisville, 69
University of Maryland, 198, 248–249, 250, 326
University of Michigan, 45, 234, 264, 329
University of Pennsylvania Press, 262, 265, 267, 269
University of Pittsburgh, 238, 254, 277, 327–328
University of Toronto (Canada), 272
Unsung Hero award, 255

V

Vanderbilt University
- Blalock, Alfred. see Blalock, Alfred—events
- Body, Issaac, 23, 24
- Brooks, Barney. see Brooks, Barney
- dogs, 197
- Harrison, Tinsley, 36, 86
- Manlove, Charles, 20–22
- Merrill, Walter, 328
- race discrimination, 20–21, 35, 36, 37, 49, 85–86, 235, 245
- Robinson, Dean, 50–51
- Rockefeller General Education Board (GEB), 35, 37, 49, 53
- rodent infestation, 49
- Tetralogy of Fallot (TOF) blue babies surgery, reaction to, 169
- Thomas, Vivien. see Thomas, Vivien—events: Vanderbilt University to Johns Hopkins University

Thomas—portrait, 276
Thomas—Tennessee pioneer proclamation, 276
Timms, Minnie Mae, 36, 259
traumatic shock. see traumatic shock
Vivien Thomas Award for Clinical Research, 276
Vivien Thomas Medical Training Program, 276
Vivien Thomas Way, 276
Waters, Samuel, 23, 24, 32, 33, 60, 64, p144
Watkins, Levi, 245
Veteran Affairs National Center, 328
Vivien T. Thomas College Advisory Program, 275
Vivien T. Thomas Fund, 275–276
Vivien T. Thomas Medical Arts Academy, 275
Vivien Thomas Award for Clinical Research, 276
Vivien Thomas Endowed Scholarship, 276
Vivien Thomas High School Research Program, 275
"Vivien Thomas, Hopkins Pioneer Surgical Technician, Dies" (newspaper article), 266
Vivien Thomas Medical Training Program, 276
Vivien Thomas Scholars Initiative, 275–276
Vivien Thomas Scholarship for Medical Science and Research, 276
Vivien Thomas Technical Leadership program, 276
Vivien Thomas Way, 276
Vivien Thomas Young Investigator award, 276
vivisectionists. see animal rights

W

Washington, D.C., 198
Washington, G.E., 16
Washington, George, 224
Washington Post, 196
Washingtonian, 268
Waters, Samuel, 23, 24, 32, 33, 60, 64, p144
Watkins, Levi
- Abernathy, Ralph, 245
- Association of Black Cardiologists, 276
- civil rights movement, 245
- defibrillator, implantable cardiac (ICD), 6, 246, 329

Eaton, Koco (Katuelle), 257
Harvard University, 245–246
HBO, 269
Johns Hopkins University, 89, 105, 223, 245–246, 329
King, Martin Luther, Jr., 245
Levi Watkins, Jr. MD Outpatient Center, 329
Montgomery Bus Boycott, 245
Something the Lord Made (television movie), 269
Tennessee State University, 245
Thomas—friendship, 245, 329
Thomas—funeral, 265–266, 277, 329
University of Alabama, 245
Vanderbilt University, 245
Welch, William H., 44
Weldon, Clarence, 194
White, Shaun, 271–272
Whitman, Walt, 75–76
Williams, Juan, 77
women's equality. *see* sex discrimination
Woods, Alan C., 138, 231–232
Woolfe, Harvey, p155
World War I, 29
World War II
  Ambrose, Stephen E., 109
  Arizona, USS, 108
  Baltimore, 91–92
  Blalock, Alfred. *see* traumatic shock
  blood drives, 114–115, 115–116
  blood plasma, p146
  D-Day (1944), 141
  death statistics, 117
  Delano, Victor, 109
  Drew, Charles, 115–116
  GI Bill, 163
  Green, Thomas, 108
  Hitler, Adolf, 1
  Johns Hopkins University, 110
  Miller, Dorrie (Doris), 109–110
  National Research Council, 107, 108–109, 114
  Office of Scientific Research and Development, 107, 168
  Patton, George S., 116–117
  Pearl Harbor attack, 106–107, 115
  Pittsburgh Courier, 110
  Pyle, Ernie, 116
  race discrimination, 91–92, 109
  Red Cross, 107–108, 114–115, 115–116
  Roosevelt, Franklin Delano, 1
  Solace, USS, 108
  Thomas, Vivien. *see* traumatic shock
  traumatic shock. *see* traumatic shock
  Victory over Europe (VE) Day, 1, 167–168
  Victory over Japan (VJ) Day, 1

Y

Yale University, 104, 277
Young, Ralph J., 214

Z

Zimmerman, Jack McKay, 220, 329
Zuidema, George
  Blalock—surgery chair fight, 234
  Johns Hopkins University surgery chair, 234, 235, 329
  Thomas—alcoholism, 237, 274
  Thomas—BS degree, 248
  Thomas—instructor promotion, 252, 329

Zuidema, George *cont'd*
  Thomas—LLD degree, 249–250, 252, 329
  Thomas—*Pioneering Research in Surgical Shock and Cardiovascular Surgery: Vivien Thomas and His Work with Alfred Blalock* (book), 266–267
  Thomas—portrait, 240, 242, 329
University of Michigan, 264, 329

Printed in the USA
CPSIA information can be obtained
at www.ICGtesting.com
CBHW080213210824
13484CB00008B/156

9 798989 332519